BIOMARKERS IN BREAST CANCER

CANCER DRUG DISCOVERY AND DEVELOPMENT

BEVERLY A. TEICHER, SERIES EDITOR

BIOMARKERS IN BREAST CANCER

MOLECULAR DIAGNOSTICS FOR PREDICTING AND MONITORING THERAPEUTIC EFFECT

Edited by

GIAMPIETRO GASPARINI, MD

Division of Medical Oncology
"San Filippo Neri" Hospital
Rome, Italy

and

DANIEL F. HAYES, MD

Breast Oncology Program
University of Michigan Comprehensive Cancer Center
Ann Arbor, MI

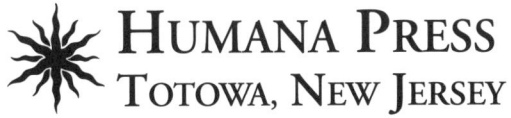

HUMANA PRESS
TOTOWA, NEW JERSEY

© 2006 Humana Press Inc.
999 Riverview Drive, Suite 208
Totowa, New Jersey 07512
www.humanapress.com

This publication is printed on acid-free paper. ∞
ANSI Z39.48-1984 (American National Standards Institute) Permanence of Paper for Printed Library Materials.

Cover design by Patricia F. Cleary.

For additional copies, pricing for bulk purchases, and/or information about other Humana titles, contact Humana at the above address or at any of the following numbers: Tel.: 973-256-1699; Fax: 973-256-8341; E-mail: orders@humanapr.com or visit our Website at www.humanapress.com

Printed in the United States of America. 10 9 8 7 6 5 4 3 2 1
Library of Congress Cataloging-in-Publication Data
Biomarkers in breast cancer : molecular diagnostics for predicting and monitoring therapeutic effect / edited by Giampietro Gasparini and Daniel F. Hayes.
    p. cm. — (Cancer drug discovery and development)
  Includes bibliographical references and index.
  ISBN 1-58829-227-4 (alk. paper) eISBN 1-59259-915-X
  1. Breast—Cancer—Molecular diagnosis. 2. Breast—Cancer—Prognosis. 3. Tumor markers. I. Gasparini, Giampietro. II. Hayes, Daniel, 1951- III. Series.
  RC280.B8B54 2005
  616.99'449075—dc22   2005001922

PREFACE

Biomarkers in Breast Cancer: Molecular Diagnostics for Predicting and Monitoring Therapeutic Effect is an updated view of the prognostic and predictive biomarkers in breast cancer written by experts in this field. This book covers the major advancements in the application of novel sophisticated molecular methods as well as the state of the art of the conventional prognostic and predictive indicators.

The first three chapters by Simon, Sweep et al., and Kimel et al. highlight the relevance of appropriate and rigorous study design and guidelines for validation studies on new biomarkers, concerning the standardization with quality control of the assay(s) used for their determination, their clinical development, and the statistical approaches. Of particular importance is the suggested optimized protocol for the HER-2/*neu* FISH assay applied by the NSABP network (*1*).

Gene expression profiling by tissue microarray is treated in depth in the following two chapters by De Bortoli and Briglia and by Kim and Paik. Recent studies conducted using this methodology have clearly documented the heterogeneous nature of invasive breast cancer within the same pathologic stage and menopausal status. These methods have clearly provided powerful new tools for more accurate individual definition of prognosis. However, much more work remains to be done before standard pathology laboratories can use tissue microarrays to perform tumor marker studies for routine clinical use.

Several individual factors are accepted or appear to be promising for standard clinical care. Of course, the use of estrogen and progesterone receptors (ER, PgR) to predict benefit from endocrine therapy represents the gold standard of tumor markers, and should be tested on every breast cancer tissue (*2*). More recently, testing for HER-2 status has also become standard to help select whether a patient with metastatic breast cancer should receive trastuzumab (*2*). Other factors that are still controversial, but are considered standard by some guideline panels, include indicators of cell proliferation as well as the urokinase-type plasminogen activator (PAI)-1 system. These are the topics of the next four chapters written by authors who are among the pioneers and worldwide experts in translational research studies in the field.

The roles of the epidermal growth factor receptor (EGFR) pathway and altered p53 in breast cancer growth and progression and as possible prognostic and predictive indicators are outlined by Ciardiello et al. and by Kandioler and Jakesz, respectively. In addition to trastuzumab, several preclinical and clinical studies suggest that other agents that disrupt the signaling pathways generated by members of the EGFR family may be effective against breast cancer. The ability to identify predictive surrogate biomarkers of response is the key for the rational selection of the patients most likely to benefit from these anti-EGFR compounds.

Moreover, it seems likely that markers of EGFR activity might provide the opportunity for monitoring therapeutic efficacy. The recent demonstration that mutation of the phosphorylation site of the receptor may be predictive of gefinitib activity in patients with non-small-cell lung cancer may represent an important step toward the right strategy for the use of such a class of new anticancer agents (3,4).

Adjuvant systemic therapy has now been clearly shown to reduce the odds of recurrence and death (5,6). However, because of the inaccuracy of currently available prognostic and predictive factors, much of adjuvant systemic therapy, especially chemotherapy, is given inefficiently, either to patients whose cancer was never destined to recur or to those patients whose cancer will recur, but for whom the therapy will not be effective. Enormous work has been directed toward prognosis, with advancements in the field of molecular biology and in the detection of occult metastatic cells distant from the tumor. Hawes et al. and Braun et al. comprehensively cover the methodology, state of the art, pitfalls, and promises of detection of early tumor cell dissemination in breast cancer patients.

Although determination of tumor biology in tissue justifiably garners much interest, the ability to test and monitor for biological changes with a simple blood test is obviously appealing. Chapters 13 and 14 deal with the clinical significance of circulating HER-2/neu and vascular endothelial growth factor (VEGF), these being among the more promising therapeutic targets for approaches based on selective molecular-targeting agents.

We hope this text offers a critical view of the modern approach to the development of surrogate biomarkers of prognosis and responsiveness to selective treatments in breast cancer. We are confident that it will provide useful reading for investigators involved either in laboratory research or in clinical development of prognostic/predictive indicators and of novel molecular-targeted therapy.

Giampietro Gasparini, MD
Daniel F. Hayes, MD

1. Paik S, Bryant J, Tan-Chiu E, et al. Real-world performance of HER2 testing—National Surgical Adjuvant Breast and Bowel Project experience. *J Natl Cancer Inst* 2002;94:852–854.

2. Bast RC, Jr, Ravdin P, Hayes DF, et al. 2000 update of recommendations for the use of tumor markers in breast and colorectal cancer: clinical practice guidelines of the American Society of Clinical Oncology. *J Clin Oncol* 2001;19:1865-1878. Erratum in: *J Clin Oncol* 2001; 19:4185–4188. *J Clin Oncol* 2002;20:2213.

3. Lynch T, Bell D, Sordella R, et al. Activating mutations in the epidermal growth factor receptor underlying responsiveness of non-small cell lung cancer to gefitinib. *N Engl J Med* 2004;350:2129–2139.

4. Paez JG, Janne P, Lee JC, et al. EGFR mutations in lung cancer: correlation with clinical response to gefitinib therapy. *Science* 2004;304:1497–1500

5. Early Breast Cancer Trialist's Collaborative Group. Tamoxifen for early breast cancer: an overview of the randomised trials. *Lancet* 1998;351:1451–1467.

6. Early Breast Cancer Trialist's Collaborative Group. Polychemotherapy for early breast cancer: an overview of the randomized trials. *Lancet* 1998;352:930–942.

CONTENTS

CONTRIBUTORS

SUHAIL M. ALI, MD • *Medical Oncology Department, Penn State Milton S. Hershey Medical Center, Hershey, PA, USA*

DINO AMADORI, MD • *Division of Oncology and Diagnostics, Pierantoni Hospital, Forli, Italy*

NICOLETTA BIGLIA, MD • *Unit of Gynecological Oncology, Institute for Cancer Research and Treatment (IRCC), University of Turin, Turin, Italy*

STEPHAN BRAUN, MD • *Breast Center Tirol, Department of Obstetrics and Gynecology, University Hospital, Innsbruck, Austria*

WALTER P. CARNEY, PhD • *Diagnostics Division, Oncogene Science/Bayer HealthCare, Cambridge, MA, USA*

FORTUNATO CIARDIELLO, MD • *Cattedra di Oncologia Medica, Dipartimento Medico-Chirurgico di Internistica Clinica e Sperimentale F Magrassi e A Lanzara, Seconda Universita degli Studi di Napoli, Naples, Italy*

RICHARD J. COTE, MD, FRCPath • *Norris Comprehensive Cancer Center, Keck School of Medicine, University of Southern California, Los Angeles, CA, USA*

MARIA GRAZIA DAIDONE, PhD • *Department of Experimental Oncology, National Cancer Institute, Milan, Italy*

MICHELE DE BORTOLI, PhD • *Department of Oncological Sciences, Institute for Cancer Research and Treatment (IRCC), University of Turin, Turin, Italy*

LAURENCE DEMERS, PhD • *Pathology Department, Penn State Milton S. Hershey Medical Center, Hershey, PA, USA*

MICHAEL J. DUFFY, PhD, FRCPath, FACB • *Department of Nuclear Medicine, St. Vincent's Hospital, Dublin, Ireland*

ROBERTA FRANCESCHINI, MS • *ABO Association c/o Centre for the Study of Biological Markers of Malignancy, Unit of Laboratory Medicine, Regional General Hospital, Venice, Italy*

GIAMPIETRO GASPARINI, MD • *Division of Medical Oncology, San Filippo Neri Hospital, Rome, Italy*

MASSIMO GION, MD • *Centre for the Study of Biological Markers of Malignancy, Unit of Laboratory Medicine, Regional General Hospital, Venice, Italy*

DEBRA HAWES, MD • *Norris Comprehensive Cancer Center, Keck School of Medicine, University of Southern California, Los Angeles, CA, USA*

DANIEL F. HAYES, MD • *Breast Oncology Program, University of Michigan Comprehensive Cancer Center, Department of Medicine, University of Michigan Health System, Ann Arbor, MI, USA*

RAIMUND JAKESZ, MD • *The Department of Surgery, University of Vienna Medical School, Vienna, Austria*

DANIELA KANDIOLER, MD • *The Department of Surgery, University of Vienna Medical School, Vienna, Austria*

CHUNGYEUL KIM, MD • *Division of Pathology, National Surgical Adjuvant Breast and Bowel Project Foundation, Pittsburgh, PA, USA*

KIM LEITZEL, MS • *Medical Oncology Department, Penn State Milton S. Hershey Medical Center, Hershey, PA, USA*

ALLAN LIPTON, MD • *Medical Oncology Department, Penn State Milton S. Hershey Medical Center, Hershey, PA, USA*

RAFFELE LONGO, MD • *Division of Medical Oncology, San Filippo Neri Hospital, Rome, Italy*

CHRISTIAN MARTH, MD • *Breast Center Tirol, Department of Obstetrics and Gynecology, University Hospital, Innsbruck, Austria*

ROBERT MASS, MD • *Clinical Scientist, Genentech, Inc., South San Francisco, CA, USA*

SABRINA MEO, MS • *ABO Association c/o Centre for the Study of Biological Markers of Malignancy, Unit of Laboratory Medicine, Regional General Hospital, Venice, Italy*

RAINER NEUMANN, PhD • *Bayer HealthCare, Leverkusen, Germany*

SOONMYUNG PAIK, MD • *Division of Pathology, National Surgical Adjuvant Breast and Bowel Project Foundation, Pittsburgh, PA, USA*

CHRISTOPHER P. PRICE, PhD • *Diagnostics Division, Bayer Health Care, Slough, United Kingdom*

ROBERTA SARMIENTO, MD • *Division of Medical Oncology, San Filippo Neri Hospital, Rome, Italy*

MANFRED SCHMITT, PhD • *Clinical Research Unit, Department of Gynecology, Technical University of Munich, Munich, Germany*

JULIA SEEBER, MD • *Breast Center Tirol, Department of Obstetrics and Gynecology, University Hospital, Innsbruck, Austria*

ROSELLA SILVESTRINI, PhD • *National Cancer Institute, Milan, Italy*

RICHARD M. SIMON, DSc • *Biometric Research Branch, National Cancer Institute, Bethesda, MD, USA*

YONGKUK SONG, PhD • *Division of Pathology, National Surgical Adjuvant Breast and Bowel Project Foundation, Pittsburgh, PA, USA*

Vered Stearns, MD • *The Sidney Kimmel Comprehensive Cancer Center, Johns Hopkins University, Baltimore, MD, USA*

Fred C. G. J. Sweep, PhD • *Department of Chemical Endocrinology, University Medical Centre Nijmegen, Nijmegen, The Netherlands*

Chris M. G. Thomas, PhD • *Department of Chemical Endocrinology, University Medical Centre Nijmegen, Nijmegen, The Netherlands*

Giampaolo Tortora, MD • *Division of Medical Oncology, Department of Molecular and Clinical Endocrinology and Oncology, Universita di Napoli Federico II, Naples, Italy*

Teresa Troiani, MD • *Division of Medical Oncology, Department of Molecular and Clinical Endocrinology and Oncology, Universita di Napoli Federico II, Naples, Italy*

I GENERAL TOPICS

1 Guidelines for the Design of Clinical Studies for the Development and Validation of Therapeutically Relevant Biomarkers and Biomarker-Based Classification Systems

Richard M. Simon, DSc

CONTENTS

INTRODUCTION
PITFALLS IN DEVELOPMENTAL STUDIES
STRUCTURED RETROSPECTIVE STUDIES
VALIDATION STUDIES
REFERENCES

SUMMARY

Standards for the development of therapeutically relevant biomarkers and biomarker-based classification systems are lacking. The literature of prognostic marker studies for breast cancer is inconsistent, and few such markers have been adopted for widespread use in clinical practice. This is problematic, as many patients are overtreated and many others are treated ineffectively. The deficiencies in clinical development of biomarkers may become more severe as DNA

Cancer Drug Discovery and Development: Biomarkers in Breast Cancer:
Molecular Diagnostics for Predicting and Monitoring Therapeutic Effect
Edited by: G. Gasparini and D. F. Hayes © Humana Press Inc., Totowa, NJ

microarrays and proteomic technologies provide many new candidate markers and therapeutics become more molecularly targeted. In this chapter we address some common problems with developmental marker studies and provide recommendations for the design of clinical studies for the development and validation of robust, reproducible, and therapeutically relevant biomarkers and biomarker-based classification systems. The design of validation studies is addressed for (1) identifying node-negative breast cancer patients who do not require systemic chemotherapy; (2) identifying node-positive breast cancer patients who do not benefit from standard chemotherapy; and (3) identifying node-positive breast cancer patients who benefit from a new molecularly targeted therapeutic.

Key Words: Biomarkers; microarrays; classification systems; clinical trial design.

1. INTRODUCTION

Breast cancer is a heterogeneous set of diseases. Although substantial progress has been made in the treatment of breast cancer, many patients are overtreated and many undergo intensive chemotherapy with little apparent benefit. The literature on prognostic factors in breast cancer, although voluminous, is inconsistent *(1)*. The process of how to develop biomarkers that are robust, reproducibly measured, and therapeutically effective has not been well established. Although many prognostic factors have been studied, treatment selection has remained based primarily on the traditional components of Tumor–Node–Metastasis (TNM) stage and hormone receptor levels. This discrepancy between an inconsistent research literature and clinical practice will become even more problematic as DNA microarray and proteomic technologies provide new markers and therapeutics become more molecularly targeted. The objectives of this chapter are to provide information that facilitates the development of biomarkers for selection of the best treatment for each patient. We use the term *biomarker* to include predictive classification systems based on protein or RNA transcript profiles measured using technology such as DNA microarrays.

2. PITFALLS IN DEVELOPMENTAL STUDIES

Most biomarkers are developed using archived tumor specimens, and many of the problems that exist in the marker literature derive from the retrospective nature of these studies. Clinical drug trials are generally prospective, with patient selection criteria, primary end point, hypotheses, and analysis plan specified in advance in a written protocol. The consumers of clinical trial reports have been educated to be skeptical of *data dredging* to find something "statistically significant" to report in clinical trials. They are skeptical of analyses with multiple end points or multiple subsets, knowing that the chances of erroneous conclusions increase rapidly once one leaves the context of a focused single-hypothesis clinical trial. Marker studies are generally performed with no written protocol, no eligibility criteria, no primary end point or hypotheses, and no defined analysis plan. The patient population is often very heterogeneous and represents individuals for whom archived specimens are available. The patients are often not treated in a single clinical trial and represent a mixture of stages. Consequently, the overall population often does not represent a therapeutically meaningful group and the biomarkers identified may be of prognostic relevance, but less likely to be of predictive relevance for selecting therapy. Often the marker may be prognostic because it is correlated with disease stage or some other known prognostic marker. Broad populations are also often heterogeneously treated and so finding that a marker is prognostic in such a population may be difficult to interpret. Prognostic markers that do not have therapeutic implications are rarely used. The heterogeneous nature of the population also often results in multiple subset analyses of more therapeutically meaningful subpopulations. With multiple analyses, the chance of false-positive conclusions increases. Many biomarker studies perform analyses for many candidate biomarkers and several end points as well as for various patient subsets. Consequently, the chance for erroneous conclusions increases multiplicatively. The multiplicity problem is even more severe when one considers that there are usually multiple ways of quantifying biomarker level and many possible mathematical models for combining biomarker measurements.

Many of the problems that have hindered the development and acceptance of predictive single-protein biomarkers also apply for biomarkers based on DNA microarray expression profiles (2). There are multiple platforms and protocols for measuring expression profiles, and microarray research studies almost never evaluate interlaboratory assay reproducibility. Microarray expression profiles in research studies are generally performed at one time so that reagent variability is minimized, and it is almost never demonstrated that the models are predictive for tumor specimens collected and assayed at other times. This is of particular concern for printed cDNA microarrays where there may be substantial variability among batches of printed slides and batches of reference RNA.

Because of the number of genes available for analysis, microarray data can be a veritable fountain of false findings unless appropriate statistical methods are utilized. For example, in comparing expression profiles of 10,000 genes for tumor specimens selected from patients who have responded to a specified treatment to those for nonresponders, the expected number of false-positive genes that are statistically significantly ($p < 0.05$)

differentially expressed between the two groups is 500. This is true regardless of whether the expression levels for different genes are correlated. Consequently, more stringent methods for assessing differential expression must be used. Some studies do not use statistical significance at all and just identify genes as differentially expressed based on fold-change statistics; that is, the ratio of the average expression level in responders to the average in nonresponders, ignoring variability entirely. Others base their analyses on visual inspection of graphical data displays. Such methods are clearly problematic.

The unstructured nature of retrospective studies of biomarkers would not be so problematic if they were followed by structured prospective validation studies that tested specific hypotheses about predictive biomarkers. Such prospective trials are rarely performed, however, because they are difficult to accomplish. Consequently, before discussing the design of such prospective trials, we will make some suggestions about a more structured approach to retrospective studies.

3. STRUCTURED RETROSPECTIVE STUDIES

There is a role for exploratory studies in which multiple biomarkers and multiple ways of combining biomarkers into predictive models are examined so long as one has an adequate way of evaluating the result. A major problem with many retrospective studies is that they attempt to use the same set of data to both develop hypotheses (biomarkers) and to test those hypotheses. This problem is particularly severe when the number of candidate hypotheses examined in the exploratory stage is large.

In trying to determine which genes are differentially expressed in comparing responders to a given therapy to nonresponders, the number of hypotheses equals the number of genes examined. The Bonferonni method of adjusting for multiple testing requires that the p value calculated for comparing expression of a specific gene i in responders to nonresponders, say p_i, be adjusted based on the number of genes (N) examined. For microarray studies, N could be 10,000 or greater. The Bonferonni method tries to eliminate all false positives. For microarray studies, less conservative methods control the number of *false discoveries* (false positives), or the proportion of claimed positives that are false positives (*false discovery rate*) *(3)*. These same ideas apply if, for example, we are examining which genes are prognostic for survival or disease-free survival on a particular treatment.

For assessing statistical significance, adjustments such as those described in the preceding paragraph can be applied to adjust for the fact that we do not have a specific hypothesis to test, but rather are in a hypothesis development mode. The adjustment is based on treating the problem as one of testing all possible hypotheses. For retrospective biomarker studies in which a number of biomarkers are examined, such adjustments to statistical significance should be applied. In many cases, however, statistical significance is not the best measure of biomarker value. A better measure is the extent to which the biomarker model enables us to predict whether the patient will respond to the treatment (4).

For binary outcomes such as response and nonresponse, the best measure of predictive accuracy is the number of correct predictions. For quantitative outcomes such as survival or disease-free survival, measurement of predictive accuracy is more complex. In many cases, it is reasonable to approximate quantitative outcomes in a binary manner: good outcome or poor outcome. In other cases, measures such as described by Korn and Simon (5) are used.

It is not valid to use the same set of data for selecting a predictive marker or developing a predictive model and for measuring predictive accuracy. The estimate of predictive accuracy computed on the same data used to select the marker or develop the model is called the *resubstitution* estimate and is known to be biased (6). The bias is extreme when the number of candidate markers is larger than the number of cases. For example, Simon et al. (6) showed that for two classes (e.g., responders and nonresponders) that have no genes that are truly differentially expressed in microarray expression profiles of thousands of genes, one can almost always find a predictive model that has a resubstitution estimate of accuracy of 100%. Such a model would be useless for future data, but would appear to give perfect predictions for the cases used to develop the model.

How can we develop a proper estimate of the accuracy of class prediction for future samples? For a future sample, we will apply a fully specified predictor developed using the data available today. If we are to emulate the future predictive setting in developing our estimate of predictive accuracy, we must set aside some of our samples and make them completely inaccessible until we have a fully specified predictor that has been developed from scratch without utilizing those set-aside samples.

To estimate properly the accuracy of a predictor for future samples, the current set of samples must be partitioned into a training set and a separate test set. The test set emulates the set of future samples for which class labels are to be predicted. Consequently the test samples cannot be used in any way for the development of the prediction model. This means that the test samples cannot be used for estimating the parameters of the model and they cannot be used for selecting the gene set to be used in the model. It is this latter point that is often overlooked.

The most straightforward method of estimating the accuracy of future prediction is the *split-sample* method of partitioning the set of samples into a training set and a test set as described in the previous paragraph. Rosenwald et al. (7) used this approach successfully in their international study of prognostic prediction for large cell lymphoma. They used two thirds of their samples as a training set. Multiple kinds of predictors were studied on the training set. When the collaborators of that study agreed on a single fully specified prediction model, they accessed the test set for the first time. On the test set there was no adjustment of the model, redefining of cutoff values, or fitting of parameters. They merely used the samples in the test set to evaluate the predictions of the model that was completely specified using only the training data.

Cross-validation is an alternative to the split sample method of estimating prediction accuracy *(8)*. Cross-validation can be used only when there is a well-defined algorithm for predictive model development. In such cases, cross-validation can be more efficient than the split-sample method for estimating prediction accuracy. There are several forms of cross-validation. Here we will describe *leave-one-out cross-validation (LOOCV)* in the context of a class predictor based on gene expression levels determined by DNA microarray analysis. LOOCV starts like split-sample cross-validation in forming a training set of samples and a test set. With LOOCV, however, the test set consists of only a single sample; the rest of the samples are placed in the training set. The sample in the test set is placed aside and not utilized at all in the development of the class prediction model. Using only the training set, the informative genes are selected and the parameters of the model are fit to the data. Let us call M_1 the model developed with sample 1 in the test set. When this model is fully developed, it is used to predict the class of sample 1. This prediction is made using the expression profile of sample 1, but obviously without using knowledge of the true class of sample 1. Symbolically, if $\underline{x}_1$ denotes the complete expression profile of sample 1, then we apply model M_1 to $\underline{x}_1$ to obtain a predicted class $\hat{c}_1$. This predicted class is compared to the true class label c_1 of sample 1. If they disagree, then the prediction is in error. Then a new training set–test set partition is created. This time sample 2 is placed in the test set and all of the other samples, including sample 1, are placed in the training set. A new model is constructed from scratch using the samples in the new training set. Call this model M_2. Model M_2 will generally not contain the same genes as model M_1. Although the same algorithm for gene selection and parameter estimation is used, since model M_2 is constructed from scratch on the new training set, it will in general not contain exactly the same gene set as M_1. After creating M_2, it is applied to the expression profile $\underline{x}_2$ of the sample in the new test set to obtain a predicted class $\hat{c}_2$. If this predicted class does not agree with the true class label c_2 of the second sample, then the prediction is in error.

The process described in the previous paragraph is repeated *n* times, where *n* is the number of biologically independent samples. Each time it is applied, a different sample is used to form the single-sample test set. During the steps, *n* different models are created and each one is used to predict the class of the omitted sample. The number of prediction errors is totaled and reported as the leave-one-out cross-validated estimate of the prediction error.

At the end of the LOOCV procedure you have constructed n different models. They were constructed only in order to estimate the prediction error associated with the model constructed by applying the algorithm to the complete set of samples. The model that would be used for future predictions is one constructed using all n samples. That is the best model for future prediction and the one that should be reported in the publication. The cross-validated error rate is an estimate of the error rate to be expected in use of this model for future samples assuming that the relationship between class and expression profile is the same for future samples as for the currently available samples. With two classes, one can use a similar approach to obtain cross-validated estimates of the sensitivity, specificity.

Leave-one-out cross-validation is applicable only in settings in which there is an algorithm for the development of a predictive model. In many studies, the analysis is less algorithmic and many kinds of prediction models are explored. For such studies, it is best to use the split sample approach of setting aside at least one third of the samples as a test or validation set. The samples in the test set should not be used for any purpose other than testing the final model developed in the training set. Specifically, the test set samples should not be used for limiting the set of genes to be considered in detail in the training set. The samples in the test set should not be accessed until a single model is identified based on training set analyses as *the* model to be tested.

LOOCV can be used to evaluate risk group predictors using survival or disease-free survival data. Suppose we wish to identify patients in a low-risk group with 10-year disease-free survival >90%. Consider the leave-one-out training set in which observation i is left out in the test set. A disease-free survival model M_i is developed for the training set. For example, the model might be a proportional hazards regression model that predicts disease-free survival based on the expression profile and/or standard prognostic factors. The model M_i is applied to the left-out specimen i to obtain a prediction of the probability that the ith patient has 10-yr disease-free survival >90%. Let $y_i = 1$ if this probability is greater than 50%. This process is repeated for all of the leave-one-out training sets. Then, the Kaplan–Meier disease-free survival curve estimate is computed and plotted for the patients predicted to be of very low risk, those with $y_i = 1$. The adequacy of the model is judged by whether the estimated 10-yr disease-free survival for the identified low-risk group is in fact in excess of 90%. An approach similar to this was used for developing a classification system based on survival for patients with renal cancer by Vasselli et al. *(9)*.

One of the common errors in retrospective studies of biomarkers is that the statistical significance of the biomarker is evaluated rather than the predictive accuracy of the biomarker *(4)*. We have indicated in the preceding how predictive accuracy can be evaluated in a manner that avoids the bias of the resubstitution estimate. But even this is not sufficient. New biomarkers are often correlated with existing prognostic factors. The retrospective study must provide strong evidence that the new marker is substantially more predictive than the currently available prognostic factors. This can be addressed by computing the split-sample or cross-validated error rate for a model consisting of current prognostic factors and then computing the split-sample or cross-validated error rate for a model consisting of current prognostic factors plus the new candidate markers. Only if the latter is substantially greater than the former with regard to a therapeutically relevant prediction will a prospective validation study be warranted.

4. VALIDATION STUDIES

Assuming that the initial study is performed properly with attention to the statistical principles described in previous section, it might be considered a phase II study, and the next step should be to conduct a phase III study that is focused on testing the specific classifier developed by the initial study *(10)*. The phase III study should be conducted with a written protocol. The phase III trial should be designed to test the biomarker classifier developed in the previous study. The classifier should be fully specified in the protocol. If the biomarker is expression profile based, the specification must include the genes used, the mathematical form of the classifier, parameter values, and cutoff thresholds for distinguishing the classes or prognostic groups.

The phase III study should attempt to perform the assays in a manner as similar as possible to the way it would be performed broadly outside of a research setting if the diagnostic classifier were adopted. Consequently, attention is required in determining whether the same platform should be used for the phase III trial as for the phase II trial. If the platform is changed, then clearly some intermediate study will be needed to translate the classification algorithm from use on the phase II platform to the platform used in the phase III trial.

Even if there is not a change in platform, an intermediate study may be required to prepare the classifier for use with multiple laboratories performing the assay. In the phase II trial all of the assays may have been performed at a single location by a research laboratory and it may be advisable to conduct the phase III trial in a manner more similar to the way it would be performed if the classifier were adopted for national use. Generally this will mean that several laboratories will be conducting the assays. Consequently, the protocol for the phase III study should specify procedures to be used for conducting the assay. It is also useful to conduct intermediate studies of interlaboratory reproducibility of the assays. Unless interlaboratory repro-

Table 1
Guidelines for Validation Studies *(10)*

1. Intra- and interlaboratory reproducibility of assays should be documented.
2. Laboratory assays should be performed blinded to clinical data and outcome.
3. An inception cohort of patients should be assembled with <15% of patients nonevaluable owing to missing tissue or data. The referral pattern and eligibility criteria should be described.
4. Treatment should be standardized or randomized and accounted for in the analysis.
5. Hypotheses should be stated in advance, including specification of prognostic factors, coding of prognostic factors, end points, and subsets of patients and treatments.
6. The sample size and number of events should be sufficiently large that statistically reliable results are obtained. Statistical power calculations that incorporate the number of hypotheses to be tested and appropriate subsets for each hypothesis should be described. There should be at least 10 events per prognostic factor examined per subset analyzed.
7. Analyses should test whether new factors add predictiveness after adjustment for or within subsets determined by standard prognostic factors.
8. Analyses should be adjusted for the number of hypotheses to be tested.
9. Analyses should be based on prespecified cutoff values for prognostic factors or cutoffs should be avoided.

ducibility is sufficiently high, it is not advisable to proceed with the phase III trial.

If the biomarker classifier was developed using a dual-label microarray platform, then use of the classifier in other laboratories requires that they use the same common reference RNA as was used for the initial study. Because different batches of the common reference will be utilized for classifying subsequent patients, calibration studies will generally be required to ensure that the expression profile of the common reference does not change and to adjust the classifier for small changes.

Conducting the validation study as a prospective trial is desirable for many reasons. One can never be sure that the patients for whom one has adequate preserved tissue are representative of the population of patients presenting for treatment. It is difficult to assure that a retrospective cohort was adequately staged and treated, and the data available may be incomplete. It is also difficult to assess whether a diagnostic procedure is practical unless it is studied in the real-time context of presenting patients who need to be evaluated and treated. Prospective accrual is also important for evaluating the diagnostic classifier in the context of real-time tissue handling. Table 1, reprinted from Simon and Altman *(10)*, indicates some important design features of prospective validation studies.

The objective of the validation trial of a predictive marker is to test the hypothesis that the marker is useful for treatment selection. This is often a more complex objective than validation of a prognostic marker, in which the objective is to determine whether the marker can separate the uniformly staged and treated patients into groups of differing outcome. There are some cases, discussed below, in which prognostic markers are also predictive markers. Our focus is on predictive markers and we will consider three breast cancer scenarios.

4.1. Identifying Node-Negative Patients
Who Do Not Require Chemotherapy

Our first scenario is a putative marker for identifying node-negative patients whose prognosis on local therapy and possibly tamoxifen is so good that they do not require chemotherapy. The retrospective study for development of such a marker would have probably been based on archived tumors of node-negative patients who did not receive chemotherapy. A tissue microarray of a large number of such specimens, with associated clinical follow-up data, can provide a valuable resource for ensuring that the marker is sufficiently promising to warrant evaluation in a prospective clinical trial if the classifier is not RNA transcript profile based. A marker of this type meets the definition of a prognostic marker, but it can also be a predictive marker if it enables us to determine which node negative patients do not require chemotherapy.

The theoretically optimal trial design would be to randomize candidate node-negative patients to receive or not receive chemotherapy and then to validate whether the marker identifies those who do not benefit from chemotherapy. The candidate node-negative patients might be those with tumors 1–3 cm in diameter without known poor prognostic features such as hormone receptor negativity. This is probably not a feasible approach, however, because chemotherapy has already been established as being effective for much of the candidate population.

An alternative study design is to withhold chemotherapy from a subset of node-negative patients selected based on marker status to be of particularly low risk. If their outcomes were sufficiently good relative to some standard, then the marker would be accepted as useful. The standard might be based on outcomes for node-negative patients that are similar with regard to standard prognostic factors in other studies. It may also be useful to compare outcome for the selected patients (M^+) to the outcome for the patients of the same series who did not have such predicted good prognosis (M^-). The latter patients would have received chemotherapy, but their outcome even with chemotherapy may not be as good as that of the M^+ patients without chemotherapy. If that is the case, then the value of the marker for withholding chemotherapy will have been demonstrated.

An alternative approach would be to randomize patients selected as low risk based on marker status (M^+) to either receive or not receive chemotherapy. The marker would be validated if the randomized trial demonstrated that there was no clinically significant benefit of chemotherapy in the selected subset of patients. This would have to be a very large clinical trial, however. The benefit of chemotherapy would be expected to reduce the hazard or recurrence only by approx 25%, and with a very low event rate this is equivalent to a very small difference in absolute disease-free survival. The randomized trial asks a different question than the strategy described in the previous paragraph. The randomized trial asks whether there is a benefit of treatment. For patients with a very good prognosis, however, a statistically significant treatment effect may be of questionable clinical significance. Consequently, the randomized trial may not answer the most relevant question.

Gasparini et al. *(11)* describe guidelines for the adoption into clinical practice of new prognostic markers for use in treatment selection for patients with node-negative breast cancer.

4.2. Identifying Node-Positive Patients Who Do Not Benefit From a Chemotherapy Regimen

Consider now a putative marker that permits the identification of patients who do not benefit from a chemotherapy regimen that has been standard treatment. Let T denote the chemotherapy regimen, and let S denote local therapy or local therapy plus tamoxifen. The retrospective study used to develop the marker may have been based on tissue from a randomized trial of T vs S. In some cases the marker may be based on finding a signature of patients who do not respond to T in metastatic disease trials.

The ideal validation trial would probably be a randomized trial of S vs T for patients with node-positive breast cancer. One could analyze such a trial by seeing whether the benefit of T vs S depended on the marker level. Such a trial would generally be impractical, however, because T or some other kind of chemotherapy is standard treatment for node-positive patients. It might be possible, however, to randomize patients to receive or not receive one or more courses of T preoperatively, and to correlate marker result with biological response to T as assessed from the surgical specimen.

A second strategy would be to use chemotherapy T on all patients after measuring the marker. One could then determine prospectively whether the marker level correlates with outcome. This is a strategy analogous to that recommended in Subheading 4.1. Here, however, one is trying to determine whether the marker identifies a group of such poor disease-free survival on standard treatment T that the chemotherapy is judged nonworthwhile even in the absence of a control group not receiving chemotherapy. This strategy may be less satisfactory for judging poor prognosis in absolute terms than it was in Subheading 4.1. for judging good prognosis.

A third strategy would be to randomize the patients to marker based vs non-marker-based therapeutic management. The non-marker-based management would assign T to all patients. The marker-based management would assign T to all except those predicted based on the marker to be nonresponsive (M-). One way of conducting such a trial is to measure the marker only for those patients assigned to marker-based management. The value of the marker is determined by comparing the outcome for the marker-based management arm to the outcome for the non-marker-based management arm. This is, however, a very inefficient trial design. Because most patients in both arms of the trial will be receiving the same treatment, the average treatment difference will be very small between the arms and a huge sample size will be required. The situation is even more problematic because it is a therapeutic equivalence trial in the sense that failure to find a statistically significant difference leads to the adoption of the new treatment approach, in this case marker-based treatment assignment.

A better design is to measure the marker on all patients, and then randomize them to marker-based treatment vs non-marker-based treatment. The evaluation of the marker can be performed by comparing outcomes for the M- patients who received chemotherapy T on the non-marker-based arm but treatment S on the marker-based arm. This will require a much smaller sample size than the design described in the previous paragraph. This design is essentially equivalent to randomizing the M- patients to T or S.

4.3. Identifying Node-Positive Patients Who Benefit From a Specific Regimen

Our third scenario is that we have a putative marker that identifies patients whose tumors are responsive to a new regimen E when the standard chemotherapeutic regimen is T. Many new therapeutics have defined molecular targets and are developed in conjunction with an assay that measures the expression of the target. The most adequate validation study is often a randomized clinical trial in which both marker-positive and marker-negative patients are randomized to either standard treatment T or T plus the new regimen E. The trial should be large enough so that the new regimen can be evaluated separately in the M+ and M- subsets. This requires about twice as many patients as if the regimen T+E were to be evaluated overall, without reference to the marker.

If the biological relationship between the marker and the therapeutic is sufficiently strong, it may be difficult to justify including marker negative patients in the study. A randomized study comparing T to T+E for M+ patients may be very efficient for demonstrating the effectiveness of the new treatment E, but it will not really constitute a validation of the marker.

The development of the therapeutic, supported by the marker assay, may, however, be more important than validation of the essentiality of the marker for selecting patients.

The least desirable alternative would be to randomize patients between T and T+E without measuring the marker. If the marker is important, then such a trial design may be very inefficient for evaluating the therapeutic E, and of course, it provides no information for validating the marker.

The scenario described here is also applicable to the development of treatment regimens in which the molecular target is not known or not known with certainty. Instead of using an assay based on the expression of the putative target, one may use a DNA microarray–based classifier developed in phase II trials of metastatic disease patients for distinguishing responders from nonresponders to the new regimen E. If tumor specimens are available from patients treated with the standard treatment T as well as those treated with the new treatment E, the classifier can be developed to identify patients who are predicted to be more responsive to the new treatment E but not to standard treatment T.

REFERENCES

1. Hilsenbeck SG, Clark GM, McGuire WL. Why do so many prognostic factors fail to pan out? *Breast Cancer Res Treat* 1992;22:197–206.
2. Simon RM, Korn EL, McShane LM, Radmacher MD, Wright GW, Zhao Y. *Design and analysis of DNA microarray investigations*. Springer, New Yok, 2003.
3. Reiner A, Yekutieli D, Benjamini Y. Identifying differentially expressed genes using false discovery rate controlling procedures. *Bioinformatics* 2003;19:368–375.
4. Kattan MW. Judging new markers by their ability to improve predictive accuracy. *J Natl Cancer Inst* 2003;95:634–635.
5. Korn EL, Simon R. Measures of explained variation for survival data. *Stat Med* 1990;9:487–504.
6. Simon R, Radmacher MD, Dobbin K, McShane LM. Pitfalls in the analysis of DNA microarray data: class prediction methods. *J Natl Cancer Inst* 2003;95:14–18.
7. Rosenwald A, Wright G, Chan WC, et al. The use of molecular profiling to predict survival after chemotherapy for diffuse large-B-cell lymphoma. *N Engl J Med* 2002;346:1937–1947.
8. Radmacher MD, McShane LM, Simon R. A paradigm for class prediction using gene expression profiles. *J Comput Biol* 2002;9:505–511.
9. Vasselli J, Shih JH, Iyengar SR, et al. Predicting survival in patients with metastatic kidney cancer by gene expression profiling in the primary tumor. *Proc Natl Acad Sci USA* 2003;100:6958–6963.
10. Simon R, Altman DG. Statistical aspects of prognostic factor studies in oncology. *Br J Cancer* 1994;69:979–985.
11. Gasparini G, Pozza F, Harris AL. Evaluating the potential usefulness of new prognostic and predictive indicators in node-negative breast cancer patients. *J Natl Cancer Inst* 1993;85:1206–1219.

2 Analytical Aspects of Biomarker Immunoassays in Cancer Research

Fred C.G.J. Sweep, PHD, Chris M.G. Thomas, PHD, and Manfred Schmitt, PHD

SUMMARY

Many difficulties associated with immuno(metric) assay kits designed for quantification of a particular biomarker arise from their variation in specificity and binding affinity of the employed antibodies. Other important sources causing varying assay results are the use of different standard preparations in these kits and the nonuniform preanalytical specimen processing procedures employed, each of which should be subjected to standardization. To improve the performance and comparability of assays, continuous interlaboratory external quality control procedures are needed. Such quality assurance

Cancer Drug Discovery and Development: Biomarkers in Breast Cancer:
Molecular Diagnostics for Predicting and Monitoring Therapeutic Effect
Edited by: G. Gasparini and D. F. Hayes © Humana Press Inc., Totowa, NJ

programs provide a forum for expert laboratory investigators to discuss technical details and to exchange laboratory issues and related practical information. This chapter addresses some of these issues and presents initial analytical validation procedures of newly developed biomarker assays, the validation of already established assay procedures for routine use on a day-to-day basis, and finally discusses some aspects on adequate (external) quality control proficiency testing.

Key Words: Biomarkers; immunoassay; cancer; tumor markers.

1. INTRODUCTION

In many cases progression of cancer growth is rather slow and often it may take years for a malignancy to manifest clinically. Because early cancer detection is required to significantly reduce cancer mortality, screening procedures are needed that are highly specific (i.e., providing almost a 100% proportion of negative test results for a tumour marker in nondiseased individuals) and sensitive enough to detect malignancies at an early stage of development. Thus, the screening procedure should give assay results above a defined cutoff value in a reasonable proportion of early stage diseased persons. As yet, there are no assay procedures available that meet such a specification, although there is a growing public interest in improving early cancer detection. Ideally, determination in biological specimens of cancer-derived analytes for a particular type of cancer not only should provide valuable information for initial diagnosis, but also should have prognostic value to guide the choice of treatment, and such a test should provide a reflection of the tumor burden of the patient, being predictive for recurrent disease after initial treatment, and of help in monitoring the course of the disease throughout time of follow-up. Each of these properties should contribute to more effective treatment of an individual patient and thus provide indispensable information for improving the quality of life and outcome of the disease by increasing disease-free and overall survival. Despite extensive research efforts in the last decades and numerous papers dealing with development and clinical testing of potentially promising biochemical markers, no assays are as yet available that are sensitive enough to convincingly detect any of the major types of cancer at the most early stage. Although an impressive number of biochemical markers with the capacity to predict disease recurrence and/or early death have been introduced, a comprehensive understanding of the tumor biological processes involved is still lacking.

1.1. Guidelines for Evaluating Clinical Value of Biomarkers

At present, cancer diagnosis is based mainly on clinical symptoms and confirmed by histomorphological findings. Application of biochemical markers in this process may have additional value but still, depending on the marker test applied, the reliability criteria may become less important. In case of screening and diagnosis ("rule-in-disease") specificity is of utmost importance (to avoid false-positive assay results leading to unfavorable and unnecessary medical examination and treatment), although it should be realized that increasing specificity of a test goes at the cost of decreasing its sensitivity (that should remain high enough to detect early-stage diseased individuals). If the purpose of the test is disease monitoring to detect recurrence during follow-up, precision should be high; providing a prognosis for treatment, the test should put emphasis on specificity and accuracy. All of these criteria are not well established and should become standard criteria for evaluation of biomarker assays and their clinical application. In line with this, Hayes et al. (1) proposed certain criteria to standardize the available biomarker information for clinical use in a biomarker utility grading system.

Currently, many biochemical markers of potentially prognostic value are intensively tested in multicenter clinical trials. Only a few of these show a benefit for predicting prognosis of node-negative breast cancer patients. To conclude that these newly developed biochemical markers have independent prognostic value over already known factors, McGuire and Clark (2) some years ago proposed strict guidelines for evaluating newly developed prognostic markers, addressing the biological role of the new factor as well as the extent of the sample size, the risk of sample bias, the appropriate testing system, the establishment of cutoff values in a training data set, and confirmation of these observations in an independent validation data set.

2. IMMUNOASSAY DESIGNS

Immunochemical assay procedures can be classified according to the kind of analysis (qualitative, semiquantitative, or quantitative), type of assay format (manual or automated) and assay system (liquid phase, solid–liquid phase, [non-]equilibrium), making use of (radioisotopic or nonisotopic) labeled markers (to detect the antigen–antibody complex) or nonlabeled markers (in which the antigen–antibody complex is detected without labeled markers). The term immunoassay refers to competitive methods while immunometric assays refer to noncompetitive, sandwich-type assay formats. As early as 1969 the first generation of binding assays emerged with development of a radioimmunoassay (RIA) for quantification of insulin antibody formation. Later, the evolution of technical developments led to nonisotopic labels (enzyme-, fluorescence, time-resolved fluoro, (chemo-) luminescence immunoassays, etc.), monoclonal antibodies, phase matrices, and two-site immunometric sandwich-type assay formats employing two or more antibodies that will bind the analyte at repetitive or different epitope binding sites. The enzyme-linked immunosorbent assay (ELISA) format is a commonly used type of two-site sandwich type assay in clinical routine work. The analyte is allowed to react noncompetitively with an excess of immobilized ("capture") antibody (coupled to a solid phase) and after addition and washing off the excess amount of sample specimen, an excess amount of marker labeled ("signal") antibody is added to bind to another epitope of the analyte. The sandwich thus formed is provided with marker label proportional to the amount of analyte present in the sample. These quantitative assay formats have several advantages: large numbers of specimens can be processed in parallel, providing reproducible results with reasonable precision, sensitivity, specificity, and accuracy. A major advantage of immunometric assay formats over semiquantitative or qualitative techniques is provided by the quantitative endpoint as measured against a defined standard, although there are limitations. Often, the analyte standard is not well defined, the assay procedure is not fully validated prior to use in patient studies, or the possibility to make comparisons to a reference method is lacking. Strict measures of quality assurance or good manufacturing practice protocols are needed to ensure proper assay performance before they should be applied.

Because early detection of small breast lesions is becoming common practice, there is an increasing demand to measure correctly biomarkers in smaller pieces of tumor specimens obtained through fine needle aspiration, core biopsies, or cryostat sections. This implies that there is an immediate need for more sensitive techniques than the standard immunoassays available to date. Alternative approaches to ELISA are proteomic methods such as MALDI and SELDI TOF mass spectrometry (MS), tandem MS, plasma resonance techniques, and antibody chip technologies. Of course the same rigorous principles of quality assurance should be applied for these new methodologies as for the more conventional immunoassays.

3. VARIABILITY IN TEST RESULTS

Assay results are often heterogeneous because of variations in specimen composition, tissue processing, design and specificity of the employed assay, as well as the statistics used for analyzing the collected data. In each of these stages, intrinsic differences in molecular forms (isoforms) of the biomarker present in the tumor tissue are augmented by external causes. The sampling procedure (e.g., fine-needle aspirate, core biopsy, or large biopsy obtained during surgery), the source of tissue (fresh or frozen), storage conditions (time, temperature, freeze–thawing cycles, etc.), and tissue processing (cytosol fraction, membrane extracts) may severely influence the final assay results (3). Likewise, this also holds true for the quantification of biological markers in serum or plasma (4).

Variable design of immuno(metric) assays results in the generation of different test results because different kits incorporate a broad spectrum of antibodies, sometimes with different antibody specificities and/or affinities. Also, the use of different standards and reference materials provided with the kits are a source of variations in test results. Furthermore, different data reduction processes and statistical techniques are used to analyze tumor marker data and this may lead to a variety of conclusions regarding the clinical interpretation. The computational data processing of laboratory results must be appropriate, uniform, and evaluated extensively *(5)*. McGuire and Clark stated that the design of confirmatory clinical studies should be identical to that of the definite study *(2)*. It is of most importance to note that this also applies to all laboratory steps including tissue storage and processing, the analytical procedures, and the subsequent data processing.

The number and diversity of biomarkers for assessment of cancer prognosis is expanding rapidly, as is the variety of analytical formats and procedures used for quantification. A substantial proportion of assays is based on immunochemical principles and there is a widespread use of nonvalidated assay formats in clinical research settings. Because many assays are poorly standardized and (external) quality control is lacking in most cases, nonvalidated assay results without provided certified guidelines for interpretation become available at a too preliminary stage of assay development. Thus, biomarker testing procedures in laboratories participating in clinical trials should be standardized and externally quality assessed. This requires settlement of quality standards of all assay reagents included in assay kits, provision of guidelines for standardized assay protocols, standardized algorithms for calculation of assay results, and statistical procedures to allow unequivocal interpretation of clinical effect measures. Finally, to ascertain continuity of reliable biomarker data generation, there is a need for guidelines toward uniform internal and external quality assessment procedures. The next sections will discuss preanalytical, analytical, and postanalytical aspects of assay performance.

4. ASPECTS OF BIOMARKER ASSESSMENT

4.1. Preanalytical Criteria

4.1.1. SAMPLING BIAS OF TISSUE SPECIMENS AND TISSUE PROCESSING

Because many tumors are heterogeneous the size of a tumor tissue specimen is important to avoid sampling bias. This bias may lead to different assay results if different areas of a tumor are analyzed (different content of tumor cells, nonmalignant cells, extracellular matrix, fat, and necrotic spots). Thus, fine needle biopsy results may differ from those obtained from a tumor tissue biopsy specimen. Selection bias may occur if frozen tissue specimens from large tumor banks are used in retrospective studies as generally in tumor banks relatively larger samples of frozen tumor tissues are overrepresented *(6)*.

The use of blood specimens requires standardization of blood collection conditions (fasting, fixed time of day, supine position), type of specimen (whole blood, serum, or plasma) and type of anticoagulant. Care should be taken to immediately transport tissue specimens or blood directly after surgery or blood collection to the laboratory in a standardized manner (time, temperature). Disintegration or extraction procedures of tissue samples should be performed according to the consensus protocols written by internationally acknowledged experts. Errors in this preanalytical phase of biomarker level quantification will affect the reliability of the final experimental data.

4.2. Analytical and Reliability Criteria

Prior to producing and subsequent reporting of test results it is the task of the laboratory to verify or establish performance specifications for each analytical procedure, irrespective whether the assay of interest has been developed in an academic institution or by a commercial company. In their instructions for use, kit manufacturers have often included disclaimers for misusing or overinterpreting the information included in their product information. It is common practice of diagnostic kit manufacturers to advice their clients that each laboratory should establish its own reference values in particular for specified populations or applications, irrespective of already available data provided by the manufacturer. The next sections deal with reliability criteria of analytic testing systems.

4.2.1. STANDARD CALIBRATION PREPARATIONS

Standards are used to prepare a standard dose response curve that relates the response reading as the independent variable to the quantity of the standard as the dependent variable. This allows calculation of the quantity of analyte from the response reading obtained for the unknown sample. It is not always possible to obtain sufficient quantities of a reasonably pure biomarker for characterization, which is the reason why in many cases arbitrary nonpurified or semipurified preparations of biomarkers are used to produce standard curves. Protein analytes may be present in different molecular forms ("isoforms") which may cause differences in affinity or other binding characteristics with antibodies. In case there are differences in affinity of the antibody for the calibrator standard and the analyte present in the unknown sample, different assay results will be obtained at different sample dilutions. For this reason we propose to analyze biological markers in at least two or three different dilutions to detect this phenomenon. This means that the suitability of a biomarker assay has to be validated for each biological specimen of concern because the procedure for the measurement of an analyte in tissue extracts is not always suitable for assaying the same analyte in plasma or serum. Stability of the standard can best be followed by longitudinal monitoring of the consecutively produced slopes of the standard dose–response curves. Thus, assays should use well-defined, well-characterized standard calibrator material with known sequence and degree of purity. Also, different kit manufacturers should adhere to internationally accepted standards and preferably use identical standards in their diagnostic kits. An important source of providing biological reference materials to the scientific community covering many areas of clinical medicine is the WHO International Laboratory for Biological Standards (National Institute for Biological Standards and Control [NIBSC], Potters Bar, UK). Finally, as an example of advancements that contribute to standardization of widely used biomarker assays, we mention the introduction of an assay procedure for prostate-specific antigen (PSA) that determines several molecular forms of PSA on an equimolar basis, and the calibration of this assay with the Stanford 90:10 Reference Material, composed of 90% PSA-ACT and 10% free-PSA *(7)*.

4.2.2. Accuracy

Definition of accuracy of an assay by the International Federation of Clinical Chemistry (IFCC) is the agreement between the best estimate of a quantity and its true value. As this quantity has no numerical value, the term inaccuracy is used. Thus, inaccuracy is the difference between the mean of a set of replicate measurements and the true value. Although the concept is clear, it has realistic value for those analytes for which a reference method is available. As no such reference values are available or even feasible for many biomarkers, the concept of (in)accuracy has limited significance, emphasizing even more the necessity of standardization of assays.

4.2.2.1. Linearity

As outlined earlier, linearity of an assay in fact refers to identity between affinity of the antibody for the calibrator standard and the analyte present in the unknown sample. This should be the case and these tests of parallelism between standard and unknown analyte can be conducted by measuring samples at different sample dilutions and multiplying the amount of analyte measured with the dilution factor. Linearity studies are used to assess and establish the working range of an assay that is in between the lowest and highest concentration that can reliably be measured with that assay. This can easily be realized by mixing two different samples in several proportions (e.g., 1:3, 1:1, 3:1). See also the National Committee for Clinical Laboratory Standards (NCCLS) evaluation protocol (EP6).

4.2.2.2. Recovery

Recovery experiments are conducted to test whether the standard of the assay and analyte in the unknown sample behave chemically identical, or to exclude whether disturbing interactions of the analyte with the matrix or other compounds of the assay will lead to different assay results. Thus, in order to obtain insight into the identity of the analyte vs the standard, or to study matrix interactions with the standard, known amounts of standard are added to samples with an already known amount of endogenous biomarker and the recovery of the added amount is calculated.

4.2.2.3. High-Dose Hook Effect

This phenomenon is a source of error specifically occurring in double determinant one-step sandwich-type assays and comprises the saturation of capture and/or signal antibodies resulting from extremely high concentrations of biomarker analyte present in the incubation medium. This leads to a falsely low concentration calculated for the analyte. High-dose hook effects can be avoided by conducting a two-step assay protocol in which the immobilized capture antibody is incubated with an appropriately diluted unknown sample and excess of unbound analyte is washed off. The assay is completed by addition of signal antibody in the second incubation step. It is also advised to analyze samples at different dilutions to check whether the assay is vulnerable for the high-dose hook effect.

4.2.2.4. Interferences

Heterophilic antibodies are an often underestimated source of error in immunometric assays. In particular the treatment of patients with monoclonal mouse antibodies for immune-imaging and immune-targeting purposes has emerged occurrence of human antimouse antibodies (HAMAs), that is, the generation of human immune globulins G and M (IgG, IgM) in the blood of these patients. These antimouse IgG or IgM may also originate from other iatrogenic animal sources, all of these interfering to variable extents with the antibodies incorporated in biomarker sandwich-type assays. For a review of HAMA occurrence and it consequences for assay methodology see Kricka *(8)*.

4.2.3. Specificity

In epidemiological terms specificity refers to the proportion of true-negative test results of a control population and in fact is similar to its definition in analytical terms where it is defined as (absence of) interference (cross-reaction) in an assay system of compounds more or less related to the analyte to be measured in that assay. Thus, specificity of immunoassays refers to the degree of interference by compounds that may resemble but differ from the analyte to be quantified. One established manner to express cross-reaction is comparison of the amount of analyte homologous for the assay with the amount of another compound tested for interference with the assay. This is performed at half the maximum response level (often referred to as $B/B_0 = 0.5$) of the linearized standard dose–response curve. The specificity of immunometric assays strongly depends on antibody characteristics because polyclonal or monoclonal antibodies or mixtures of both are applied in different testing kits. Specificity will be highest with monoclonal antibodies because these are directed against one epitope on the analyte molecule. Many tumor-associated antigens have epitopes also common to other proteins present in a variety of many other tissues. Because epitope mapping data of antibodies is not often documented, investigators have to check cross reactivity of a number of compounds related structurally or biologically to the assay's analyte.

4.2.4. SENSITIVITY

In epidemiological terms, sensitivity refers to the proportion of true-positive test results of a diseased population. Analytically, sensitivity may be defined as the limit of detection of the analyte in the assay, that is, the lowest concentration of analyte significantly different from zero, also called the analytical sensitivity. The limit of quantification at which a test can be reliably measured with a coefficient of variation of less than 20% is called the functional sensitivity. It is recommended to report clinical assay results not below the functional sensitivity limit that can easily be retrieved from the precision profile of an assay that is constructed by plotting the coefficients of variation of replicate measurements of all the samples assayed against the concentrations of the obtained results. Data on sensitivity should be provided by the kit manufacturer and checked by the investigator on first use of a kit. One of the goals of immunoassay methodology is to optimize continuously the lower detection limits of assays in order to settle clinically relevant cutoff points. Defining such low thresholds requires a high degree of reproducibility of assay results, that is, precision.

4.2.5. PRECISION

According to the IFCC, precision is defined by the agreement between replicate measurements. As is also the case with accuracy, precision has no numerical value, the reason why the use of imprecision is more practical, although not commonly used. The imprecision is the standard deviation or coefficient of variation of the results of a set of replicate measurements.

The precision of a biomarker determination varies depending on whether duplicate determinations are performed in one sample, different samples in the same batch, or in different batches, and so forth. Obviously, the estimate of the precision used to assess the validity of experimental results must be related to the assay conditions in the definite study. For instance, if the concentration of a biomarker in malignant vs nonmalignant tissue of the same patient is determined in one assay run, the statistical significance of relevant difference is referred to the intraassay precision of the method. On the other hand, when a marker is monitored over a long time of observation (follow-up), samples will be assayed in different batches of test kits and the interassay precision is the more relevant parameter. For validation of an assay, at least the intrasample, intraassay precision performance should be investigated. The precision profile is an ideal tool to assess this (see below). The NCCLS offers a practical evaluation protocol (EP5) for evaluating the precision performance of an assay.

4.2.6. MINIMAL CONSISTENCY CRITERIA

Apart from the aforementioned assay characteristics that should be assessed by the investigator once a new kit is introduced into the laboratory, assay performance may be hampered by day-to-day, performer-to-performer, and batch-to-batch variability. Run-to-run performance errors may be reduced by daily consistency testing of the calibration curve, the precision profile, and data on quality control specimens. Charting of standard dose–response curve characteristics comprises at least the calibrated slope; y-intercept, correlation coefficient, analyte concentration at 50% response (ED_{50}), and minimum detectable analyte concentration. The shape of this curve defines the quality of the performed assay and offers a basis for selection of the working range of the assay, while it also quite easily allows to detect unreliably scattering duplicates.

4.3. Postanalytical Criteria

Once an assay has been performed the results of unknown samples must be derived from the obtained response parameters by calculating the analyte concentrations from the standard dose–response curve. Numerous computerized algorithms are available, but irrespective of the choices made, it is highly advisable to use the same statistical approach to process assay data, especially if one participates in or conducts a multicenter study. Each laboratory should establish its own reference values to circumvent population sampling errors and biological variation.

5. QUALITY ASSURANCE (QA)

Defined protocols for (internal and external) quality control (QC) should be part of routine practice in the laboratory. QA not only comprises the analytical process as such (QC), but it also regards the total of the managerial, technical, and interpretative aspects and is intended to prevent, monitor, and correct mistakes in the laboratory chain process. Reasonable quality management requires knowledge about the level of quality that is needed. It is useless to implement and adhere to too strict control rules because this may cause unnecessary, false rejection of assay runs. Ideally, an adequate control procedure should be based on a definition of quality requirements weighing acceptable error against needed clinical decision levels.

5.1. Internal and External QC

Every biomarker assay should include control sample procedures to check the validity of the unknown sample results. Control samples and comparison of their results against control limits should always be integral part of a complete assay procedure.

5.1.1. QC Samples

QC samples are stabilized specimens and available in liquid or lyophilized form because freshly collected sample materials are not always available and unstable for long-term QC use. Important requirements of QC preparations are that they should be time and temperature resistant with little or no vial-to-vial variation, homogeneous, similar in matrix structure to the test material, available at concentrations that cover the physiological range expected in the experimental material, and available in sufficient quantities. Unfortunately these requirements are not always achieved. For serum assays, large pools of serum can be established, aliquoted, and made available to laboratories. However, many manufacturers nowadays supply reference samples on a non-serum–based matrix, and in some cases this yields assay results different from those of true native serum samples. Thus, control samples should resemble as close as possible the analyte fractions representative of those routinely encountered in patient specimens.

5.1.2. Monitoring of Daily Performance

At least two samples of different concentrations of control material should be included in each assay run to make multirule/decision control procedures possible, for example, by applying Westgard evaluation rules for internal QC (IQC) *(9)*. Thus, repeated measurement of control samples allows to determine imprecision of the assay system. In addition to the use of IQC for day-to-day assay monitoring, the long-term trend in assay performance should be regularly checked in order to detect any shift or drift. Obviously, there should be agreed criteria for batch rejection. Levey–Jennings charts *(10)* are practical tools to evaluate the controls simply by plotting the individual values on a chart and compare these with a predefined mean with signaling limits (e.g., ± 2 SD). The chart patterns bring different kinds of technical problems (random error, systematic error, etc.) to light, and are also useful, simple tools for investigators or supervisors to decide whether or not assay results are within (or beyond) acceptable ranges and whether the data can be reported. Lot-to-lot variation errors of commercial reagents can be reduced by prescreening of critical reagents and be rejected before use if not consistent.

For external QC (EQC) purposes, preparations distributed by a reference laboratory should be included in assay runs if available. In proper EQC programs, the obtained data of control samples should be submitted to an external organization for statistical evaluation. These programs serve to monitor long-term assay performance within each participating laboratory. Moreover, they provide comparison of assay results between laboratories and between different assay designs or brands, if available. This enables the organization to assess systematic errors between laboratories just by comparing the reported mean values of the individual laboratories with the mean of the total or reference group (all laboratory trimmed mean).

5.1.3. EXTERNAL QUALITY ASSESSMENT (EQA) DOES NOT COVER ALL PROCESS STEPS

EQA based on lyophilized tumor tissue extracts or blood specimens does not allow any conclusion with regard to preanalytical, methodological issues such as variation in tissue collection, transport from operating theater to the laboratory, sample storage conditions, homogenization of tissue, and extraction procedures, as the use of external controls covers only reproducibility of the analytical assay procedure and subsequent computation of data. Providing proper instructions and careful observation of the results obtained is the only feasible way to monitor (between-hospital) variations in sample treatment conditions. Because most clinical trials are carried out on a multicenter basis, the interlaboratory QC is very important but the obtained deviations are most probably underestimations of true differences. Therefore, all steps in the procedure from taking biopsies to reporting assay results to the clinician including the preanalytical items should be conducted according to strict protocol guidelines.

5.2. Normalization of Assay Results

Long-term QA trials on steroid hormone receptors (estrogen receptors [ERs] and progestin receptors [PgRs]) assays by the Receptor and Biomarker Group of the European Organisation for Research and Treatment of Cancer (RBG EORTC) have shown that even highly experienced laboratories, with excellent intralaboratory between-run performance, can have difficulties in directly comparing their results with those of another institution. As variation among laboratories in general appeared to be not random (11), a high interlaboratory coefficient of variation (CV) does not necessarily mean inconsistencies in performance of all individual laboratories. These systematic differences in ER and PgR test results pave the way for calibration (see Fig. 1). However, normalization can be achieved only when a marker is homogeneous with only one molecular form present. The presence of more molecular forms of the analyte will yield a broad range of data, especially when different immuno(metric) assays (with varying sets of antibodies, each with other affinities to these molecular forms of the analytes) are used.

6. CONCLUSIONS

An important issue in applying (pre-)clinical immuno(metric) testing kits is that different kits in many cases generate different assay results in the same tumor specimen owing to variation in test design, antibody specificity

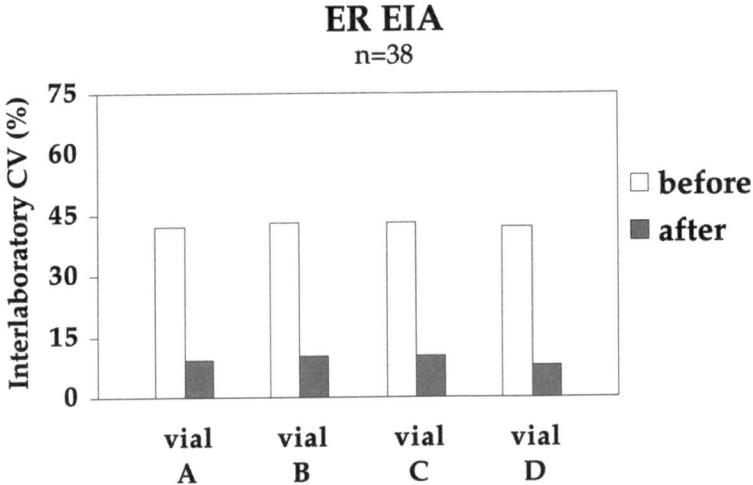

Fig. 1. Interlaboratory CV before (*open bars*) and after normalization of the observed values using a common fifth QA vial (Vial E, gray bars) in estrogen receptor enzyme immunoassay (EIA). Normalization substantially reduces the interlaboratory CVs from 45% to <15%.

and affinity between different kits (or even within a kit from one manufacturer between lots or batches), and use of different calibrators. Although of potential interest, newly explored biomarkers in our view should therefore not be included in large clinical studies unless the assay procedures are carefully evaluated, and common assay protocols, common standards, and QC preparations allowing proper EQA established. At first, such a parameter should be examined in a single expert laboratory. In addition, we strongly advice that in multicenter studies the laboratory performance to be scrutinized prior to generating results from patients in clinical trials.

Hayes proposed criteria for implementing biomarkers in clinical practice, and he defined levels of evidence (LOE) and levels of utility (1). For the highest level (LOE-1) large consistent meta-analysis and validation in a prospective clinical trial should be conducted. Recently, in case of urokinase-type plasminogen activator (uPA) and its inhibitor PAI-1 the level of evidence type-1 was reached, based on the results of a prospective randomized node-negative breast cancer therapy trial (12) and a meta-analysis combining most of the published data sets (13). The therapy trial was under strict external QC by the Receptor and Biomarker Group of the EORTC. The participating laboratories received meticulous instructions on how to run the assays, participated in workshops, used common assays, and were subject of EQC (14). They thus can be regarded as experienced and qualified, which most likely contributed to the success of this trial as well.

Although considerable progress has been made for some analytes as exemplified above for uPA and PAI-1, standardization of biomarker assay protocols, and development of proficiency testing programs for biomarkers, should be an ongoing process. Only the stringent application of QC systems enables a consistent assessment of the prognostic and/or predictive power of biomarkers.

REFERENCES

1. Hayes DF, Bast RC, Desc CE, et al. Tumor marker utility grading system: a framework to evaluate clinical utility of tumor markers. *J Natl Cancer Inst* 1996;88:1456–1466.
2. McGuire WL, Clark GM. Prognostic factors and treatment decisions in axillary-node-negative breast cancer. *N Engl J Med* 1992;326:1756–1761
3. Benraad ThJ, Geurts-Moespot J, Grondahl-Hansen J, et al. Immunoassays (ELISA) of urokinase-type plasminogen activator (uPA): report of an EORTC/BIOMED-1 workshop. *Eur J Cancer* 1996;32A:1371–1381.
4. Dittadi R, Meo S, Fabris F, et al. Validation of blood collection procedures for the determination of circulating vascular endothelial growth factor (VEGF) in different blood compartments. *Int J Biol Markers* 2001;16:87–96.
5. Biganzoli E, Boracchi P, Daidone MG, Gion M, Marubini E. Flexible modelling in survival analysis. Structuring biological complexity from the information provided by tumor markers. *Int J Biol Markers* 1998;13:107–123.
6. McGuire WL. Breast cancer prognostic factors: evaluation guidelines. *J Natl Cancer Inst* 1991;83:154–155.
7. Stamey TA, Chen Z, Prestigiacomo AF. Reference material for PSA: the IFCC standardization study. International Federation of Clinical Chemistry. *Clin Biochem* 1998;31:475–481.
8. Kricka LJ. Human anti-animal antibody interferences in immunological assays. *Clin Chem* 1999;45:942–956.
9. Westgard JO, Barry PL, Hunt MR, Groth T. A multi-rule Shewart chart for quality control in clinical chemistry. *Clin Chem* 1981;27:493–501.
10. Levey S, Jennings ER. The use of control charts in the clinical laboratory. *Am J Clin Pathol* 1950;20:1059–1066.
11. Geurts-Moespot J, Leake R, Benraad ThJ, Sweep CGJ. Twenty years of experience with the steroid receptor External Quality Assessment program—the paradigm for tumour biomarker EQA studies (review). *Int J Oncol* 2000;17:13–22.
12. Jänicke F, Prechtl A, Thomssen C, et al. Randomized adjuvant chemotherapy trial in high-risk, lymph node-negative breast cancer patients identified by urokinase-type plasminogen activator and plasminogen activator inhibitor type 1. *J Natl Cancer Inst* 2001;93:913–920.
13. Look MP, van Putten WLJ, Duffy MJ, et al. Pooled analysis of prognostic impact of urokinase-type plasminogen activator and its inhibitor PAI-1 in 8377 breast cancer patients. *J Natl Cancer Inst* 2002;94:116–128.
14. Sweep CGJ, Geurts-Moespot J, Grebenschikov N, et al. External quality assessment of trans-European multicentre antigen determinations (ELISA) of urokinase-type plasminogen activator (uPA) and its type-1 inhibitor (PAI-1) in human breast cancer tissue extracts. *Br J Cancer* 1998;78:1434–1441.

3   Tissue Microarrays

State of the Art, Pitfalls, and Promises

Chungyeul Kim, MD
and Soonmyung Paik, MD

SUMMARY

In this chapter various methods for tissue array construction are compared and protocols for constructing tissue arrays in multicenter trial setting are provided. Listing of all available arrays for breast cancer including commercial and public sources are provided in the appendix.

Key Words: Cancer; multicenter clinical trial; tissue array; tissue microarray.

Cancer Drug Discovery and Development: Biomarkers in Breast Cancer: Molecular Diagnostics for Predicting and Monitoring Therapeutic Effect
Edited by: G. Gasparini and D. F. Hayes © Humana Press Inc., Totowa, NJ

1. INTRODUCTION

Although it is possible to examine multiple markers on individual cases by serial sectioning of paraffin blocks, at some point it becomes too costly and time consuming. Tissue microarray (TMA) solves this problem of throughput. Once constructed, assay cost is reduced by more than 100-fold, so screening of multiple markers becomes a reality. Screening 100 cases for 70 markers will require staining and reading of 7000 individual slides, whereas tissue array will reduce this to only 70 slides.

Some of the obvious advantages of using TMA include:

1. Large number of cases assessed simultaneously for numerous markers.
2. Reduced amount of archival tissues.
3. Reduction in cost and time.
4. A large number of TMA sections containing different types of tissues, such as a panel of normal tissues, tumors, xenografts, or cell lines, can be produced for testing and optimization of pretreatment conditions, antibody titers, and detection systems.
5. Same control tissues can be placed directly on the actual study slides. This helps in ensuring the specificity and sensitivity of immunohistochemistry (IHC).
6. Reproducibility of the staining reaction, as well as the speed and reliability of the interpretation, is improved, as all the tissues are on the same slide.
7. Consecutive slides can be stained with hematoxylin and eosin (H&E) for morphology or with other antibodies against the same or other molecular targets. This permits comparison of multiple targets in virtually identical, histologically highly controlled regions of the tissues.

As there are many excellent reviews on technical aspects of TMA *(1–4)*, this chapter focuses on topics related to TMA construction in multicenter trial setting and practical guidelines.

2. EVOLUTION OF THE TISSUE ARRAY METHOD

Like any technology, tissue array development has proceeded through almost two decades of evolution *(1)*. In 1986 Battifora described a novel method of creating a block that contains tissue from many cases *(5)*. The creation of this Multitumor (Sausage) Tissue Block involved the tedious process of removing portions of tissue from paraffin blocks, deparaffinization, rehydration to 50% ethanol, and cutting it into 1-mm thick slices and then further into slender rods to produce cross-sectional areas of about 1 mm². These rods were wrapped with small intestine of small animals such as rabbits, and processed into a single paraffin block. The resulting Sausage

Table 1
Comparison of Two Widely Used Tissue Array Methods

	Allred (7)	Kononen (1)
Number of cores per array	Up to 60	Up to 500
Diameter of the cores	2–6 mm	0.6–2 mm
Representation of the original block	Good	Need at least two to three cores if using 0.6 mm
Initial investment	Skin biopsy punch at under 2 USD (Miltex, York, PA)	Manual arrayer at over 10,000 USD (Beecher Instruments, Sun Prarie, WI)
Donor block after sampling	Large prominent hole evident	Very little damage to the donor block
Sectioning	Easy	Learning curve

block could be used to screen tissue specific monoclonal antibodies. However, the poor control over the specific location of each component case inside the Sausage limited the value of this strategy as a tool to screen a cohort with clinical follow-up. In 1990 Battifora et al. improved this approach by creating a checkerboard tissue block method in which tissues are evenly distributed in a checkerboard arrangement, and therefore readily identified by their position in the resulting sections (6). However, this method still suffered from the need to go through the tedious process of deparaffinizing the samples as well as the requirement for custom construction of specimen molds with grid pattern. In the same year, Lampkin and Allred devised a novel method of creating a tissue array without the need to deparaffinize the donor samples by using a skin biopsy punch of 3–6 mm in diameter, resulting in up to 40 samples per array (7). Further improvement of this method has resulted in a method that used 2-mm diameter skin biopsy punch resulting in an array containing 60 cores. In 1998, Kononen et al. improved this method further by reducing the core diameter to 0.6 mm, using a high-throughput manual device (1). Owing to affordability of the instrument and increased density of the array, the tissue array has become widely accepted as a high-throughput screening method for candidate molecular markers.

3. WHICH ARRAY METHOD AND IN WHAT DENSITY?

Table 1 summarizes comparison of the two most popular arraying methods. While the method developed by Kononen et al. can generate much higher density array, in reality it may be unnecessary to put so many cores into one array block. Design of an array with more than 100 cores often results in the need for creating subarrays or subsections within the array, which creates problems when navigating between the cores, especially when using fluorescence markers. However, the Kononen method may be preferable to the Allred method because the latter leaves a large hole in the donor block. This defect may create legal or political problems with the pathology department from which the block was provided.

3.1. Beecher Instruments Manual Arrayer

The original commercialized version of the method described by Kononen et al. has popularized the use to tissue array (1). This simple device uses a micrometer to move the recipient block in a precise manner. It has two vertical arms with 0.6-mm punches. The donor punch is slightly bigger in diameter so that the tissue core squeezes into the smaller sized hole in the recipient block. The cores are seeded slightly above the recipient block surface and then later pressed, after incubation at 37°C, so that the height of the seeding can be adjusted to an even surface level.

3.2. Improvements on Beecher Arrayer

When creating a high-density array, the center of the block tends to bulge significantly owing to the increased volume (the diameter of the donor core is slightly larger than that of the recipient hole). In his excellent review of the tissue array technique, Jensen has suggested that keeping the recipient block at approx 100°F using two heating strips attached to the recipient block holder will prevent the problem (2). This compression effect can be resolved, which greatly improves the quality of the array.

3.3. Advanced Tissue Arrayer
(Chemicon International, Temecula, CA)

The Advanced Tissue Arrayer device has one advantage over the Beecher Instrument arrayer—adjustable locking Z-height ensures that the top of every tissue sample is delivered precisely to the top of the array block. However, this instrument costs more than five times the Beecher arrayer, and a well-trained histologist or operator will not have problems with height adjustment using the Beecher arrayer. As with the Beecer instrument, during high-density seeding, the center of the block will bulge and require pressing.

3.4. Automated Arrayer ATA-27
(Beecher Instruments, Sun Prarie, WI)

The Automated Arrayer ATA-27 is a high-throughput system that generates three replica arrays containing one core each from 100 cases in about

4 h. Based on a precision XYZ robot, it allows convenient walkaway mapping on a video screen. The only drawback stems from its small footprint that allows loading of only 20 cases at a time. Theoretically the array generated using this automated system should be much superior to manually constructed ones owing to its Z-axis control—that is, control of the depth of seeding of cores into the array block. However, because it also creates a compression effect, this potential advantage is lost. Although one could heat the recipient block, as described by Jensen for manual arrayer, the block holding mechanism and moving parts in the ATA27 make it difficult to attach a heating strip. One solution has been to heat the entire enclosed environment to 37°C using an air heating system. However, temperatures higher than this cause the donor blocks to soften and the tissue core push through the block.

4. HOW MANY CORES PER CASE ARE ADEQUATE?

A potential drawback of testing a marker in a TMA is that a small core may not be representative of the whole tumor, given the likelihood of heterogeneity. Heterogeneity of the marker expression may not be captured if only one core is sampled especially for 0.6-mm core sampling. Camp et al. examined the correlation between cores and whole sections and came to the conclusion that sampling of two cores are sufficient for breast lesions *(8)*. Zhang et al. found even one 0.6-mm core adequately represents the whole section *(9)*. However it is a safe practice to sample three cores from random spots of each tumor case. In our practice, we routinely sample three cores and seed them into three separate arrays. For initial marker screening we use one core. Promising markers are then validated using all three cores.

5. CONSTRUCTION OF THE ARRAY
IN THE MULTICENTER TRIAL SETTING

5.1. Handling of Donor Blocks—
Cutting, Staining, and Mapping of the Region of Interest

The standard operating procedure (SOP) for TMA construction at the National Surgical Bowel and Breast Project (NSABP) Division of Pathology Laboratory is as follows:

1. Align blocks to microtome knife with Histo-Collimator (Richard-Allan Scientific).
2. Cut one tape section with Paraffin Tape-Transfer System (Instrumedics).
3. Stain with H&E and map the region of interest/core sampling target with red Sharpie permanent marker.
4. Overlay the H&E slide to the original block to mark the core sampling target with red Sharpie permanent marker.

5. Sort the blocks according to the thickness of the tissue in the block.
6. Recipient array block is heated to 100°F before arraying.
7. Construct the array with three spleen cores as position marker on one corner.
8. Seed 100 cores in each array block containing one core from each 100 cases. Three replica arrays are generated.
9. Incubate the array block at 37°C for 10 min before pressing with the glass slide to level the surface of the array block.

Alignment of the block surface to the microtome knife can be quite varied, posing a serious problem to the histologist. Significant time may be wasted orienting the block to the knife. More importantly, several sections of tissue may be lost before a good-quality section can be cut. Use of a microtome equipped with a Histo-Collimator (product no. 755130. Richard-Allan Scientific, Kalamazoo, MI) can largely eliminate this problem. Using an optical alignment method, the Histo-Collimator allows correct alignment of the block surface to the angle of the microtome knife.

Mapping of the region of interest, especially small areas such as normal lobule, can be difficult and often inaccurate when using routinely processed H&E stained sections, because fatty breast tissue expands or becomes deformed in the water bath before the section is picked up on the glass slide. To solve this problem, we have been using the Paraffin Tape-Transfer System (Instrumedics, Hackensack, NJ) that bypass the water bath step completely. First, a plastic tape is attached to the block surface and a section is cut. The section is mounted on the tape and laminated on a special slide coated with UV curable acrylic, which is cured by brief exposure to UV light. The tape is then removed using an organic solvent and the slide is stained with H&E. This procedure will produce an H&E slide that is an exact match to the original tissue in the paraffin block allowing precise mapping of the region of interest for core sampling. We use red colored permanent marker pen to mark the region of interest for two reasons. First, it is readily identifiable for sampling and second, after core transfer to the array block and during sectioning, the red colors on the core provide visual landmarks to evaluate the quality of the array. By combining Histo-Collimator with Paraffin Tape-Transfer System, the mapping of the donor blocks can become a highly efficient process.

5.2. Handling of Refusal to Submit Blocks

The major benefit of TMA construction is to facilitate analysis of large numbers of tissues while preserving time, money, and tissue resources. Thus, TMA preparation is ideal for tumor marker studies in large cooperative groups, such as the NASBP. However, in such an organization, individual institutions may be reluctant to share paraffin blocks. One solution is to provide an alternative to block submission. For example, NASBP accepts submission of a 2-mm core plus a minimum of 10 unstained sections as an alternative to block submission. This strategy has received favorable feedback from the membership. A skin punch biopsy device used for the Allred method (Miltex 2-mm skin biopsy punch) is provided to each member institution on request and the device is shipped back after sampling the tissue without the core extraction from the device to minimize the end user time and effort. We create Allred arrays from these cores, cut and H&E stain, map it, and resample three 0.6-mm cores from them.

6. ANALYSIS SYSTEM

Several systems have been developed to aid in navigation and scoring of assay results for tissue microarray. Table 2 summarizes some of the commercial systems that can be used for navigation. Depending on the need of the institution or investigators, there are wide variety of system choices. At this point ACIS (ChromaVision, San Juan Capistrano, CA) seems to provide the most tested algorithm for immunohistochemistry (IHC) marker analysis. This system has the advantage of being available in most large pathology departments in the United States. Access and image analysis can be accomplished through Web interface systems, such as the BLISS system (Bacus Laboratories, Lombard, IL) and ScanScope (DakoCytomation, Glostrup, Denmark).

Kemp et al. have described an image analysis system that is based on double-immunofluorescence staining with the marker of interest and epithelial cell markers. In this system, tumor epithelial cells can be automatically detected, and therefore staining intensity of only the epithelial cells is measured quantitatively. This has resulted in scoring that has a wider dynamic range than the usual IHC analysis (10).

7. SOME UNTAPPED APPLICATIONS OF TMA

7.1. Use in the Clinical Laboratory

In a typical reference laboratory setting, batch processing of clinical cases using a tissue array would be quite possible. In this case, the reference laboratory might conduct a new TMA periodically (e.g., once a week), prepare slides for IHC for the markers of interest, analyze them, and report the data back to the individual caregiver for routine clinical use. The remaining TMA would then be available for future research studies. Such a strategy is currently employed in some cancer agencies regional laboratories in Canada for immunohistochemical markers such as estrogen receptor (ER) and for fluorescence *in situ* hybridization (FISH) for HER2. While objectivity and reproducibility of the IHC could be questionable, studies have

Table 2
Commercially Available TMA Analysis Systems

System	Hardware	Mapping of cores	Image analysis	Fluorescence capability	Remote viewing through Web interface	Remote image analysis through Web interface
BLISS (Bacus Laboratories, Lombardi, IL)	Remote pathology station based on motorized microscope and Web slide server	Semiautomatic, interactive Each core image is a montage of six image files	Has proven track record of developing CAS 200 system	No	Yes	Yes
ACIS (ChromaVision, San Juan Capistrano, CA)	Motorized microscope based image analysis station Auto slide feeder	Semiautomatic, interactive	Has proven track record for HER2 IHC and CISH scoring	No	No	No
ScanScope (DakoCytomation, Glostrup, Denmark)	Remote pathology station, scanner based	Semiautomatic, interactive Can save individual core images as TIFF or JPEG file format for exporting to other programs	Under development	No	Yes	Under development
ARIOL (Applied Imaging, New Castle Upon Tyne, UK)	Motorized microscope based image analysis station Auto slide feeder	Semiautomatic, interactive	High-throughput image analysis system	Yes	No	No
Icys Research Imaging Cytometer (Compucyte, Cambridge, MA)	Laser scanning cytometer	Mapping using low power scan mosaic	Dedicated three-channel laser scanning of three fluorescent dyes Highly quantitative	Yes	No	No

demonstrated the feasibility of improving this with pixel-based image analysis system such as ACIS from Chromavision.

7.2. Survey of Amplicons

One interesting potential use of tissue microarray is in combination with array-based comparative genomic hybridization. Recently Pollack et al. *(11)* and Hyman et al. *(12)* have conducted a comprehensive survey of amplifications and deletions in the breast cancer genome and correlated the results with gene expression levels using the same cDNA microarray chips. Both groups found significant contribution of gene amplification in the transcriptional activity of the cancer genome. These genes are obviously good candidates for prognosticators as well as therapeutic candidates. Hyman et al. have examined one of these amplified genes *HOXB7*, by FISH on tissue microarray and found it to be prognostic *(12)*. However, they did not go further to screen all of the described amplicons. It would be feasible to construct FISH probes for each one of these amplified and overexpressed genes and screen them rapidly on tissue microarrays. FISH is in general more objective than immunohistochemistry because it relies on spot counting—therefore such markers may turn out to be clinically useful ones.

8. LIMITATIONS AND FUTURE PERSPECTIVES

When the tissue array method was first introduced, it was expected to revolutionize the development of cancer marker studies. However, progress has been slow, for at least two reasons: (1) difficulty and high cost of creating antibodies that work for immunohistochemistry and (2) lack of availability of tissue resources with solid clinical outcome data. One effort to resolve the latter problem is the Cooperative Breast Cancer Tissue Resource (CBCTR), established by the National Cancer Institute of the United States. Based on distributed tissue banks of paraffin blocks in the United States, CBCTR not only provides individual tissue sections but also makes tissue microarray arrays of various designs from breast cancer available. One of the most valuable arrays from CBCTR has been the "progression array" containing cores from various lesions through the presumed stages of breast cancer progression. However, the CBCTR has not developed tissue arrays for prognostic or predictive marker studies. Recently the NSABP has decided to release tissue microarrays generated from NSABP clinical trials to the scientific community, using NCI as an honest broker. Availability of the first array containing 2000 cases from NSABP trial B-28, in which node-positive breast cancer patients who all received adjuvant doxorubicin and cyclophosphamide (AC) were randomly assigned to receive paclitaxel or not, was announced in 2003. While individual laboratories may not be able to develop IHC for 100 different markers at once, 100 laboratories in the world perhaps can share this burden and achieve the same aim. It is hoped that other clinical trial groups and banks will follow similar steps to make their resources as widely as possible.

9. APPENDIX: AVAILABLE TISSUE ARRAYS

9.1. Commercial Sources

As listed in Table 3, many companies now offer both multiorgan site arrays as well as breast cancer specific arrays.

9.2. CBCTR Tissue Array (http://www-cbctr.ims.nci.nih.gov/)

This is currently the best resource to investigate the role of a candidate marker on breast cancer progression once the assays have been optimized for paraffin sections and arrays using in-house or commercially available arrays. The National Cancer Institute (NCI) Cooperative Breast Cancer Tissue Resource (CBCTR) is funded by the NCI to supply researchers with primary breast cancer tissues with associated clinical data. The CBCTR has designed a breast cancer TMA that can be used to investigate differences in prevalence of potential markers in three stages of invasive breast cancer: node-negative, node-positive, and metastatic disease. All of the invasive cases are primary breast cancers with a principal histology of ductal cancer accessioned through the CBCTR. The arrays were designed by National Cancer Institute statisticians to provide high statistical power for studies of stage specific markers of breast cancer.

Each TMA block consists of 288 0.6-mm cores taken from paraffin-embedded specimens that represent 252 breast cancers and normal breast specimens plus 36 controls. Each array is created in quadruplicate to address possible tissue heterogeneity: four cores are taken from each specimen block, with one core per specimen appearing in each of the four replicate array blocks. The information provided for each case on the array are: tumor size, Tumor–Node–Metastasis (TNM) stage, number of nodes positive, grade, age at diagnosis, and race.

The 252 normal breast and breast cancer cores appearing on each TMA block include:

NODE-NEGATIVE BREAST CANCER: 64 cores.

NODE-POSITIVE BREAST CANCER: 64 cores.

METASTATIC BREAST CANCER: 64 cores.

DUCTAL CARCINOMA IN SITU (DCIS): 20 cores (10 from individuals without an invasive disease component and 10 from individuals with invasive disease represented elsewhere on the TMA).

NORMAL BREAST TISSUE: 40 cores (20 from individuals without breast cancer and 20 from individuals with breast cancer represented elsewhere on the TMA).

Table 3
List of TMAs from Commercial Sources

Company	Website	Product	Core	Clinical data	Composition
Ambion	http://www.ambion.com	LandMark high-density breast tissue microarrays	260 Cases	Stage, surgery type, tumor size, node status, histologic type, age, and sex	Mixed infiltrating ductal carcinoma, lobular carcinoma, and matched benign tissue
		LandMark low-density breast tissue microarrays	72 Cases		
Clinomics	http://www.clinomicslabs.net	HD-BR-1 LD-BR-1	200 Cases 60 Cases	Complete pathology data, medication history, outcome, and follow-up data	Representing virtually all stages of breast cancer, from DCIS through stage IV, includes matched normals, benign disease (e.g., fibrocystic disease), and clinically defined normals.
Biogenex	www.biogenex.com	High-density tissue microarray	200 (0.6-mm diameter)	Age, sex, organ, morphology, tumor size, origin (biopsy/surgery)	
		Low-density tissue microarray	50 (1.2-mm diameter)		
Chemicon	http://www.chemicon.com	Chemicon select tissue array	6 (2-mm diameter)	N/A	Four cancer, two normal tissue

(continued)

Table 3 (*continued*)

Company	Website	Product	Core	Clinical data	Composition
Ardais	http://www.ardais.com	Standard breast cancer array	50 (1-mm diameter)	Associated clinical data	Tumors are different histological grades from various stage groups; 3 Stage I, 13 stage II, 14 stage III, 10 stage IV
Zymed	http://www.zymed.com	MaxArray™ breast carcinoma tissue microarray	60 (1.5-mm diameter)	N/A	Tissue cores 1–2 and 4–49 are infiltrating ductal breast adenocarcinoma, tissue core 3 is breast mucinous carcinoma, tissue cores 50–54 are medullary carcinoma, tissue cores 55–57 are ductal carcinoma in situ (DCIS), tissue cores 58–59 are tubular breast cancer, and tissue core 60 is infiltrating nodular adenocarcinoma
Abcam	http://www.abcam.com/	Receptor Grid™ tissue array—breast	70	N/A	Mixed breast cancer, fibroadenoma, and normal breast tissue
Gentaur Imagenex	http://www.gentaur.com/ http://www.imgenex.com/	CB1 IMH-304 (CB) human, breast cancer	60 (2mm) 60	N/A Age, sex, organ, diagnosis, T stage, LN, ER, PR, p53	N/A 34 infiltrating ductal carcinoma, 2 DCIS, 1 papillary carcinoma, 1 lobular carcinoma, 1 medullary carcinoma, 1 signet rig cell carcinoma, 12 metastatic breast carcinoma in lymph node, 10 normal breast tissue

The 36 control cores appearing on each TMA block include:

NORMAL NON-BREAST TISSUE: 16 cores (4 cores from each of the following tissue types: kidney, endometrium, prostate, and appendix). CELL LINES: 20 cores (5 cores from each of the following cell lines: HT-29, PC-3, MCF-7, and T-47D). These cell lines have previously been characterized with regard to expression of a variety of markers of interest in breast cancer.

9.3. NSABP
(National Surgical Adjuvant Breast and Bowel Project): (http://www.nsabp.pitt.edu)

NSABP conducts large phase III clinical trials and started offering tissue arrays constructed from its trials to general scientific community through NCI. The first available array is constructed from 2000 cases enrolled in its trial B-28, which addressed the question of adding sequential paclitaxel to four cycles of adriamycin plus cyclophosphamide. NSABP plans to offer tissue arrays from other protocols as they are constructed. These arrays are great resources for studying marker-by-treatment interaction questions, although they suffer from being inherently underpowered.

REFERENCES

1. Kononen J, Bubendorf L, Kallioniemi A, et al. Tissue microarray for high-throughput molecular profiling of tumor specimens. *Nat Med* 1998;4:844–847.
2. Jensen TA. Tissue microarray: advanced techniques. *J Histotechnol* 2003;26: 101–104.
3. Jensen TA, Hammond E. The tissue microarray—a technical guide for histologists. *J Histotechnol* 2001;24:283–287.
4. Simon R, Mirlacher M, Sauter G. Tissue microarrays. *BioTechniques* 2004;36: 98–105.
5. Battifora H. The Multitumor (Sausage) Tissue Block: novel method for immunohistochemical antibody testing. *Lab Invest* 1986;55:244–248.
6. Battifora H, Mehta P. The checkerboard tissue block. An improved multitissue control block. *Lab Invest* 1990;63:722–724.
7. Lampkin SR, Allred DC. Preparation of paraffin blocks and sections containing multiple tissue samples using a skin biopsy punch. *J Histotechnol* 1990;13: 121–123.
8. Camp RL, Charette LA, Rimm DL. Validation of tissue microarray technology in breast carcinoma. *Lab Invest* 2000;80:1943–1949.
9. Zhang D, Salto-Tellez M, Putti TC, et al. Reliability of tissue microarrays in detecting protein expression and gene amplification in breast cancer. *Mod Pathol* 2003;16:79–84.
10. Camp RL, Dolled-Filhart M, King BL, Rimm DL. Quantitative analysis of breast cancer tissue microarrays shows that both high and normal levels of

HER2 expression are associated with poor outcome. *Cancer Res* 2003;63: 1445–1448.

11. Pollack JR, Sorlie T, Perou CM, et al. Microarray analysis reveals a major direct role of DNA copy number alteration in the transcriptional program of human breast tumors. *Proc Natl Acad Sci USA* 2002;99:12963–12968.

12. Hyman E, Kauraniemi P, Hautaniemi S, et al. Impact of DNA amplification on gene expression patterns in breast cancer. *Cancer Res* 2002;62:6240–6245.

II   ASSAYS FOR GENE EXPRESSION AND POST-TRANSLATIONAL PROTEIN ABNORMALITIES

4   Gene Expression Profiling with DNA Microarrays

Revolutionary Tools
to Help Diagnosis, Prognosis,
Treatment Guidance,
and Drug Discovery

Michele De Bortoli, PHD and Nicoletta Biglia, MD

CONTENTS

SUMMARY

DNA microarrays are small solid supports on the surface of which DNA probes for thousands of genes have been orderly arrayed. Hybridization of labeled RNA from tissues or tumors allows evaluation of the relative amount of any specific mRNA present in the samples, depicting its gene expression profile. During development and progression of breast cancers, specific genetic programs are activated, which can be assayed on DNA microarrays. Studies performed

Cancer Drug Discovery and Development: Biomarkers in Breast Cancer:
Molecular Diagnostics for Predicting and Monitoring Therapeutic Effect
Edited by: G. Gasparini and D. F. Hayes © Humana Press Inc., Totowa, NJ

so far show that the gene expression profile of a tumor defines its biology, its invasive and metastatic potential, and its responsiveness to treatments. Classification of breast cancer by expression profiling appears a very powerful approach, outperforming all commonly used methods of classification. However, much work has to be done before microarray will give robust information for clinical decisions and become routine practice.

Key Words: DNA microarrays; gene expression profiling; breast cancer.

1. INTRODUCTION

A modern view of genetics is that the genomes of all organisms, most spectacularly those of Metazoa, are made of—rather than genes—genetic programs, that is, ensembles of genes that coordinately specify developmental phases, cell types, tissue and organ morphogenesis, and cellular responses to endogenous and exogenous stimuli.

The genomic era has led to the complete description of the DNA sequence of a number of organisms, from *Escherichia coli* to humans—in other words the complete chemical structure of genetic materials, represented as huge strings of A, T, C, and G, stored and accessible in public databases (*www.ncbi.nlm.nih.gov*, to cite the most popular). Saying that we know the complete DNA sequence of some organisms does not mean that we know what the sequence means, even though, at an increasing rate, DNA sequences in databases become annotated with functional information. Genome sequencing was one fundamental step to move on to functional genomics, that is, to understand the functions of all the genes, to unreveal regulatory networks and perhaps to discover many unsuspected genetic languages and functions.

DNA microarrays are tools to analyze genetic programs. Hybridization of the entire messenger RNA (mRNA) pool expressed by a tissue to DNA microarrays, containing probes to theoretically all the genes of an organism, allows to evaluate in a single analytical step which genes and to which extent they are transcribed, that is, in technical terms, the gene expression profile. This gives an immediate and complete picture of genome activity in a specific biological situation, or an estimate of the difference between two biological situations. For example, one of the first published applications of DNA microarrays was the analysis of genome activity changes during metamorphosis in *Drosophila (1)* or during sporulation in yeast *(2)*. These kinds of experiments give remarkable results and open the way to completely new studies, for example, to analyze regulatory sequences of coregulated genes to discover common regulatory pathways, to find the coordinated actions by which cells respond to pathogens or drugs, or to describe changes in genomic structure and expression that accompany tumorigenesis and cancer progression. Several articles, indeed, have reported gene expression profiles of human and experimental tumors and provided exceptionally interesting, albeit preliminary, evidence on the genetic reprogramming during cancer development, progression, and response to treatments.

This chapter deals with the use of gene expression profiling in breast cancer, showing that it will represent an unprecedented powerful tool for reclassifying breast cancers to formulate prognosis, predict and monitor response to treatments, and provide information on the pathogenetic mechanisms relevant to designing new therapeutic interventions. At the same time, we will try to make the focus on the number of steps that are necessary before applying these tools to patient care.

2. HOW A MICROARRAY EXPERIMENT WORKS: THE TECHNICAL PRINCIPLE

Genomics and microarrays have pervaded the scientific literature so extensively during the past 5 yr that probably no further description is necessary. Some excellent reviews have been published (3–6). In brief, a microarray is a physical support (nylon filters, plastics, glass slides) presenting on the surface an ordered array of hundreds or thousands of DNA sequences, representing probes (i.e., the complementary sequence) for each mRNA species, that is, primary gene products. To produce a gene expression profile, the RNA is extracted from tissues or cells, labeled, and hybridized to the array. Hybridization, which is highly specific, produces labeled spots whose intensity is proportional to the level of expression of that particular sequence (gene) in the sample. In the very first applications of this methods, nylon membranes were spotted with one to a few hundred cDNA probes using vacuum manifolds or spotters and hybridization of radioactively labeled RNA was evaluated by densitometry. Evolution of this technique has produced DNA microarrays or DNA chips, usually made of microscope glasses on which cDNA or oligonucleotide probes representing up to 50,000 human genes are orderly arrayed. Fluorochrome-labeled sample RNA hybridizing to the array gives fluorescent spots that are quantitatively measured by laser scanning.

2.1. DNA Chip Technology

Today there are three main alternative techniques for microarray production and two principal approaches for hybridization. The historically first approach is represented by the robotic spotting of probes onto the surface of microscopic glasses. This was introduced by Pat Brown's laboratory (7) and is widely used at present both by biotech companies and in university facilities. Probes are usually cDNA fragments (200–1000 bp) produced by polymerase chain reaction (PCR) from collections of clones or—more recently—chemically synthesized oligonucleotides, 50–70 bases in length, representing relevant parts of the genes. These chips may accommodate up to 50,000 spots/cm^2. The second approach, which was pioneered by Affymetrix, makes use of oligonucleotide probes, 20–25 nt in length, that are directly synthesized on a microscope glass using a photolithographic technique, at a very high density (up to 300,000 different oligos/cm^2) *(8)*. Third, chemical synthesis of oligonucleotides, up to 70 nt in length, on solid supports is realized, at densities of up to 50,000 different sequences per slide, with an ink-jet technology from Rosetta Inpharmatics *(9)*.

2.2. Samples

Sample preparation, always based on the production of copies of mRNA (cDNA) by reverse transcriptase enzymes, also presents alternatives. The most popular method is the dual-color fluorogenic technique, in which two different fluorochromes (most often the cyanines Cy3-red and Cy5-green) are incorporated in cDNA during or after reverse transcription, the first in the interrogated sample and the second in a reference sample (e.g., RNA from tumor labeled with Cy3 and RNA from normal tissue labeled with Cy5). The two samples are then cohybridized to the microarray and a two-color image is rescued, in which the ratio between colors directly reflects the ratio of abundance of any particular mRNA species in the sample vs control experiment, that is, it gives a measure of differential expression. In alternative, a single-labeled RNA is hybridized to the array. This is the case of radioactive labeling, when using DNA arrays made on nylon or plastic membranes, or when using short oligonucleotide probes, as in the case of Affymetrix chips. In this case, incorporation of a small label (e.g., biotin) during RNA copy production is preferred, followed by posthybridization fluorogenic staining, for example, with fluorochrome-conjugated avidin.

Significant technical advancements were achieved toward nanoscale sample preparation. In fact, the main limitation for microarray analysis is the requirement of relatively large amounts of good-quality RNA. Techniques of linear amplification were developed that allow sample preparation, good for microarray hybridization, from as little as 10 ng of RNA *(10)*. A T7 promoter sequence is attached at the 5'-end of the first cDNA strand during reverse transcription, then the final double-stranded cDNA template is used for in vitro transcription by T7-RNA polymerase, producing several copies of complementary RNA (cRNA). This method was shown to amplify the mRNA in a quasilinear fashion, thus allowing gene expression profile analysis in very small amount of tissue, as, for example fine-needle biopsies or laser-dissected tissue specimens *(11,12)*.

2.3. Data Analysis

The primary outcome of a microarray experiment is a fluorescence image. Spot quantitation produces a long list of hybridization values that needs interpretation. The computational analysis of these results is a very important part of the story, and in parallel with technical advances in microarray production and hybridization methods, several computational tools and packages have been developed, allowing spot quantitation, background subtraction and normalization, data storage and retrieval, and higher-level analysis, that is, statistical as well as clustering analysis. Statistics is applied to measure the significance of variations seen among different samples analyzed (e.g., cells treated with the drug X in triplicate vs triplicate untreated controls). In the case of microarrays, considering each gene as a single entity and applying common statistical difference tests would mean losing much of the information that combinatorial analysis can provide. Thus, dedicated statistics should be developed, one example of which is the widely used and publicly available SAM analysis, and further developments *(13)*. The second step is represented by clustering analysis, that is, the search for genes that are coregulated in a given biological situation and/or samples that show similar gene expression patterns. There are many different methods to produce clustering, but in any case a measure of similarity is used to place each gene (and/or experimental point) into a single group or a rank within a hierarchy. Outputs are ordered lists of value but are more commonly displayed as a two-color matrix *(14)* using false-color scales to show different levels of expression or sample/reference expression ratio.

One important aspect of data analysis is data validation which, at least in the studies conducted so far, has been systematically performed by analyzing either the mRNA levels of selected genes among those resulting from microarray analysis, using established methods, such as real-time quantitative reverse transcriptase-PCR (RT-PCR), Northern blotting or RNase protection assay, or by immunohistochemistry/*in situ* hybridization. It is very important to note that in all published studied, a general consistency of expression data obtained with microarrays was found, demonstrating the general robustness of this technique.

3. DNA MICROARRAY ANALYSIS OF BREAST TUMORS

Gene expression profiling in breast cancer is being used to address a number of questions, such as which genes are activated (or down-regulated) during progression through the different stages, or which are the genes that are associated with metastatic potential, which are those that mark responsiveness to certain treatments (such as antiestrogens), and so forth. One preliminary and important question was: Because breast cancer is characterized by a high level of heterogeneity, can gene expression profiles help classify cases in a clinically useful fashion? Preliminary studies showed, in fact, that different breast carcinoma–derived cell lines display distinctive gene expression patterns under in vitro manipulation and that those patterns can be recognized in human breast tumors *(15)*.

The first study, performed with a sufficiently wide microarray (8102 human genes) and with a reasonably large number of breast tumors, confirmed this hypothesis and gave many important insights *(16)*. This article by Perou et al. was entitled "Molecular portraits of human breast tumours" to suggest immediately that a gene expression profile is a multicomponent characteristic that is *individual* but at the same time allows recognition of similarities among samples, exactly as we do when we recognize people and discriminate members of the same family by *resemblance*. This is an essential property of microarray analysis, that is, results are valid *per se*, independently of the function of every single gene that compose the profile, in the same way as recognizing people in most cases does not require concentrating on any single character, but just appreciating (integrating) the sum of all the characters. The breast tumor specimens analyzed in this study, in fact, gave individual profiles of expression, but easily recognizable as belonging to well-defined groups. First, in the study there were 22 coupled samples, that is, taken from the same patients, either primary tumor vs lymph node metastasis or tumors biopsied before and after doxorubicin chemotherapy. This allowed a remarkable conclusion: the tumors from the same individual were always much more similar to each other than to any sample from different patients. Second, tumors could be grouped together on the basis of similarity of their expression profiles to specific cell lineages, that is, luminal, basal, and myoepithelial cells. These observations, confirmed in successive studies, suggest that cell lineage, as related to the clonal origins of a cancer, is the fundamental determinant of the expression profile. Individual tumors are the result of microevolutionary processes, during which mutations in the genome have been selected by the environment ("host"), rendering the cells able to escape "normality," that is, the number of controls and checkpoints that normal cells in a normal organism exert toward each other. As in all evolutionary processes, there is no particular order in the history of genetic alterations and selection steps, so that similar end points can be attained following different pathways. This is reflected, in clinical terms, by the differences shown by individual cancers, in terms of histological appearance, local advancement, metastatic capability, time to relapse, sensitivity to chemical treatments, and so forth. In other words, it is conceivable that each tumor constitutes an individual entity from genetic and molecular aspects, exactly as members of a population do, and this underlies clinical variability.

3.1. Pathogenesis and Progression

As mentioned earlier, the epigenetic point from which tumor cells start to deviate (i.e., the cell lineage) remains recognizable as such in the expression profile. This has been clearly demonstrated also for other types of cancer, such as leukemias and liver cancers (*see* ref. *17* and references therein). In other words, gene expression profiles can "trace" the evolutionary history of a tumor. This point has been reinforced by more recent studies addressing the important point whether genome activity changes during progression from atypical ductal hyperplasia to invasive tumors. The group leaded by Dennis Sgroi developed a laser-capture microdissection technique, coupled to RNA amplification, that allowed gene expression profiling using 12,000-gene (12K) microarrays on different sections from the same tumor, showing pathologically discrete stages, in comparison to normal adjacent tissue samples *(12)*. Results showed that the different stages of progression are very similar to each other in the same patient. Furthermore, the different synchronous stages of tumor within an individual patient clustered more closely to one another than to their respective stages from other patients. These data confirm that alterations in gene expression pattern, as compared to normal tissue, are present in the earliest stage of tumor development and are remarkably stable during progression. This implies that the structural changes leading to tumor development imprint in a quite stable manner genome activity in tumor cells, in other words that the genetic point of origin can determine the final expression pattern. This question was directly addressed on the experimental model systems by Desai et al. *(18)*, by examining mammary carcinomas from six transgenic animal lines carrying different oncogenic constructs. This study demonstrated that the gene expression profiles are determined by the signal transduction pathway activated by any particular oncogene. *ras*, *neu*, and Polyoma Middle T clustered together since they all converge on the *ras*/MAPK pathway, while *myc* or SV40 Large T-induced tumors showed distinct expression patterns. The same conclusion was reached in a study by Shan et al. *(19)* showing that mammary tumors induced in rat by two different carcinogens, dimethylbenz[*a*]-anthracene and 2-amino-1-methyl-6-phenylimidazol[4,5-*b*]pyridine, display very distinctive gene expression profiles, notably associated with indistinguishable histology.

Many studies during the last two decades have reported the diverse genetic alterations that are detectable in tumor cells, comprising point-mutations, translocations, loss of heterozygosity (LOH), and amplifications. Some of these alterations are very relevant to breast cancer, for example, amplification of the *erb*-B2 oncogene. Any individual tumor at diagnosis presents a number of alterations, in patterns that until now, and with few exceptions (*erb*-B2, for instance), were not traced to any clinically relevant condition. One important question is whether the pattern of genetic alterations has a major impact on gene expression. cDNA microarray analysis allows this question to be addressed directly. In fact, the DNA extracted from tumors can be fragmented, labeled with one fluorescent dye, cohybridized together with normal DNA from the same donor, and labeled with a second fluorochrome, to the same cDNA microarrays used for parallel gene expression profiling on RNA from the same tumor. Using this approach, Pollack et al. *(20)* and Hyman et al. *(21)* were able to show that gene copy number indeed has a major impact on gene expression, at least for a number of loci. The pattern of gene amplification or deletion was consistent with previous cytogenetic studies of breast cancer. In the first study, which was done on 6.7K mapped human genes, it was observed that 62% of the genes showing high-level amplification displayed moderate or elevated expression, and that the range of amplification is generally reflected in the level of expression. Overall, it was found that 12% of all the variation in gene expression can be attributed directly to underlying variation in gene copy number *(20)*. In the second study, using microarrays featuring probes for 14K mapped human genes, it was confirmed that gene amplification or loss had substantial effects on gene expression, identifying 270 genes whose expression level was directly linked to gene copy number *(21)*.

These articles demonstrate that microarray analysis can give very important information on the pathogenetic mechanism and also define genetic alterations in subsets of tumors that, because they produce stable expression changes, represent important potential targets for drug development.

3.2. Classification, Prognosis, and Prediction

In the aforementioned articles, it was quite clear that human breast tumors show distinctly different gene expression profiles that, at the same time, bear resemblance with the cell lineage from which they most likely originated. This does not sound as a completely new concept, as it represents the principle of the common pathological classification. Under the light microscope, indeed, the appearance of a tumor often resembles the normal cell of origin, especially when some immunohistochemical marker is used in combination, such as cytokeratins.

Hierarchical clustering of gene expression profiles leads to a classification of breast tumors that follows in part that resulting from classical pathological or biochemical markers but, importantly, also suggest new categories and new subclassifications. Indeed, it is possible to identify groups of genes whose expression profile, or "signature" correlate with any "dominant" condition of the tumor. For example, the main discriminant in the biology of breast cancer, that is, the presence of steroid receptors, can be easily and clearly distinguished by a "signature" that possibly reflects many estrogen-responsive genes *(16,22–24)*. The same was true also for tumors containing an amplified *erb*-B2 oncogene, which were easily recognized by gene signature *(16,20)* and linked to several other coamplified genes *(25)* and to fatty acid metabolism *(26)* by data mining of microarray results. Specific gene expression signatures were also observed for hereditary breast cancer, with distinct signatures for *BRCA1* and *BRCA2* tumors *(27)*. In addition, microarray profiling was shown very effective in discriminating different groups in non-*BRCA* hereditary cancers, paving the way to discovery of the genetic lesions behind these *(28)*.

The sum of the observations reported in the preceding also justifies the hypothesis that tumors at diagnosis have distinguishable properties characterizing their future behavior. This represents a very important issue, which was addressed in the past, in breast as well as in other cancers, by the use of single biochemical or genetic markers, or based on the clinicopathological data. The fact that tumors with different expression patterns may represent clinically different classes with distinct risks of metastasis can be addressed with retrospective studies. In a further analysis of data already published from a 8,1K microarray analysis of locally advanced breast cancer *(16)*, Perou et al. found that the classes of tumors, previously defined on the basis of gene expression signatures, that is, normal-like, basal-like, luminal-like, *erb*-B2+, could be subdivided into further clusters by limiting the analysis to the most significant 456 genes and applying a new significance analysis procedure *(29)*. Interestingly, these new subgroups showed different frequencies of mutation to *TP53* gene and different survival *(29)*. The relatively small cohort of patients analyzed in this study and the fact that most of them were at stage III undergoing different treatments made it difficult to generalize the findings. However, in a more recent study performed using a much larger microarray platform, these finding were substantially confirmed. Van't Veer et al. *(22)* used microarrays developed at Rosetta Inpharmatics, containing oligonucleotide probes for 25K human genes, to profile gene expression in breast tumors from 117 young patients. A supervised hierarchical clustering algorithm was able to identify a gene expression signature strongly predictive of a short interval to distant metastasis ("poor prognosis" signature) in 78 patients with lymph node-negative disease. Further analysis showed that 70 genes were sufficient to correctly predict the clinical outcome in these patients. On the basis of these results, this analysis was successively extended to a cohort of 295 consecutive patients, comprising both lymph node-positive and -negative cases *(30)*. The "poor prognosis" signature was displayed by 180 patients, with an average overall 10-yr survival rate of 54.6% vs 94.5% (50.6% vs 85.2% for disease-free survival) shown by patients with the complementary "good prognosis" signature. Importantly, these highly significant differences hold true when patients were analyzed according to lymph node status. The prognostic power of gene expression signatures was stronger than any other clinicopathological parameters in predicting disease outcome. This study was the first to demonstrate that breast cancer classification based on gene expression profiling can outperform current classification methods and give concrete help in selecting patients for adjuvant therapy *(31)*.

A further issue that can be addressed by microarray analysis is prediction of response to therapies. In a very interesting study, Sotiriou et al. *(11)* determined 7.6K gene expression profiles on fine-needle aspirates (FNAs) taken from patients eligible for neoadjuvant chemotherapy. The analysis was repeated at surgery and hierarchical clustering not only confirmed the individuality and stability of gene expression profiles (successive FNAs from the same patient or the FNA and surgical biopsy from the same patient always clustered together), but also demonstrated that microarray analysis before treatment can predict the response to chemotherapy. In addition, the authors were also able to identify a small group of genes whose expression changes during chemotherapy, suggesting a new way to monitor response.

Of course, one of the main interests in breast cancer management is to define hormonal responsiveness of tumors, since the presence of estrogen receptors (ERs) and progestin receptors (PgRs) identifies tumors that can benefit from antiestrogenic treatment with limited precision (60–70%). This is a more difficult issue to address, because retrospective, uniformly treated, evaluable cohorts of patients are hardly available or not at all. For this reason, most of the studies concentrated either on the ability of gene expression profiles to identify correctly the ER/PgR status in breast tumors, or focused on "in vitro" model systems, in which gene expression changes following estrogenic or antiestrogenic treatments can be measured. In all the studies on breast tumors reported in the preceding, the main clustering pattern clearly distinguished ER^+ from ER^- tumors, providing further proof-of-concept. Conversely, various "in vitro" studies have evidenced large sets of genes whose expression is regulated by estrogen or antiestrogens *(32–37)*. These results must be validated by studying the expression of these genes in patients in whom genuine antiestrogenic response can be assessed, such as in the advanced set. Interestingly, the expression pattern of a handle of genes identified in such an "in vitro" experiment *(37)* is enough to correctly detect the ER status of breast tumors *(24)*. At the same time, these types of studies may elucidate a number of pathways that are activated in hormone-unresponsive tumors, giving insights into new targets for drug development.

4. CURRENT DEBATES

It is evident that the major advantage of gene expression profiling is given by *combinatorial analysis*. Previous work attempting to define biochemical or genetic markers that could help the clinical management of breast cancer was concentrated on single variables. When facing a complex disease such as breast cancer, featuring great clinical variability and molecular heterogeneity, it is expected that single markers may show only very partial association with tumor characteristics. Gene expression profiling, indeed, takes into account thousands of variables at the same time and singles out the individual *groups* of genes that associate with a relevant feature: none of them, individually, will show significant association with the parameter considered, but the *sum* of these does. It is noteworthy that the most important (to date) set of genes found for breast cancer, that is, the 70 genes described by Van de Vijver et al. to discriminate the risk of metastasis *(30)*, do not comprise any of the most popular genes previously proposed as prognostic markers. In this study, the authors started with a microarray featuring probes for 25,000 human genes. Of these, approx 5000 were found with significant variations in at least 3 of the initial 117-tumor cohort. Of these, 231 genes were found associated with clinical outcome and, finally, an iterative exclusion procedure narrowed the number of predictor genes down to 70 *(30)*. This is a quite common feature of this kind of study. The power of microarray analysis is given by the possibility of exploring an enormous number of features, which increases the possibility of finding a group that is significant for the question addressed.

This consideration also introduces another commonly discussed point: why measuring RNA and not proteins? One good reason is that proteomic analysis reveals a limited number of proteins (the most abundant) and require large amounts of tissue. Protein aficionados would say that the mRNA level that can be measured in a cell has little to do with the final protein product and that many posttranslational steps influence significantly the activity of a protein, in a way that the mRNA level and/or structure cannot predict. These considerations are welcomed when expression profiling is made to identify a prevalently expressed gene or genes that can be targeted for drug development or for diagnostics. However, if what we are looking for is a *profile*, the question is probably not relevant. Of course, if there is no mRNA, no protein is expected, unless an extraordinarily stable product was formed from mRNA existing prior to the analysis. The presence of an mRNA does not guarantee the protein, either. However, such cases, in which the mRNA is not translated, are quite anecdotal and often limited to very special contexts, as in the case of oocytes. Huge divergences between mRNA and protein level are also limited to special cases, such as structural or particularly abundant proteins. The extremely interesting field of proteomic analysis will integrate, rather than be in opposition, with gene expression profiling.

Another very common discussion is analysis of microdissected cancers vs whole tumor. Of course, in the case of breast cancer, large variability exists in the nontumoral component, so that the question is perfectly justified. However, many authors argue that the diverse cellular components of a tumor contribute to the tumor biology and should be evaluated as a whole. Indeed, in many studies carried out using nonmicrodissected tumors, genes belonging to lymphocytes, macrophages, adipocytes, stromal cells, and other cell types are clearly visible *(16,22)*. Apparently, however, this does not mask or hamper the identification of gene expression signatures relevant for clinical associations.

The modern success of RNA analysis on DNA microarrays is eventually linked to its relative ease, reproducibility, robustness, and feasibility and to the amount of information obtained, as compared to other approaches available to date. Once operators become acquainted with RNA extraction, handling, and storage, in fact, probe labeling, hybridization, and data analysis are sufficiently robust and produce satisfactory results most of the time. Analysis of RNA also presents the enormous advantage provided by nucleic acid biochemistry, that is, the possibility of using nanoquantities of material, given that amplification, (i.e., replication) of nucleic acid sequences is always possible with high fidelity. The linear RNA amplification technique allows microarray analysis in a number of relevant applications, notably on laser-captured tissues and on FNA. Laser-capture microdissection allows not only analysis of purified tissue or tumor components, but also comparison of different normal and tumor cells in the same biopsy, for example, different pathological stages concurrently present in the same tumor (normal, hyperplastic, *in situ*, invasive) *(12)*. Fine-needle biopsies, instead, allow evaluation of gene expression profiling before surgery, for example, when a neoadjuvant protocol can be employed, thus permitting a view of gene expression changes during chemotherapy *(11,23,37)*.

Of course, before microarray analysis of breast cancer can become a routine practice, many steps have to be performed and many questions addressed. The first important concern, even more than the kind of microchip (probes, genes) on which an analysis is performed, is given by the kind of reference RNA to which comparison is made. In fact, all the studies published to date used different references, either normal mammary tissues *(12)*, a pool of RNA from a series of cell lines *(15,16,29)*, or a pool of all tumor RNAs *(22,30)*. This poses a series of problems both when comparing results from different laboratories and also in absolute terms. For example, pooling mRNA from many different cell lines can dilute out to very low levels some less abundant, cell-specific mRNA species, thus resulting in abnormal enhancement of the sample-to-reference ratio in some cases, or to unsignificant (and therefore excluded) fluorescence signals in other cases. The debate on the optimal reference RNA is now open and must lead to common reference standards in the near future *(38–41)*. The kind of microarray for analysis is also a question to address. In fact, studies in which different platforms were compared demonstrated a certain degree of discrepancy. Different microarrays use very different probes, for example, 5' vs 3' cDNA fragment, derived from different EST libraries, or oligonucleotide probes directed to different regions of the mRNA, and this may represent a serious problem if genes possess alternative splicing forms. Thus, comparison of microarray studies deserves relevant further work.

It is quite easy to foresee that in the next few years microarrays will expand to cover the entire set of mRNAs encoded by the human genome and that exploration in breast cancer, as well as in cancer in general, will follow the same trend. Initial estimates of the number of genes in our genomes were oriented toward 100,000–150,000, considering the organism complexity and the number of proteins needed. However, the Human Genome Project showed that the actual number of genes is much smaller, currently estimated to be approx 35,000. The reason for this is that vertebrate genomes have evolved alternative splicing to encode subtly different proteins using the same gene. A current estimate is that more than 50% of human genes will encode multiple mRNA and proteins by alternative splicing. It is then likely that future microarrays will accommodate probes for all the splicing forms of all the gens, to allow a complete picture of the encoding capability of our genomes. In parallel, public repositories of data from microarray analysis will be developed, allowing researchers to compare their own data with those of others, and even to mine other investigators' data with new algorithms and data mining tools.

As already exemplified with regard to published studies, genome-wide expression profiling of breast cancer will provide relatively small dedicated sets of genes associated with peculiar characteristics of the tumor. These sets will be useful for prognosis, prediction of response, response monitoring, and prediction of the site of metastasis. It is very likely that biotech companies will develop dedicated microarrays, with hundreds—rather than thousands—of gene probes, to answer specific clinical questions and to perform complete pathological characterization of breast tumors.

As always during transfer of biological knowledge to medicine and industry, extensive technical advances and support implementations are needed, as well as brainstorming among the operators in connection with the new algorithms, bioinformatics, and development of new analytical tools.

REFERENCES

1. White KP, Rifkin SA, Hurban P, Hogness DS. Microarray analysis of *Drosophila* development during metamorphosis. *Science* 1999;286:2179–2184.
2. Chu S, DeRisi J, Eisen M, Mulholland J, Botstein D, Brown PO, Herskowitz I. The transcriptional program of sporulation in budding yeast. *Science* 1998;282: 699–705. Erratum in: *Science* 1998;282:1421.
3. Lockhart DJ, Winzeler EA. Genomics, gene expression and DNA arrays. *Nature* 2000;405:827–836.
4. Young RA. Biomedical discovery with DNA arrays. *Cell* 2000;102:9–15.
5. Phimister B, ed. The chipping forecast. *Nat Genet* 1999;21(Suppl):1–60.
6. Hughes TR, Shoemaker DD. DNA microarrays for expression profiling. *Curr Opin Chem Biol* 2001;5:21–25.

7. Schena M, Shalon D, Davis RW, Brown PO. Quantitative monitoring of gene expression pattern with a complementary DNA microarray. *Science* 1995;270: 467–470.

8. Fodor SP, Read JL, Pirrung MC, Stryer L, Lu AT, Solas D. Light-directed, spatially addressable parallel chemical synthesis. *Science* 1991;251:767–773.

9. Blanchard AP, Kaiser RJ, Hood LE. High-density oligonucleotide arrays. *Biosens Bioelectr* 1996;6/7:687–690.

10. Wang E, Miller LD, Ohnmacht GA, Liu ET, Marincola FM. High-fidelity mRNA amplification for expression profiling. *Nat Biotechnol* 2000;18:457–459.

11. Sotiriou C, Powles TJ, Dowsett M, et al. Gene expression profiles derived from fine needle aspiration correlate with response to systemic chemotherapy in breast cancer. *Breast Cancer Res* 2002;4:R3(1–8).

12. Ma XJ, Salunga R, Tuggle JT, et al. Gene expression profiles of human breast cancer progression. *Proc Natl Acad Sci USA* 2003;100:5974–5979.

13. Storey JD, Tibshirani R. Statistical significance for genomewide studies. *Proc Natl Acad Sci USA* 2003;100:9440–9445.

14. Eisen MB, Spellman PT, Brown PO, Botstein D. Cluster analysis and display of genome-wide expression patterns. *Proc Natl Acad Sci USA* 1998;95:14863–14868.

15. Perou CM, Jeffrey SS, van de Rijn M, et al. Distinctive gene expression patterns in human mammary epithelial cells and breast cancers. *Proc Natl Acad Sci USA* 1999;96:9212–9217.

16. Perou CM, Sorlie T, Eisen MB, et al. Molecular portraits of human breast tumours. *Nature* 2000;406:747–752.

17. Liu ET. Classification of cancers by expression profiling. *Curr Opin Genet Dev* 2003;13:97–103.

18. Desai KV, Xiao N, Wang W, et al. Initiating oncogenic event determines gene-expression patterns of human breast cancer models. *Proc Natl Acad Sci USA* 2002;99:6967–6972.

19. Shan L, He M, Yu M, Qiu C, Lee NH, Liu ET, Snyderwine EG. cDNA microarray profiling of rat mammary gland carcinomas induced by 2-amino-1-methyl-6-phenylimidazo[4,5-*b*]pyridine and 7,12-dimethylbenz[*a*]anthracene. *Carcinogenesis* 2002;23:1561–1568.

20. Pollack JR, Sorlie T, Perou CM, et al. Microarray analysis reveals a major direct role of DNA copy number alteration in the transcriptional program of human breast tumors. *Proc Natl Acad Sci USA* 2002;99:12963–12968.

21. Hyman E, Kauraniemi P, Hautaniemi S, et al. Impact of DNA amplification on gene expression patterns in breast cancer. *Cancer Res* 2002;62:6240–6245.

22. van't Veer LJ, Dai H, van de Vijver MJ, et al. Gene expression profiling predicts clinical outcome of breast cancer. *Nature* 2002;415: 530–536.

23. Pusztai L, Ayers M, Stec J, et al. Gene expression profiles obtained from fine-needle aspirations of breast cancer reliably identify routine prognostic markers and reveal large-scale molecular differences between estrogen-negative and estrogen-positive tumors. *Clin Cancer Res* 2003;9:2406–2415.

24. Sorbello V, Fuso L, Sfiligoi C, et al. Quantitative real-time RT-PCR analysis of eight novel estrogen-regulated genes in breast cancer. *Int J Biol Markers* 2003;18:123–129.

25. Dressman MA, Baras A, Malinowski R, et al. Gene expression profiling detects gene amplification and differentiates tumor types in breast cancer. *Cancer Res* 2003;63:2194–2199.

26. Kumar-Sinha C, Ignatoski KW, Lippman ME, Ethier SP, Chinnaiyan AM. Transcriptome analysis of HER2 reveals a molecular connection to fatty acid synthesis. *Cancer Res* 2003;63:132–139.

27. Hedenfalk I, Duggan D, Chen Y, et al. Gene-expression profiles in hereditary breast cancer. *N Engl J Med* 2001;344:539–548.

28. Hedenfalk I, Ringner M, Ben-Dor A, et al. Molecular classification of familial non-BRCA1/BRCA2 breast cancer. *Proc Natl Acad Sci USA* 2003;100:2532–2537.

29. Sorlie T, Perou CM, Tibshirani R, et al. Gene expression patterns of breast carcinomas distinguish tumor subclasses with clinical implications. *Proc Natl Acad Sci USA* 2001;98:10869–10874.

30. van de Vijver MJ, He YD, van't Veer LJ, et al. A gene-expression signature as a predictor of survival in breast cancer. *N Engl J Med* 2002;347:1999–2009.

31. van't Veer LJ, Dai H, van de Vijver MJ, et al. Expression profiling predicts outcome in breast cancer. *Breast Cancer Res* 2002;5:57–58.

32. Omoto Y, Hayashi S. A study of estrogen signaling using DNA microarray in human breast cancer. *Breast Cancer* 2002;9:308–311.

33. Inoue A, Yoshida N, Omoto Y, et al. Development of cDNA microarray for expression profiling of estrogen-responsive genes. *J Mol Endocrinol* 2002;29:175–192.

34. Bouras T, Southey MC, Chang AC, et al. Stanniocalcin 2 is an estrogen-responsive gene coexpressed with the estrogen receptor in human breast cancer. *Cancer Res* 2002;62:1289–1295.

35. Levenson AS, Kliakhandler IL, Svoboda KM, et al. Molecular classification of selective oestrogen receptor modulators on the basis of gene expression profiles of breast cancer cells expressing oestrogen receptor alpha. *Br J Cancer* 2002;87:449–456.

36. Cicatiello L, Scafoglio C, Altucci L, et al. A genomic view of estrogen actions in human breast cancer cells by expression profiling of the hormone responsive transcriptome. *J Mol Endocrinol* 2004;32:719–795.

37. Assersohn L, Gangi L, Zhao Y, et al. The feasibility of using fine needle aspiration from primary breast cancers for cDNA microarray analyses. *Clin Cancer Res* 2002;8:794–801.

38. Kim H, Zhao B, Snesrud EC, Haas BJ, Town CD, Quackenbush J. Use of RNA and genomic DNA references for inferred comparisons in DNA microarray analyses. *BioTechniques* 2002;33:924–930.

39. Puskas LG, Zvara A, Hackler L Jr, Micsik T, van Hummelen P. Production of bulk amounts of universal RNA for DNA microarrays. *BioTechniques* 2002;33:898–900, 902, 904.

40. Dudley AM, Aach J, Steffen MA, Church GM. Measuring absolute expression with microarrays with a calibrated reference sample and an extended signal intensity range. *Proc Natl Acad Sci USA* 2002;99:7554–7559.

41. Lee PD, Sladek R, Greenwood CM, Hudson TJ. Control genes and variability: absence of ubiquitous reference transcripts in diverse mammalian expression studies. *Genome Res* 2002;12:292–297.

III

ASSAYS FOR DNA ABNORMALITIES

5   Assays for Gene Amplification

State of the Art, Pitfalls, and Promises

Chungyeul Kim, MD,
Yongkuk Song, PHD,
and Soonmyung Paik, MD

CONTENTS

Cancer Drug Discovery and Development: Biomarkers in Breast Cancer:
Molecular Diagnostics for Predicting and Monitoring Therapeutic Effect
Edited by: G. Gasparini and D. F. Hayes © Humana Press Inc., Totowa, NJ

SUMMARY

Since the approval of trastuzumab for the treatment of *HER2*-positive breast cancer *(1)*, there has been an active debate as to the reproducibility and validity of the FDA-approved assays that detect *HER2* abnormalities in the tumor tissue. In this chapter, various clinical assays are compared focusing on practical issues.

Key Words: Gene amplification; trastuzumab; *HER-2* testing; breast cancer.

1. IMPORTANCE OF GENE AMPLIFICATION IN BREAST CANCER

Recent studies using combination of cDNA array based expression profiling and comparative genomic hybridization have elucidated the role of gene amplification in the transcriptional program of breast cancer. In the study by Pollack et al. *(2)*, copy number alteration and expression levels across 6691 mapped human genes were examined in 44 locally advanced breast cancer and 10 breast cancer cell lines. The data from this study suggest that at least 12% of all the variation in gene expression among the breast cancer is directly attributable to underlying variation in gene copy numbers. The total number of genomic alterations (gains and losses) correlated significantly with high grade ($p = 0.008$), negative estrogen receptor (ER) ($p = 0.04$), and *p53* mutation ($p = 0.0006$). Of 117 high-level amplifications (representing 91 different genes), 62% (representing 54 genes) were found to be associated with at least moderately elevated mRNA levels, and 42% (representing 36 different genes) with highly elevated mRNA levels. In a similar effort, Hyman et al. examined the correlation between copy number changes and expression levels in 14 breast cancer cell lines using a cDNA microarray of 13,824 genes *(3)*. They found 44% of highly amplified genes resulting in overexpression and 10.5% of overexpressed genes being amplified.

Together these results suggest a profound role of gene amplification in transcriptional control of gene expression in breast cancer and provide a rationale for pursuing amplified genes as a preferred target for developing therapeutics and diagnostics.

2. *HER2* GENE AMPLIFICATION IN BREAST CANCER

HER2 was originally cloned as a gene that is amplified with homology to human epidermal growth factor receptor gene. Since Slamon et al. demonstrated the clinical significance of the *HER2* gene amplification *(4)*, numerous studies largely replicated their original findings using a variety of methods ranging from immunohistochemistry to Southern blotting technique.

It is noteworthy that many genes are included in the *HER2* amplicon. These include v-*erbA*/thyroid hormone receptor-α (THRA1), the retinoic acid receptor α (RARA), the MLNs 50, 51, 62 steroidogenic acute regulatory protein related protein (MLN 64/CAB-1), peroxisome proliferator–activated receptor binding protein (PBP/PARBP/TRAP-220), growth factor receptor-bound protein 7 (GRP7), homebox genes 2 and 7 (*HOXB2* and *HOXB7*), junction plakoglobin (JUP), dopamine and cAMP-regulated phosphoprotein (32 kDa in size) (DARPP-32), thyroid hormone receptor associated protein complex component 100 (TRAP-100), titin cap protein (TCP), CDC2 related protein kinase-7 (CrkRS), Aiolos, gastrin, 17β-hydroxysteriod dehydrogenase type 1 (HSDl7B1), and topoisomerase IIα (topoIIα, encoded by *TOP2A*), all of which have been shown to be coamplified in the portion of the *HER2*-amplified tumors *(5)*. High-resolution mapping of tumors with *HER2* amplification with these gene-specific probes may provide additional insight as to the complex behavior of *HER2*-positive tumors such as differential response to trastuzumab.

3. WHAT IS THE BEST SOURCE OF ASSAY MATERIALS FOR *HER2*?

Trastuzumab, a humanized monoclonal antibody directed against extracellular domain of *HER2*, is perhaps the most successful targeted therapy second to tamoxifen *(1)*. Because it is difficult to get tissue from many of the metastatic sites at the time of presentation as an advanced disease, the question arises as to whether one can use an archived paraffin block from the primary index tumor as a surrogate for *HER2* status of the metastatic lesion. There are only a handful of studies addressing this question of concordance between primary and metastatic lesions, and most of them compared primary and concurrent lymph node metastases. The only true study of concordance comparing primary index tumor with metachronous distant metastases was reported by Niehans et al. *(6)*. They examined *HER2* status by immunohistochemistry in 14 autopsy cases (2–9 yr after primary) and found 100% concordance between primary tumors and metastases. In a survey of 56 matched primary and metastatic sites in the node assessed by Herceptest immunohistochemistry, Masood and Bui observed nearly identical staining results between the two *(7)*. The largest study is by Simon et al. *(8)*. In their study, using tissue microarray constructed from 125 cases of breast cancer with nodal metastasis, only 9 cases produced metastasis with partially or completely discordant *HER2* status. Among these only two cases exhibited a complete discordance of *HER2* status (i.e., all samples of the metastases were *HER2* negative). The remaining seven cases exhibited partial discordance (i.e., at least one of their metastases had both *HER2*-positive and -negative samples). These data seem to justify the use of any tumor tissue, regardless of whether they are from primary index tumor, metastatic lymph node, or other metastatic site, as a source of material for *HER2* testing. However, owing to the paucity of data for comparing the *HER2* status of index tumor vs systemic metastases, more extensive survey using fluorescence *in situ* hybridization (FISH) is required. Furthermore, if use of trastuzumab in the adjuvant setting is approved, it will be important to examine what happens to the *HER2* status of recurrent tumor cells.

4. WHICH IS THE BEST ASSAY PLATFORM FOR THE DETERMINATION OF *HER2* STATUS?

Because overexpression of *HER2* is almost always attributable to gene amplification *(2)*, one could use assays for protein expression and gene amplification to cross-validate the assays. Thus, there are many available options for the determination of *HER2* status, including immunohistochemistry (IHC), enzyme-linked immunosorbent assay (ELISA), FISH, chromagenic *in situ* hybridization (CISH), and quantitative polymerase chain reaction (qPCR). Each assay has its own advantages as well as disadvantages. The availability of so many options obviously has created confusion among clinicians who are not familiar with the biology of *HER2*.

The most widely used assay for clinical decision making is FISH. FISH is a method in which a fluorescence-labeled DNA probe is directly hybridized to the tissue section and hybridization signals are numerically recorded. In normal cells, because of the presence of two alleles, one each from each parent, one expects to see two distinct signals, whereas in tumor cells with amplification of the target gene numerous signals are seen. In the most popular clinical FISH assay for *HER2* developed by Vysis (PathVysion *HER2* assay), an alpha satellite probe for chromosome 17 labeled with a different color is used to rule out polysomy of chromosome 17 in which the *HER2* gene resides (Fig. 1).

There are two aspects to be considered in making a choice for which assay is to be used for clinical studies. First, one has to consider which test provides better predictability for trastuzumab response. Obviously none of the available assays is ideal, as the response rate of FISH-positive cases to first-line trastuzumab monotherapy is below 50% *(9)*. Dissection of the *HER2* amplicon and signaling pathways may eventually provide better predictors. However, currently, one must use non-ideal tests investigating *HER2* itself. Available data regarding which clinical *HER2* assays are better correlated with clinical response to trastuzumab therapy are not very clear. Much of the confusion is caused by the fact that the IHC assay used in comparison of IHC vs FISH for clinical efficacy in the analysis of pivotal trial data was the Clinical Trials Assay (IHC with both CB-11 and 4D5 antibodies), which is no longer available. Because concordance between Herceptest, an FDA-approved IHC kit, and the CTA was only about 78%,

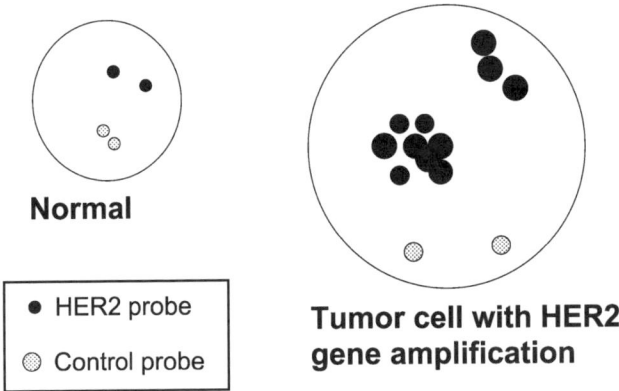

Fig. 1. FISH using Vysis PathVysion assay.

Table 1
H0649g Overall Response Rate
to Single-Agent Trastuzumab (Herceptin)
According to CTA (IHC) or FISH Results

	CTA 3+ (%)	CTA 2+ (%)
FISH (+)	22	11
FISH (–)	0	0

Table 2
H0648g Overall Response Rate
to Chemotherapy vs Trastuzumab + Chemotherapy (T+C)

	CTA 3+ T + C (%)	CTA 3+ Chemotherapy (%)
FISH (+)	55	28
FISH (–)	62	55

it is difficult to extrapolate the pivotal trial data to Herceptest or other IHC assays. However, the data from the pivotal trial for trastuzumab strongly suggest that in the absence of gene amplification as measured by FISH, the benefit from trastuzumab therapy is limited or nonexistent (Tables 1 and 2) (http://www.fda.gov/ohrms/dockets/ac/01/briefing/3815b1_08_ HER2%20FISH.doc). Therefore further studies are necessary to answer this question. There are no published data regarding the correlation between gene dosage and trastuzumab response in those cases with gene amplification—although logic dictates that such correlations should exist. In summary, the available data suggest that FISH appears to be the assay of choice for predicting response to trastuzumab therapy, but it is clearly not the ideal test.

Other issues to be considered include assay reproducibility, reliability, and practicality. Because most of the treatment decisions for metastatic case are based on analysis of the archived primary index tumor tissue, there is a need for reliable and accurate methods to detect *HER2* abnormalities in archived formalin-fixed paraffin-embedded tissue. This requirement essentially eliminates candidates such as ELISA, Northern blot, and Southern blot methods, all of which are better performed on frozen tissue. Although FISH appears to be more accurate and reproducible, complete automation is difficult for FISH. Furthermore, scoring and interpretation of FISH results is time consuming for the pathologists. There is also a consistent assay failure rate of about 5% for FISH. On the other hand, IHC is completely automated and image analysis systems such as ACIS (Chromavision) or ARIOL (Applied Imaging) are now available to help interpret the results. In addition, IHC costs 10–20 times less than the FISH assay. Therefore many laboratories and agencies have now adopted a tiered approach using both IHC and FISH. This is based on the experience by many laboratories that there is a near-perfect correlation between 3+ IHC (by essentially any method using any antibody) and gene amplification by FISH, and between 0 or 1+ IHC and no amplification by FISH. This leaves only 2+ IHC cases that must be confirmed by FISH testing. Dowsett et al. compared the assessment of *HER2* by IHC (HercepTest) and FISH in 426 breast carcinomas from patients being considered for trastuzumab therapy *(10)*. The tumors were sent in from 37 hospitals and tested in three reference centers. Only 2/270 (0.7%) IHC 0/1+ tumors were FISH positive. Six of 102 (5.9%) IHC 3+ tumors were FISH negative. Five of the six had between 1.75 and 2.0 *HER2* gene copies per chromosome 17 and the sixth had multiple copies of chromosome 17. Thirteen percent of tumors were IHC 2+ and overall 48% of these were FISH positive, but this proportion varied markedly between the centers. Sixty IHC-stained slides selected to be enriched with 2+ cases were circulated among the three laboratories and scored. In 20 cases there was some discordance in scoring. Consideration of the FISH score in these cases led to concordance in the designation of positivity/negativity in 19 of these 20 cases. These data support an algorithm in which FISH testing is restricted to IHC 2+ tumors in reference centers.

This tiered approach is a quite reasonable compromise owing to much less cost and personnel efforts involved. One caveat for this tiered system is that it will work only when qualified laboratories do initial IHC screenings, as the US clinical trial groups learned through their painful experiences from their clinical trials for trastuzumab.

5. REPRODUCIBILITY OF *HER2* ASSAYS— US COOPERATIVE CLINICAL TRIAL GROUP EXPERIENCE

In the United States, the National Adjuvant Breast and Bowel Project (NASBP) is conducting clinical trial B-31, in which node-positive patients are randomized to standard AC-T regimen or the same regimen plus trastuzumab for 1 yr. In this trial original eligibility was based on 3+ IHC results or amplification by Vysis PathVysion assay, reported by any laboratories in the United States or Canada. Owing to patient safety concerns, a central assay for initial 100 cases enrolled into the trial whose blocks become available was preplanned in the protocol. To prevent any bias in assay performance, a third-party commercial reference laboratory was used to perform central assays using both Dako Herceptest (FDA-approved IHC assay) and Vysis PathVysion assay (FDA-approved FISH assay). Results from 104 cases were ultimately evaluated *(11)*. Surprisingly, 19/104 (18%) of the cases were negative by both FISH and IHC (3+) when assayed in the central laboratory. Examination of the data according to where the original assays were performed demonstrated a striking trend between poor concordance and laboratories that handle small assay volumes. Only one of 29 cases from large-volume laboratories (that assay 100 or more cases per month) were incorrectly classified as 3+ by IHC. In contrast, 18 of 75 (24%) cases deemed *HER2* positive by small-volume laboratories were negative by both central IHC and FISH. This result was observed regardless of whether FDA-approved Herceptest or other IHC assays were used.

An additional 27 cases were entered based on FISH by local laboratories. When subjected to central assays, all 27 cases were validated to have gene amplification. Seventeen of these cases were entered by small-volume laboratories and 10 from large-volume laboratories. Therefore, we concluded that the FISH assay is in general more reproducible than IHC assays. Based on these findings, protocol eligibility was modified to accept 3+ IHC results only when reported by approved or high-volume laboratories and FISH results by any laboratories. To test the validity of this modification, we conducted a central review of cases entered after the implementation of the eligibility changes. The results confirm our previous findings. Of 240 cases entered after the amendment, only 6 of 133 cases entered based on gene amplification by FISH performed by local laboratories were negative by central FISH. In 1 of 133 cases, a hybridization signal could not be obtained. Among 107 cases that were entered based on 3+ IHC results reported by approved laboratories, 2 were negative by central FISH, with assay failure in 3 cases. Among 6 cases entered by FISH and negative on central assay, 3 had an original *HER2*/Control probe ratio of under 3, suggesting caution when dealing with cases with a ratio under 3. Although our experience suggests reliability of FISH assay in general, the experience of the Intergroup in its trastuzumab trial is completely different *(12)*. Tumor specimens from the first 119 patients enrolled in its protocol N9831 were centrally tested; 74% were found to be HercepTest 3+ and 66% were found to have *HER2* gene amplification. In contrast to NSABP experience, only 6 of 9 (67%) of the specimens submitted by local laboratories as FISH positive could be confirmed by central assays.

6. OPTIMIZATION OF FISH FOR OLD FORMALIN-FIXED PARAFFIN-EMBEDDED TISSUE SPECIMENS

Although commercial FISH probes are very expensive, one can use DenHyb (Insitus Biotechnologies, Albuquerque, NM) to dilute the probe by approx 1:10 and still obtain comparable results. We have found that this hybridization mix is extremely cost-effective when commercial probes are used (we use 1:15 dilution of the probe mix in Den Hyb for PathVysion kit).

Because *HER2* testing is usually performed using the original primary tumor rather than a metastatic specimen, archived paraffin blocks are often used as test material. In our experience, older blocks have a significant higher failure rate even when we used the Vysis PathVysion *HER2* FISH assay per manufacturer's instructions. However, we have found three generic ways of improving the signal, especially from archived tissue. One is to include a formalin postfixation step during pretreatment before hybridization—this may work especially well for cases with poor fixation. The second method is to increase the incubation time in sodium thiocyanate solution. We generally use longer incubation according to the age of the block with up to 1 h for 30-yr-old blocks. A third method is to use antigen retrieval in pH 4.0 sodium citrate buffer.

In this regard, Anderson et al. have reported a new pretreatment procedure to increase the sensitivity of the FISH assays, with a decrease in assay failure rate from 20% to 10%. Although this protocol is much more complicated than the manufacturer's protocol, it improves the hybridization of older samples *(13)*. Our in-house optimized protocol for Vysis PathVysion *HER2* assay is provided in Table 3.

7. CHROMOGENIC *IN SITU* HYBRIDIZATION

FISH suffers from two main problems. First, it requires fluorescence microscopy (with special filter sets if using PathVysion) and digital photomicrography for clinical reporting and archiving. Second, pathologists need to identify the area of interest (e.g., delineating the invasive vs *in situ* component), which can be time consuming. Therefore, development of an *in situ*

Table 3

Optimized Pretreatment Protocols for Vysis PathVysion HER-2 FISH Assay According to Representative NSABP Protocols

	NSABP Protocols (accrual period)			
Steps	B-31 (2000–present)	B-28 (1995–1998)	B-14 (1982–1988) and B-20 (1988–1993)	B-04 (1971–1974)
Deparaffination	3X xylene for 5 min, 2X 100% EtOH for 1 min at RT	Identical	Identical	Identical
Acid treatment	0.2 N HCl for 10 min, dH₂O for 3 min	0.2 N HCl for 20 min, dH₂O for 3 min	0.2 N HCl for 30 min, dH₂O for 3 min	0.2 N HCl for 40 min, dH₂O for 3 min
Pretreatment	Vysis pretreatment solution at 80°C for 20 min, dH₂O for 3 min	Vysis pretreatment solution at 80°C for 40 min, dH₂O for 3 min	Vysis pretreatment solution at 80°C for 60 min, dH₂O for 3 min	Vysis pretreatment solution at 80°C for 60 min, dH₂O for 3 min
Protease treatment	Vysis Protease I solution at 37°C for 5 min, dH₂O for 3 min	Vysis Protease I solution at 37°C for 15 min, dH₂O for 3 min	Vysis Protease I solution at 37°C for 20 min, dH₂O for 3 min	Vysis Protease I solution at 37°C for 30 min, dH₂O for 3 min
Fixation	10% buffered formalin for 10 min at RT, dH₂O for 3 min	Skip	Identical	Identical
Dehydration	EtOH series (70, 85, 100%) for 1 min at RT, air dry	Identical	Identical	Identical

hybridization method that questions a colorimetric signal may provide an alternative that would be favored by pathologists.

Tanner et al. have reported a CISH protocol based on hybridization of tissue target DNA with a subtracted fluorescein-labeled probe. Signal amplification is detected using an antifluorescein antibody, and a colorimetric reaction results in brown diaminobenzidine precipitation *(14)*. Subtracted probe technology used in this protocol (subtracting repetitive sequences using subtraction PCR) has the potential advantage over the direct labeled BAC probe used in the PathVysion FISH kit of having less background owing to elimination of repetitive sequences. Furthermore, this method is less expensive, as it employs a PCR amplifiable template for probe generation. CISH produces results very comparable to those obtained with FISH, with 95–100% concordance rate. In our study of 81 cases, identical results for both methods were found in 26 cases (10 amplified, 16 nonamplified) *(15)*. One case was misinterpreted as overexpressed by CISH because of background precipitate. In 4 cases, CISH suggested low-level amplification. Three of these cases subsequently were found to have chromosome 17 polysomy. Therefore, cases with chromosome 17 polysomy and those with background staining may be misinterpreted as amplification signals. However, the clinical consequences of misclassification of polysomy cases are unknown.

Using material from the NSABP B31 trial, we observed hybridization signal from only 60/81 cases. Forty-nine were scored positive for gene amplification by CISH and 11 negative. Among 49 positive cases, 47 were positive by FISH and 2 negative. Among 11 cases negative by CISH, 8 were also negative by FISH and 3 were positive. The overall concordance rate was 92%. In another cohort of 123 evaluable cases from NSABP trial B-15, 88 cases were positive by CISH. Among these, 83 were also positive by FISH. Among 35 cases negative by CISH, 30 were also negative by FISH. Again the concordance rate was 92%. This concordance rate of <100% could simply reflect the fact that we have not fully optimized the assay for the multicenter-derived materials in our trials. Therefore, other published data may be more relevant to general use of CISH.

8. REAL-TIME PCR

Real-time reverse transcriptase-PCR (RT-PCR) permits quantification of DNA. In theory, this method might combine the advantages of nucleic acid and protein measurement. Milson et al. reported results of analysis of 336 cases with real-time PCR method to quantify the copy number changes of the *HER2* gene over a reference gene (β-globulin) *(16)*. Real-time PCR gave *HER2/neu* gene doses of 10 for SKBR3 cells and 2 for T47D cells with coefficients of variation (CV) of <3% for within-run and <6% for between-run analysis. Examination of 97 breast tumors found a correlation of

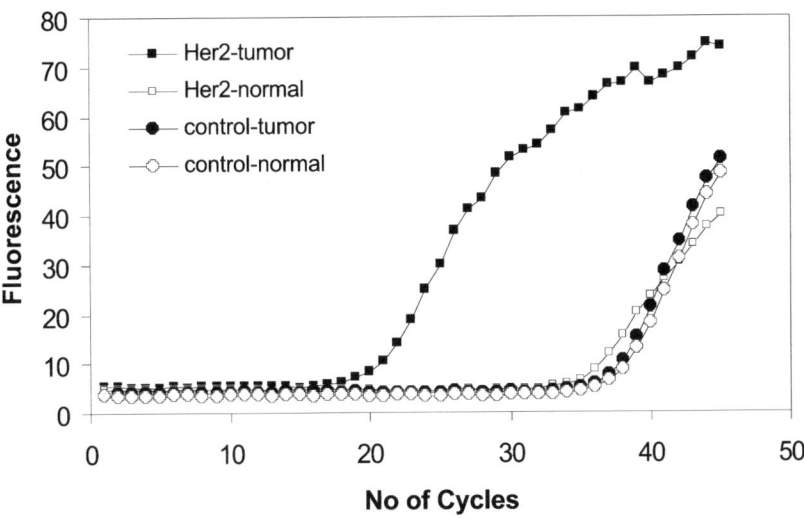

Fig. 2. An example of real-time PCR profile of *HER2* vs control gene in breast cancer specimen with *HER2* amplification.

$r = 0.974$ between the real-time PCR and quantitative PCR methods. IHC and PCR results agreed for 234 of the subsequent 294 samples analyzed (79% concordance). A subset of 10 discrepant samples was microdissected. After microdissection, all 10 were positive by PCR, thus resolving the discrepancy. We have developed real-time PCR methods based on both TaqMan probes and Cybergreen dye and both work well for formalin-fixed paraffin-embedded tissue. Figure 2 shows representative results from a breast cancer with *HER2* gene amplification. One of the major drawbacks of the real-time PCR method is the compression of the dynamic range in comparison to FISH. Only two cycle differences may be observed, even in the presence of a 5- to 10-fold difference in gene copy number. Because of this problem, the assay has to be performed with high precision and quality control. However, owing to the possibility of complete automation using high-throughput devices for PCR, good reproducibility and portability, and low cost per specimen, real-time PCR does have a good potential for clinical assay. Survey of other amplicons also would be possible with relative ease using this approach.

9. COMPARATIVE GENOMIC HYBRIDIZATION (CGH)

Although probably not a good candidate to become a clinical assay, CGH does provide valuable information regarding the status of genome-wide changes in *HER2*-amplified breast cancer. Isola et al compared conventional CGH with FISH and IHC in the same cases *(17)*. The concurrence for *erb*-B2 detection between FISH and IHC was 90%; between FISH and CGH it was 82%, and between IHC and CGH it was 84%. An increased number of losses of 18q and gains of 20q was found in *erb*-B2-positive tumors. *erb*-B2-amplified tumors as detected by FISH, IHC, or CGH had twice as many CGH-defined chromosomal alterations (means of 11.8, 11.0, and 12.7, respectively) as the nonamplified tumors (means of 6.8, 7.0, and 5.6, respectively). Array CGH provides higher resolution than conventional CGH, but in our hands it suffers from the compressed dynamic range when compared to FISH. Therefore actual copy number determination may be difficult.

10. CONCLUSIONS

Currently, the tiered approach for using FISH only for IHC 2+ cases seems to be well justified as long as IHC is performed by experienced laboratories with proper quality control measures. CISH is a promising alternative to FISH. Further dissection of the *HER2* pathway needs to be pursued to develop more sensitive predictors of response to trastuzumab. Investigation of the clinical significance of amplicons other than *HER2* seems to be warranted, based on their contribution to transcriptional control of genes in breast cancer cells.

REFERENCES

1. Slamon DJ, et al. Use of chemotherapy plus a monoclonal antibody against HER2 for metastatic breast cancer that overexpresses *HER2*. *N Engl J Med* 2001;344: 783–792.
2. Pollack JR, et al. Microarray analysis reveals a major direct role of DNA copy number alteration in the transcriptional program of human breast tumors. *Proc Natl Acad Sci USA* 2002;99:12963–12968.
3. Hyman E, et al. Impact of DNA amplification on gene expression patterns in breast cancer. *Cancer Res* 2002;62:6240–6245.
4. Slamon DJ, et al. Human breast cancer: correlation of relapse and survival with amplification of the HER-2/neu oncogene. *Science* 1987;235:177–182.
5. Jarvinen TA, Liu ET. *HER-2/neu* and topoisomerase IIalpha in breast cancer. *Breast Cancer Res Treat* 2003;78:299–311.
6. Niehans GA, et al. Stability of *HER-2/neu* expression over time and at multiple metastatic sites. *J Natl Cancer Inst* 1993;85:1230–1235.
7. Masood S, Bui MM. Assessment of *Her-2/neu* overexpression in primary breast cancers and their metastatic lesions: an immunohistochemical study. *Ann Clin Lab Sci* 2000;30:259–265.
8. Simon R, et al. Patterns of *her-2/neu* amplification and overexpression in primary and metastatic breast cancer. *J Natl Cancer Inst* 2001;93:1141–1146.
9. Vogel CL, et al. First-line Trastuzumab monotherapy in metastatic breast cancer. *Oncology* 2001;61(Suppl 2):37–42.

10. Dowsett M, et al. Correlation between immunohistochemistry (HercepTest) and fluorescence in situ hybridization (FISH) for *HER-2* in 426 breast carcinomas from 37 centres. *J Pathol* 2003;199:418–423.

11. Paik S, et al. Real-world performance of HER2 testing—National Surgical Adjuvant Breast and Bowel Project experience. *J Natl Cancer Inst* 2002;94:852–854.

12. Roche PC, et al. Concordance between local and central laboratory *HER2* testing in the breast intergroup trial N9831. *J Natl Cancer Inst* 2002;94:855–857.

13. Andersen CL, et al. Improved procedure for fluorescence in situ hybridization on tissue microarrays. *Cytometry* 2001;45:83–86.

14. Tanner M, et al. Chromogenic in situ hybridization: a practical alternative for fluorescence in situ hybridization to detect *HER-2/neu* oncogene amplification in archival breast cancer samples. *Am J Pathol* 2000;157:1467–1472.

15. Gupta D, et al. Comparison of fluorescence and chromogenic in situ hybridization for detection of *HER-2/neu* oncogene in breast cancer. *Am J Clin Pathol* 2003;119:381–387.

16. Millson A, et al. Comparison of two quantitative polymerase chain reaction methods for detecting *HER2/neu* amplification. *J Mol Diagn* 2003;5:184–190.

17. Isola J, et al. Genetic alterations in ERBB2-amplified breast carcinomas. *Clin Cancer Res* 1999;5:4140–4145.

IV TISSUE PREDICTIVE BIOMAKERS

6 Cell Kinetics

Maria Grazia Daidone, PhD, Rosella Silvestrini, PhD, and Dino Amadori, MD

CONTENTS

INTRODUCTION
MEASUREMENT OF CELL PROLIFERATION
CONCLUSIONS
REFERENCES

SUMMARY

Cell proliferative activity represents one of the biological processes most widely investigated because of its association with tumor progression, and in the past years many laboratories have set up and compared different approaches to measure the proliferation of tumor cells for clinical use. Although available results suggest that the majority of proliferation indices may help clinicians in treatment decision making, their clinical usefulness is still controversial owing to some unresolved technical issues linked to preanalytical and analytical aspects and, most importantly, to interpretation of results. However, some laboratories have dedicated considerable time and effort to develop and optimize reproducible methods and standardized methodologies to quantify cell proliferation in clinical tumors, to assess laboratory performance and reproducibility, and to validate preliminary results. Prospective randomized clinical studies have demonstrated the prognostic and predictive significance of breast cancer proliferative activity in different clinical situations.

Cancer Drug Discovery and Development: Biomarkers in Breast Cancer: Molecular Diagnostics for Predicting and Monitoring Therapeutic Effect
Edited by: G. Gasparini and D. F. Hayes © Humana Press Inc., Totowa, NJ

Novel prospective, multicenter, randomized clinical trials of adjuvant chemotherapy are ongoing to test the utility of cell kinetics to define therapy options for patients with negative or one to three positive nodes presenting rapidly proliferating tumors considered at high risk of relapse. The results will probably help to better establish the predictive role and clinical usefulness of proliferation indices for their transferral to general oncology practice.

Key Words: Assay standardization; cell kinetic-based clinical trials; posttreatment variations; prognostic and predictive relevance.

1. INTRODUCTION

Cell proliferation represents a fundamental biological process because of its involvement in determining growth and in maintaining homeostasis of tissues. The proliferative activity of a tissue can be considered as the result of a complex and dynamic equilibrium of its cell subpopulations. Cells progress through four consecutive phases of the cell cycle, $G_1 \to S \to G_2 \to M$, under the control of regulatory elements. Cytoplasmic proteins, organelles, and RNA are synthesized in the G_1 and G_2 phases, DNA is replicated during the S phase, and then cells either undergo the mitotic (M) phase or leave the cell cycle and enter a state of quiescence (G_0). The activity of cell cycle regulators is modulated according to stimulatory or inhibitory growth signals and is subject to strict control in normal cells, whereas in cancer cells a variable degree of independence from such stimuli seems to occur. In particular, the activation of oncogenes, probably associated with the inactivation of tumor suppressor genes, is responsible for the induction of stimulatory signals as well as for the disruption of checkpoints that ensure an orderly progression through the cell cycle *(1,2)*.

The proliferative activity of the tumor cell population, which is closely linked to disease progression, has emerged from clinically oriented research as an increasingly important feature to complement clinicopathological staging for a more accurate prediction of risk of relapse (in different clinical and pathological situations), and has contributed to defining the phenotype of highly aggressive tumors. Thus, in view of biological intertumor heterogeneity, increasing efforts have been made in the past decade to obtain as much cell kinetic information as possible from individual clinical lesions to improve knowledge of tumor biology and potential aggressiveness and to provide clinicians with information on the clinical utility of proliferation markers assessed in large consecutive case series.

To render cell kinetic determination feasible in consecutive series of patients, investigators have turned their attention to specific aspects of the complex phenomenon of proliferation and growth. In particular, kinetic characterization has focused on some specific proliferating cell compartments, that is, on cells that transit through the cell cycle that are generally responsible for tumor growth, and more susceptible to the action of therapeutic agents.

Biologists and pathologists have used several approaches to determine cell proliferative fraction, in accordance with their professional backgrounds *(3)*. Such approaches are based on different rationales and employ different morphometric, immunocytochemical, cytometric, or autoradiographic methods, with inherent advantages and disadvantages. They are designed to analyze and quantify either the whole proliferating fraction or discrete fractions of cells in specific cell cycle phases, mainly in the S and M phases. From a methodological viewpoint, common requirements for clinically useful proliferation markers include technical and biological effectiveness in terms of ability to describe a specific biological phenomenon and to provide results that are informative, reliable, accurate, and reproducible in intra- and interlaboratory settings, at an acceptable cost and obtainable easily and quickly when needed for clinical decision making.

In breast cancer, retrospective correlative studies have indicated that proliferative activity is generally unrelated to clinicopathological stage *(4)*, but at the same time strongly and persistently indicative of risk of relapse and death *(5)*, even in the presence of prognostic information provided by other important pathobiological features. Evidence is also emerging of an association between cell proliferation and response to systemic treatments. Preliminary investigations on the clinical usefulness of cell proliferation have been carried out retrospectively on large, generally monoinstitutional case series, and quality control programs have been activated to guarantee the reproducibility of laboratory determinations *(6)*. Following these initial developments, prospective randomized controlled trials were recently planned to assess the clinical usefulness of proliferation markers, that is, whether they provide information that will affect choice of treatment and improve clinical outcome *(7,8)*. Available results indicate a chemotherapy benefit for node-negative breast cancer patients at high risk of relapse as they present with rapidly proliferating tumors, but the relationship between cell proliferation and response to specific treatments is in need of further validation in large, prospective, proliferation-based studies.

2. MEASUREMENT OF CELL PROLIFERATION

Initially, measurement of the proliferative activity of human tumors was considered with scepticism because it took into account only a fraction of the entire tumor cell population in a single tissue sample obtained at only one time in tumor life, which generally corresponded to surgical intervention for diagnosis and/or tumor removal. Today, currently used proliferation indices assessed by morphometry, immunocytochemistry, flow cytometry, or incorporation techniques have become widely accepted to determine and quantify the whole proliferative fraction or discrete fractions of cells in specific cell cycle phases on consecutive series of clinical tumors, including breast cancers *(3,9)*.

2.1. Phase-Specific Markers

These include proliferation markers measuring the only two phases of the cell cycle in which cells are detectable on the basis of morphological or phenomenological aspects or as a result of their capacity to incorporate DNA precursors.

2.1.1. MITOSIS

Quantification of cells in the mitotic phase *(10)* is currently expressed as the number of mitotic figures per 10 high-power fields (mitotic activity index [MAI]) or, when corrected for field size and area fraction of the neoplastic epithelium, as standardized mitotic index (volume fraction-corrected mitotic index, or M/VV index, giving the result in mitotic figures per mm^2 of neoplastic epithelium). Both methods of expressing the presence of mitotic figures provide comparable results, but the standardized mitotic index (SMI) has consistently shown smaller interobserver variations. These indices, which have long been employed as diagnostic and prognostic tools in the study of tumor pathology, are important components of all histological grading systems and are routinely used by pathologists. They do not require special processing or staining procedures or the fragmentation of tumor tissues. However, although an increased mitotic activity is a frequent finding in aggressive tumors, the validity of these measurements as markers of tumor proliferative activity will remain controversial *(11)* until they are standardized or until interlaboratory reproducibility is guaranteed. In fact, mitotic figure counting represents a simple, rapid, and highly feasible approach even for very small tumors, which, however, can be affected by biological and technical factors, and by intra- and interobserver variability owing to the subjective identification of mitotic figures. Although the latter weaknesses can be virtually eliminated by providing precise descriptive criteria for the morphological identification of mitoses, such as those developed by the Amsterdam group *(12)*, technical aspects, including type and time of fixative, section thickness as well as drawbacks related to definition of high-power fields and total number of tumor cells can compromise the interstudy comparability of results. Finally, in addition to problems related to intratumoral heterogeneity and to the poor resolution of the cell kinetics parameter caused by the relatively short time of the M phase (40–60 min) compared to the duration of the entire cell cycle (40–50 h), metaphase arrest may also represent a final stage of cell life.

2.1.2. S-Phase

The quantitative determination of cells in the S phase initially based on the active incorporation of labeled ([^{3}H]thymidine) or halogenated DNA precursors (bromo- or iododeoxyuridine) *(13)* was successively paralleled by flow or image cytometry of cells with an S-phase DNA content *(14)*. Incorporation measurements, which are performed with autoradiographic or immunohistochemical techniques, require fresh material, aspirates, and surgical or bioptic specimens, and must therefore be prospectively planned. The fraction of S-phase cells is quantified and expressed as the percentage of DNA precursor-incorporating cells over the total number of tumor cells. The main advantages of these approaches, which are considered complex, are the high accessibility and, as *in situ* procedures, the possibility to discriminate tumor from nontumor cells to overcome bias related to tumor heterogeneity. Thymidine labeling index (TLI) is not affected by type or time of fixation, gives clear-cut and unequivocally positive images of reduced silver grains, and permits determinations of labeled cells even after lengthy preservation of archival paraffin blocks.

The main limitation of these approaches is the requirement of fresh tumor material with a sufficient number of viable cells, which has been partially overcome by the availability of kits for TLI (distributed by Euroframe, Asti, Italy) and for bromodeoxyuridine (distributed by Amersham) labeling index (BrdULI) determination, which guarantee the standardization of the first methodological steps and facilitate their use in institutions without adequately equipped laboratories.

The cytometric quantification of nuclear DNA content, which generally provides information on total DNA content and gross genomic abnormalities, can be used to quantify cells in the different cell cycle phases, in particular in the S phase, based on the knowledge that S-phase cells have a variable DNA content ranging from the presynthetic phase $G_{0/1}$ *(2n)* to the postsynthetic G_2 phase *(4n)*. The utilization of dyes that specifically bind DNA, such as propidium iodide, ethidium bromide, mitramycin, 4',6-diamidino-2-phenylindole (DAPI), acridine orange, and Hoechst 33258 allows a quantitation of nuclear DNA content by flow cytometry on isolated nuclei or cell suspensions, or by image static cytometry on cytohistological specimens. Both approaches give a frequency histogram of DNA content, which reflects the cell cycle. The fractions of cells in the different phases are quantified by computerized cell cycle analysis. In addition to S-phase cells, the fraction of cells in the S+G_2M phases is also considered by some authors as a more complete proliferation index that defines the proportion of cells in the cell cycle excluding only those in the $G_{0/1}$ phase. The most diffuse approach for the evaluation of the S-phase cell fraction is flow cytometry (FCM-SPF), the main advantage of which consists in a rapid, potentially objective evaluation of a large number of cells obtained from surgical specimens, biopsy or fine-needle aspirates, effusions, and bone marrow aspirates. The main drawback, which is common to all the non-*in situ* techniques, is the impossibility to discriminate tumor from nontumor cells. This automated technique received a major impetus in the late 1980s, with the development of procedures to perform flow cytometry in solid tumors using material from formalin-fixed paraffin-embedded blocks *(14)* or from frozen tumor specimens. The use of the latter material also guarantees more reproducible information on specimens that have been in storage for some time and accrued from different centers. The feasibility of FCM-SPF is potentially high, but the quality of results can be affected by methodological factors. To make results reproducible and comparable among the different centers, standardization of assay methodologies, cell cycle analysis techniques, and cutoff points for classifying and interpreting FCM-S from DNA histograms, as well as strict quality control, are mandatory.

Recently, a concerted effort was carried out and developed by US, French, and Swedish investigators to optimize the prognostic strength of flow-cytometric DNA measurements and to test the validity of the proposed adjustments *(15)*. This study, performed on about 1400 patients with node-negative breast cancer, emphasized the complexity of the interpretation of DNA ploidy histograms and quantification of S-phase cells, which are so closely related to each other that they provide non-independent prognostic information when considered in association. Following 10 adjustments to the two measurements, which involved both DNA ploidy reclassification and S-phase calculation, the association between the two flow cytometric measurements has been reduced and their confounding technical correlation eliminated, thus permitting them to become independent prognostic factors in a single model.

2.2. Antigen-Related Markers

These approaches involve the determination of enzymes (DNA polymerase α, thymidine kinase), antigens (Ki67/MIB-1, KiS1, KiS2, cyclin-PCNA), or structural alterations (AgNOR, that is, argyrophilic nucleolar organizer regions) *(16–21)*, which in some instances represent the natural evolution and the integration of morphological and functional determinations, and provide information on the overall fraction of proliferating cells, that is, the growth fraction of the tumor. However, available information on their clinical relevance, albeit interesting, has been questioned, especially for solid tumors, and indicates the need for methodological verification and standardization through quality control assessments *(10)*.

Among proliferation-associated antigens, Ki67 has long been regarded as the most reliable marker of proliferating cells. The expression of Ki67 antigen, detectable by Ki67 antibody, was first identified in phytohemagglutinin-stimulated lymphocytes and described as putatively expressed only by proliferating cells *(18)*. Its main drawback is that it can be detected only in acetone-fixed frozen sections. However, the recent availability of a series of reagents (MIB-1, Ki-S1, and Ki-S5), which recognize Ki67 proliferation antigen and can be used on formalin-fixed paraffin-embedded material following antigen retrieval with pretreatment in a microwave oven or in a pressure cooker *(10)*, has overcome the fixation-related constraint and opened up interesting perspectives for assessing the clinical utility of MIB-1 index on consecutive large series of cancers.

2.3. Comparability and Standardization of the Different Proliferation Indices

The indices most frequently used to quantify the proliferative rate of clinical tumors (mitotic figures, FCM-SPF, TLI, and Ki67/MIB-1) can be determined on viable, frozen, or paraffin-embedded tissues using different detection techniques, which may also involve DNA histogram modeling software. Each approach has inherent advantages and disadvantages, including different feasibility rates, which appear to depend on the availability of fresh tumor tissue for TLI or BrdULI, and on data analysis and interpretation in tumors with multiple cell subpopulations for FCM-SPF. These differences in biological and technical aspects could be one of the main causes of the inconsistency of results among laboratories, which may help to explain the reasoning behind the caution raised by the American Society of Clinical Oncology against the routine use of proliferation indices in breast cancer, notwithstanding the large number of studies demonstrating the prognostic relevance of the different tumor proliferation indices. Prospective studies, associated with an evaluation of laboratory effectiveness in terms of presence of quality assurance programs and methods comparison, could provide definitive information on the clinical utility of proliferation markers.

2.3.1. REPRODUCIBILITY OF THE MEASUREMENTS AND QUALITY CONTROL PROGRAMS

Efforts have been made to standardize methodologies and interpretation criteria to improve reliability, accuracy, and reproducibility of results within and among the different laboratories and to promote and maintain quality control programs to provide clinicians with a network of qualified laboratories for currently employed proliferation indices. In particular, it is worth mentioning that all the prospective randomized phase III trials of chemotherapy vs observation in node-negative breast cancer, activated in the last decade to test the clinical utility of identifying high-risk patients on the basis of high tumor cell proliferation (by MAI, TLI, or FCM-SPF), have been paralleled by the activation of quality control programs for preanalytical and analytical phases of cell kinetic determination *(6,12,22–25)*.

INTRA-LABORATORY   INTER-LABORATORIES

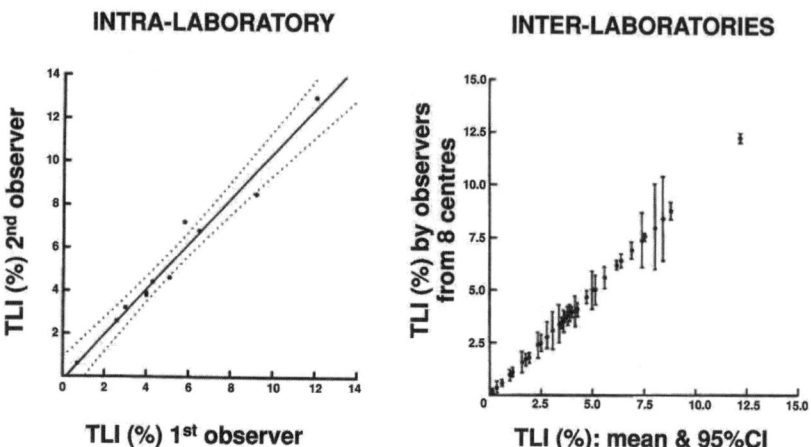

TLI (%) 1st observer   TLI (%): mean & 95%CI

Fig. 1. Reproducibility of TLI determination within a single laboratory (intra-laboratory) and among eight different laboratories (interlaboratory) participating in the Italian Network for Quality Assessment of Tumor Biomarkers *(6)*.

The external quality control assessment of TLI determination has been extended nationwide in Italy *(22)* to ensure its reproducibility, and is currently used in multicenter clinical protocols. This initiative focuses on the assessment of the reproducibility of histoautoradiographic evaluation of samples and, in accordance with previously defined standard operating procedures for sample scoring, is based on (1) sample identification and selection by the coordinating laboratory; (2) circulation of samples among the participating laboratories; (3) TLI evaluation; and (4) data collection and analysis by an independent Statistical Unit. Results *(6)* to date have demonstrated satisfactory levels of intra- and interlaboratory reproducibility (Fig. 1), with an improvement in the performance of participating laboratories to more than three runs.

2.3.3. ASSOCIATION BETWEEN PROLIFERATION INDICES: BASIC RESULTS AND CLINICAL STUDIES

The different indices of proliferation have not always proven to be associated with one another in terms of biological or clinical significance when comparatively analyzed in the same case series. In fact (Table 1), moderate or poor correlation coefficients have generally been observed between proliferation indices detecting cells not only in different but also in the same cell cycle phase, and slightly varying sensitivity and specificity rates have been reported for different proliferation indices when related to clinical outcome on the same case series *(21,26–49)*. However, at present only one study *(29)* has been specifically planned to simultaneously challenge the prognostic

Table 1
Comparison Between Different Proliferation Markers

	SPF		Ki67/MIB-1		MI-M/V	
	No. of cases (No. of studies)	r	No. of cases (No. of studies)	r	No. of cases (No. of studies)	r
TLI/BrdULI	1078 (6)	0.54	1482 (7)	0.29	541 (2)	0.27–0.81
SPF			1835 (23)	0.42	611 (3)	0.42
Ki67/MIB-1					1046 (7)	0.49

MI, Mitotic (figure) index/count; M/V, volume/corrected mitotic index; r, median correlation or regression coefficients.

Space constraints do not permit us to mention all the articles whose results contributed to the data reported in the table.

capability of BrdULI, MI, or MIB-1 on the same series of stage I–III breast cancers, and its results support the importance of MI evaluation over the other proliferation markers.

2.3.3.1. Association With Risk Profiles

Initial studies investigated the association between cell kinetic markers and the most important conventional prognostic factors, such as the extent of the disease at diagnosis, that is, at the time of clinical detection. Information is available for TLI on 14,147 primary breast cancers collected and characterized in a single institution, the National Cancer Institute (Istituto Nazionale Tumori) of Milan, over a 25-yr period (1975–2000). Proliferative activity was only weakly related to tumor size, as large tumors (>2 cm) were slightly more frequent in the highest proliferation class, whereas it was unrelated to nodal involvement (Fig. 2). Conversely, in undifferentiated tumors and in premenopausal women or in women younger than 50 yr of age, high cell proliferation was more frequently observed (Fig. 2). However, such associations, although statistically significant, are relatively weak. A direct association was much stronger with biomarkers that are indicative of an unfavorable clinical outcome, such as aneuploid DNA content, a weak or absent bcl-2 expression, absence of steroid hormone receptors, and p53 accumulation (Fig. 3). Moreover, when considering the association between proliferation and traditional prognostic factors for breast cancer including tumor size, patient age, histological grade, estrogen and progesterone receptors (ER, PgR), the more unfavorable factors that are detected in a tumor, be it node negative or node positive, the more likely it is to be rapidly proliferating. In fact, when four or more unfavorable factors (i.e., size >2 cm, age <50 yr, ER-negative, PgR-negative, grade 3) were simultaneously present, even in the absence of axillary lymph node involvement, tumor proliferative activity was very high in about 30–40% of cases

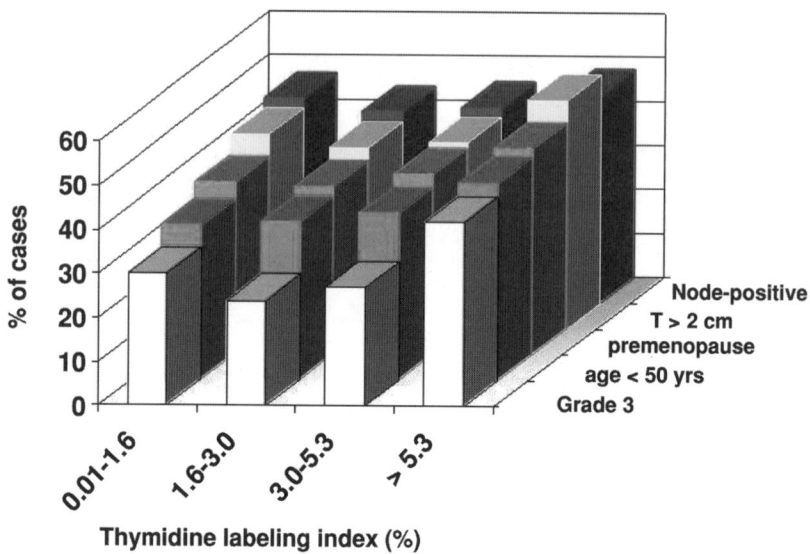

Fig. 2. Unfavorable clinicopathological factors (including patient age and menopausal status, tumor size, axillary lymph node involvement, histological grade) as a function of TLI in 14,147 primary breast cancers.

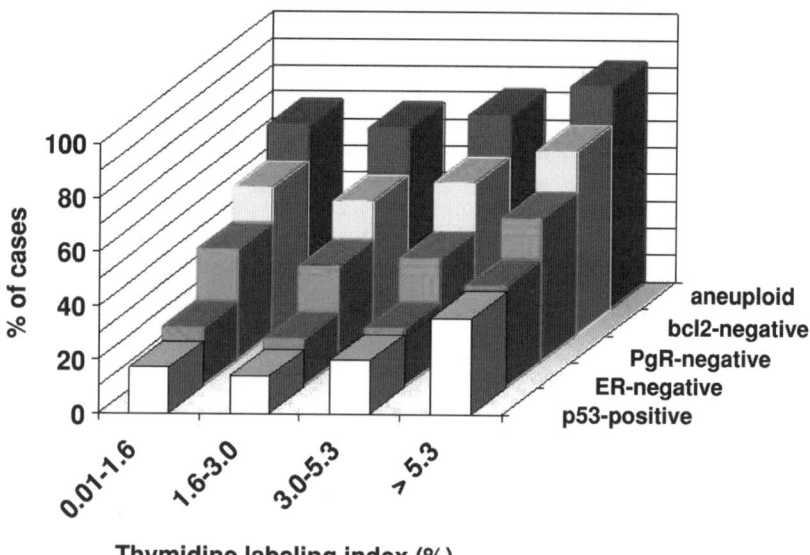

Fig. 3. Unfavorable biological factors (including DNA-ploidy, estrogen and progesterone receptor [ER and PgR] status, bcl-2 and p53 expression) as a function of TLI in 14,147 primary breast cancers.

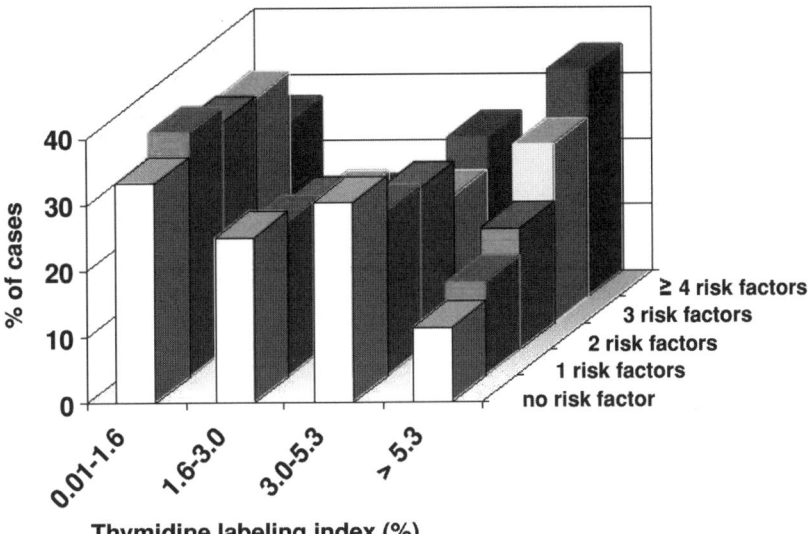

Fig. 4. Relationship between the simultaneous presence of unfavorable clinicopathological and biological factors (including tumor size >2 cm, patient age <50 yr, ER-negative, PgR-negative, histological grade 3) and TLI in node-negative primary breast cancers.

(Fig. 4). Conversely, the highest proliferation class proved to have only 10–13% of cases with no or only one unfavorable factor, which were more frequent (33 and 36% of cases, respectively) in the lowest proliferation subset.

2.3.3.2. Prognostic Significance

Translational research into human tumors has been developed along two main lines: (1) the search for markers to use as a complement to clinicopathological staging to identify patients at minimal risk of relapse or those who are destined to relapse and progress regardless of treatment and (2) the prediction of patients who are likely to respond or develop resistance to a specific treatment. At present, cell proliferation indices are used to identify patients at high risk of relapse or death (who need aggressive treatments) and those with an indolent disease (who are potentially curable by locoregional treatment alone). In fact, the majority of published articles identified in the PubMed database using *breast cancer* and the name of each *proliferation index* as search terms indicate a direct association between high proliferation indices and the probability of relapse, mainly in distant sites, and death in univariate analysis (Table 2), both in patients subjected to locoregional therapy alone until relapse or in those given adjuvant systemic treatments after radical or conservative surgery. This finding has been

Table 2
Prognostic Value of Proliferation Indices in Breast Cancer

	No. of studies[a] with worse outcome for rapidly proliferating tumors			
	No systemic treatment		Different systemic treatments	
	Relapse	Death	Relapse	Death
TLI, BrdULI				
Univariate analysis	10/10	7/8	8/9	7/7
Multivariate analysis	9/9	7/7	4/4	4/4
FCM-SPF				
Univariate analysis	18/20	8/10	23/26	19/22
Multivariate analysis	10/10	5/5	14/14	13/13
Ki67, MIB-1				
Univariate analysis	4/5	3/3	14/16	10/11
Multivariate analysis	2/2	2/2	6/6	3/3
MI, MAI, M/V				
Univariate analysis	2/3	2/2	15/15	11/11
Multivariate analysis	2/2	1/1	8/8	7/7

[a]Identified by a computerized literature search performed by PubMed using *Breast cancer* and the name of each of the *proliferation indices* as search terms, on all available original English articles that were selected for inclusion when they reported data on the relationship between proliferation indices and clinical outcome, retrospectively evaluated in univariate and/or multivariate analyses on independent case series of at least 100 patients with a minimum follow-up of 4 yr.

BrdULI, Bromodeoxyuridine labeling index; FCM-SPF, flow-cytometric S-phase cell fraction; MAI, mitotic activity index; MI, mitotic index; M/V, mitotic activity (volume/corrected MI); TLI, [^{3}H]thymidine labeling index.

confirmed for all the proliferative indices and regardless of the criteria used to classify tumors as slowly or rapidly proliferating. In all these phase I and II exploratory investigations, carried out over the last two decades without *a priori* study design or prospective definition of specimen collection procedures (studies providing level of evidence [LOE] III according to the Tumor Marker Grading Utility System *[50]*), such an association was generally maintained in multivariate analyses including patient age and menopausal status, tumor size, regional lymph nodal status and histological/cytological findings or biological markers associated with differentiation, hormone responsiveness, neo-angiogenesis, and genomic alterations *(30–32,35,42,51–80)* (Table 3). In particular, phase-specific proliferation indices, including mitotic figure counts, maintained their predictivity for disease-, event-, or relapse-free survival and for overall or cancer-specific survival even in the presence of information provided by histological or nuclear grade, despite the fact that all grading systems included the proliferative information provided by the mitotic index *(35,69,73,75,77,78)*.

From such an overview it also emerged that, in the presence of other clinical and pathobiological factors, proliferation indices contributed to a better prognostic definition within subsets of patients with an intermediate tumor size (1–2 cm) *(55)*, or those classified at an intermediate risk of relapse *(5)* according to the criteria adopted in the 1998 St. Gallen International Consensus Conference on the Treatment of Primary Breast Cancer *(81)* and integrating patient age, tumor size, histological grade, and steroid hormone receptors (Fig. 5). These findings were confirmed in a large clinical trial conducted by Intergroup (INT 0102), with the maximum level of evidence (LOE I) as it was a prospectively randomized study, in which a low FCM-SPF identified patients with ER/PgR-positive tumors of ≤2 cm who would have a clinical outcome similar to that of women whose tumors were too small for biochemical ER/PgR assay *(82)*, and who could be subjected to locoregional treatment alone.

In keeping with these observations are the findings obtained on a series of 2670 patients with histologically node-negative operable breast cancers who underwent radical mastectomy (38.6% of cases) or conservative surgery plus radiotherapy (61.4% of cases) and axillary lymph node dissection at the National Cancer Institute of Milan from 1975 to 1996, and who did not receive any systemic postoperative therapy until new disease manifestation was documented. In this case series, which was consecutive with respect to TLI determined at the time of diagnosis and in which very small (≤1 cm) and large (>2 cm) tumors accounted for 12.2% and 34.6% of cases, respectively, pathological tumor size was a strong predictor of both 10-yr relapse (size 1–2 cm vs ≤1 cm; HR = 1.33, 95% CI, 1.04–1.69; two-sided $p = 0.0217$; size >2 cm vs ≤1 cm; HR = 1.82, 95% CI, 1.42–2.33; two-sided $p = 0.0001$) and death (size 1–2 cm vs ≤1 cm; HR = 2.11, 95% CI, 1.36–3.28; two-sided $p = 0.0009$; size >2 cm vs ≤1 cm; HR = 3.75, 95% CI, 2.42–5.81; two-sided $p = 0.0001$). In patients with very small tumors, relapse-free survival was predicted only by cell proliferation (high vs low TLI, HR = 2.04, 95% CI, 1.23–3.28; two-sided $p = 0.005$), even in the presence of information provided by patient age and other tumor biological features, such as steroid hormone receptors or p53 and bcl-2 expression. Similar findings were observed for intermediate size tumors (1–2 cm, accounting for 53.2% of cases) in which, in addition to TLI, bcl-2 expression proved to be associated with prognosis (high vs low TLI, HR = 1.31, 95% CI, 1.03–1.68; two-sided $p = 0.03$; low vs high bcl-2, HR = 1.36, 95% CI, 1.07–1.75; two-sided $p = 0.014$). Conversely, when the 10-yr probabilities of disease outcome were plotted against continuous values of TLI, the relationship between relapse-free survival and cell proliferation appeared to be differ-

Table 3
Prognostic Value of Proliferation Indices by Multivariate Analysis in Patients
with Early Breast Cancer Subjected to Only Surgery ± Radiotherapy Until Relapse

Author (ref.)	Stage	No. of cases	Follow-up (yr)	Proliferation Index	Other factors considered for survival analyses	p value Relapse	p value Death
Medri (51)	N–	378	5	TLI	A, T, HG, ER, PgR, MVD	0.08	
Paradiso (52)	N–	101	5	TLI	A, T, HG, ER, PgR	0.04	
Silvestrini (53)	N–	215	5	TLI	A,T, ER	0.004	0.035
Courdi (54)	N–	167	8	TLI	A, T, HG, ER, PgR	0.037	
Silvestrini (55)	N–	1800	8	TLI	A, T, ER, PgR	0.006	0.014
Meyer (30)	N–	414	10	TLI	A, T, ER, nuclear size	NS	0.095
Cooke (56)	Mixed	164	8	TLI	T, N, HER-2/neu		NS
Tubiana (57)	Mixed	125	15	TLI	T, HG	<0.05	0.05
Aubele (58)[a]	I	329	8	SPF	Morphometric features, ploidy	NS	
Sigurdsson (59)	N–	250	4	FCM-SPF	A, T, ER, PgR, ploidy	0.03	0.0001
O'Reilly (60)	N–	169	5	FCM-SPF	T, HG, ER, ploidy	0.05	0.045
Brown (42)	N–	314	6	FCM-SPF	A, T, ER, PgR, cell type, surgery, treatment, Ki67, ploidy	0.006	
Harbeck (61)	N–	125	6.5	FCM-SPF	T, HG, ER, PgR, PAI-1, uPA, cathepsin D, p53, HER-2/neu	NS	
Merkel (62)	N–	280	6.5	FCM-SPF	T, HG, NG	NS	0.05
Winchester (32)	N–	198	6.5	FCM-SPF	A, T, HG, NG, ER, MAI, ploidy	0.03[b]	
Baslev (63)	N–	421	7	FCM-SPF	A, T, HG, ER, PgR, no. of examined N	NS	NS
Stal (64)	N–	152	8	FCM-SPF	A, T, ER	0.035	
Isola (65)	N–	289	8.5	FCM-SPF	T, HG, ER, ploidy, p53, HER-2/neu		0.0001

Study	N status	n	Cutoff	Method	Prognostic factors	p1	p2
Bosari (66)	N–	136	9	FCM-SPF	Peritumoral lymphatic and vessel invasion, ploidy	NS	
Johnson (67)	N–	100	9	FCM-SPF	T, HG, ploidy, HER2/neu		0.03
Lipponen (36)	N–	180	10	FCM-SPF	T, HG, histotype, MI, M/V, ploidy		NS
Peirò (31)[a]	N–	115	10	SPF	A, T, HG, NG, ER, tubule formation, vascular invasion, necrosis, desmoplasia, inflammatory reaction, MI, ploidy	0.03	NS
Witzig (68)	N–	265	12.5	FCM-SPF	A, T, HG, NG, ER, no. of examined N, histotype, ploidy	0.05	NS
Joensuu (69)	N0	123	5	FCM-SPF	T, HG, ER, PgR, nuclear pleomorphism, mitotic count	NS	NS
Klintenberg (70)	Mixed	210	5.5	FCM-SPF	ER, N, clinical stage, ploidy	0.038	
Arnelov (71)	Mixed	158	6	FCM-SPF	T, HG, N, pathological stage, ploidy	0.020	
Stanton (72)	Mixed	201	8	FCM-SPF	A, T, ER, N, ploidy, HER-2/neu		NS
Eskelinen (35)	Mixed	148	9	FCM-SPF	A, T, HG, ER, PgR, N, histotype, nuclear pleomorphism, intraductal growth, treatment, M/V, ploidy	0.022	0.003
Fisher (73)	Mixed	377	10	FCM-SPF	A, T, HG, clinical N	0.04	0.08
Toikkanen (74)	Mixed	223	25	FCM-SPF	A, T, HG, N, histotype, tumor margin, tubule formation, nuclear pleomorphism, necrosis, intraductal growth, MAI		0.02
Ladekarl (75)	N–	98	9	Mitotic count	A, T, HG, ER, histotype	0.03	
Kato (76)	N–	200	10	Mitotic count	T, HG, tumor necrosis, lymphatic and blood vessel invasion, p53, HER-2/neu, PCNA	NS	NS
Lipponen (36)	N–	180	10	Mitotic count	T, HG, histotype, SPF, ploidy	NS	

(continued)

Table 3 (continued)

Author (ref.)	Stage	No. of cases	Follow-up (yr)	Proliferation Index	Other factors considered for survival analyses	p value Relapse	p value Death
Aaltomaa (77)	N−	294	13	Mitotic count	A, T, HG, histotype, tumor margin, tubule formation, necrosis, intraductal growth	0.005	NS
Clayton (78)	N−	378	20	Mitotic count	A, T, HG, NG, ER, lymphatic invasion, skin/muscle invasion, nucleoli		<0.001
Joensuu (69)	N0	161	5	Mitotic count	T, HG, ER, PgR, nuclear pleomorphism, SPF		<0.0001
Eskelinen (35)	Mixed	216	9	Mitotic count	A, T, HG, ER, PgR, N, histotype, treatment	0.010	NS
Toikkanen (74)	Mixed	223	28	Mitotic count	A, T, NG, N, histotype, tumor margin, tubule formation, nuclear pleomorphism, necrosis, intraductal growth, SPF, ploidy		NS
Brown (42)	N−	618	6	Ki67	A, T, ER, PgR, cell type, surgery, treatment	0.0005	
Iacopetta (79)	N−	263	6	MIB-1	Tumor size, histological grade, ER, PgR, p53, HER-2/neu	NS	NS
Harbeck (40)	N−	100	6.5	MIB-1	T, HG, ER, PgR, PAI-1, uPA, cathepsin D, p53, HER-2/neu	NS	NS
Pinder (80)	Mixed	177	12	MIB-1	T, HG, N	0.05	

A, Patient age; HG, histological grade; MVD, microvessel density; N, axillary nodal status; NG, nuclear grade; NS, not significant; T, tumor size.
[a]Image cytometry.
[b]Diploid tumors.

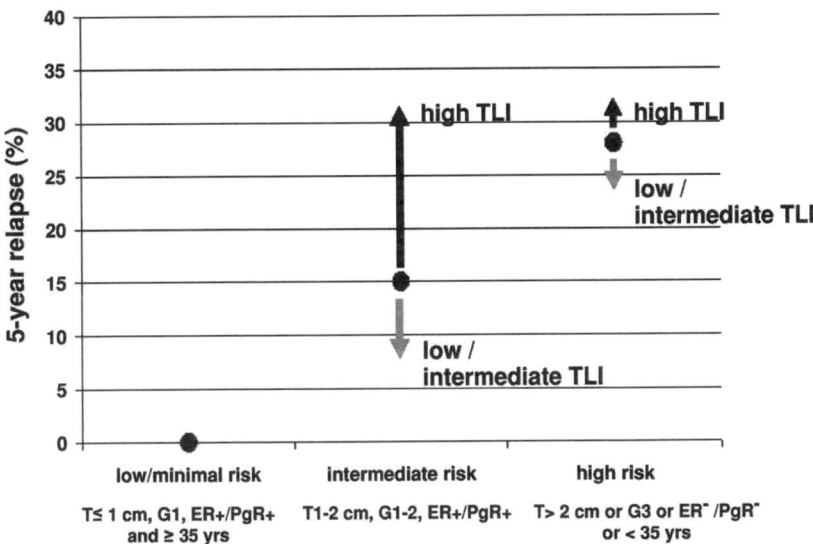

Daidone & Silvestrini, JNCI Monographs, 30, 2001

Fig. 5. Prognostic contribution, in terms of 5-yr relapse probability (%), provided by TLI (≤3%, gray line; > 3%, black line) to risk categories of node-negative breast cancers based on patient age, tumor size, histological grade, and ER and PgR status *(80)*. Dots represent the 5-yr relapse probabilities (%) calculated for risk categories. *Arrows* indicate the 5-yr relapse probabilities (%) calculated as a function of tumor proliferation classes (according to TLI) within each risk category. Overall analysis performed on 543 cases *(5)*.

ently modulated as a function of tumor size (Fig. 6). In fact, a direct inverse relationship between relapse-free survival probability and TLI values was observed in the subset of patients with very small tumors and was also paralleled by the pattern of relationship observed for women with intermediate-size (1–2 cm) tumors, whereas in those with large tumors, relapse-free survival sharply decreased from about 70% to about 45% by raising the TLI cutoff value to 3%, after which this relationship remained almost constant.

2.3.3.3. Predictivity of Response to Specific Treatments

The second objective of translational research in breast cancer, that is, the identification of patients who are likely to respond or develop resistance to a specific treatment, has not provided conclusive results on the role of proliferation indices. The reason for this is probably the generally modest study design, which is not appropriate for investigating the relevance and utility of biomarkers within the context of clinical treatment protocols. In fact, the ideal method to assess the role of any biological variable as a

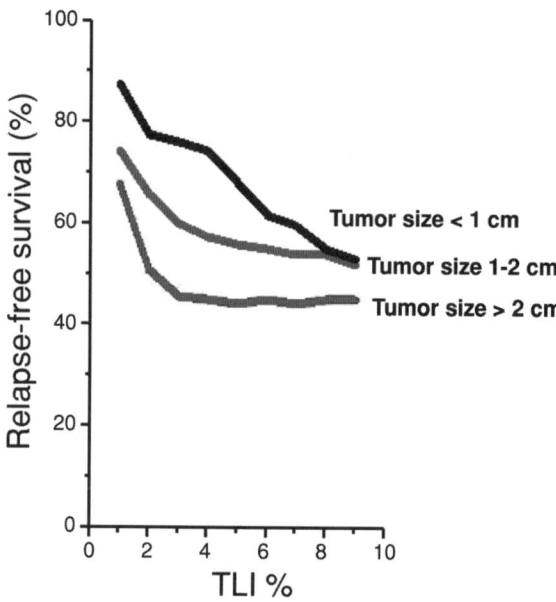

Fig. 6. Relationship between values of TLI and percentage probability of 10-yr relapse-free survival as a function of pathological tumor size in 2670 node-negative operable breast cancer patients not receiving any postoperative systemic adjuvant therapy.

predictor of response to a specific treatment would entail its prospective evaluation in a randomized clinical study specifically designed to analyze biomarker predictivity, or to compare systemic treatments with locoregional therapies. However, to date, only a small number of prospective, high-powered studies addressing the issue of the clinical utility of proliferation markers has provided conclusive results (presented and discussed in Section 2.3.3.4.). Conversely, most of the available results have been retrospectively derived from studies performed mainly in an adjuvant setting, in which the advantage of a long-term follow-up has been counterbalanced by a marked heterogeneity in technical and analytical procedures for biomarker determination on tumor specimens collected for a variety of reasons and available for evaluating proliferation indices without any *a priori* study design.

In advanced lesions, in general, a benefit from intensive polychemo-therapy, including S-phase–specific agents, has been observed for rapidly *(83–85)* rather than slowly proliferating tumors. A greater benefit for patients with rapidly proliferating tumors has also been observed, albeit not consistently, in adjuvant settings for node-positive resectable cancers *(86–90)*. Within the context of prospective randomized-clinical trials, a benefit from cyclophosphamide, methotrexate, and fluorouracil (CMF) on long-term clinical outcome has been observed *(88)* for both subgroups, although more evidently *(87,90)* in patients with rapidly proliferating tumors, but also independently of proliferative activity *(89)*. The former finding has been ascribed to a higher efficacy of polychemotherapy, including antimetabolites, in killing dividing cells. In addition to the type of drugs used, treatment schedule has also been proven to affect the relationship between cell kinetics and clinical outcome. In fact, in a randomized treatment protocol aimed to compare the efficacy of alternating vs sequential regimens of doxorubicin and CMF in node-positive breast cancer patients, the benefit of sequential administration was evident mainly in patients with low to intermediate proliferative tumors *(91)*. This result was explained by a partial synchronization of cells in the G_2–M phases following the administration of high dose intensity doxorubicin and the subsequent presentation of a large fraction of S-phase cells to antimetabolites included in the CMF regimen.

Recently, neoadjuvant chemotherapy protocols have been used as an ideal model for translational studies aimed at analyzing the predictivity of biological variables for short- and long-term clinical end points and at monitoring, at cellular and molecular levels, the effect of treatment by sequential determinations of biomarkers within a single tumor, in the presence of only intralesional heterogeneity *(92)*. Overall, proliferative activity appears to provide information on tumor biological changes and is sensitive enough to reflect, at the cellular level, the biological downstaging induced by treatment, with relevant implications on long-term follow-up. In fact, significant changes observed after chemotherapy generally consisted in a reduction in proliferative activity *(93–97)*. Tumor shrinkage proved to be less frequent in patients with pretreated slowly proliferating tumors *(93–99)*, while a favorable long-term clinical outcome was generally *(99)* observed for patients with posttreated slowly proliferating tumors *(96,100)*.

A reduction in the proliferative rate associated with a higher probability of tumor shrinkage and a more favorable outcome for patients with posttreated slowly proliferating tumors was also observed following neoadjuvant antihormonal treatment *(101,102)*. A higher response rate was observed for patients with slowly rather than with rapidly proliferating tumors *(103)*, even in the ER$^+$ subset *(104,105)*. These findings, which held true regardless of PgR status, indicate that slowly proliferating metastatic ER$^+$ breast cancers benefit from tamoxifen, whereas rapidly proliferating tumors largely escape endocrine control, even if they are ER$^+$, that is, traditionally considered hormone responsive. Therefore, in addition to a lack of estrogen receptors, a high proliferative activity represents a limiting factor for response to endocrine therapy. Furthermore, evidence of a major benefit from endocrine therapy for slowly proliferating tumors has also been confirmed in adjuvant settings *(106–108)*, although contrasting results are also present in the literature *(109)*.

However, it must be remembered that these data were obtained mainly from retrospective clinical analyses, with a LOE III *(50)*, and are insufficient to be able to draw definitive conclusions on the predictive role of proliferation indices or to use for therapeutic decision-making (endocrine therapy or chemotherapy). Moreover, they are only suggestive of qualitative relationships, and appropriately designed prospective studies are needed to confirm and validate preliminary results to define whether the improved clinical outcome for patients with ER$^+$, slowly proliferating cancer is the result of a natural indolence or of a specific susceptibility to endocrine treatment, and to evaluate whether the benefit of polychemotherapy with S-phase–specific agents in patients with rapidly proliferating tumors is attributable to a quantitative relationship between drug effect and fraction of sensitive S-phase cells. Recently, the determination of cell proliferation was prospectively planned within the context of adjuvant and neoadjuvant treatment protocols in which the evaluation of the usefulness of biological information represented a secondary objective of the clinical study. Even though such studies are not specifically designed to test the predictivity of proliferation indices, it is likely that they will improve the quality of information on their predictive accuracy and provide a definitive evaluation of the clinical usefulness of a cell kinetic characterization.

2.3.3.4. Clinical Utility

All previous findings demonstrate that the various proliferation indices could provide, with a variable level of specificity and sensitivity, information to identify patients (1) at minimal risk of relapse; (2) destined to relapse and progress regardless of treatment; (3) likely to respond or develop resistance to a specific treatment. However, it is only in the past few years that these results, albeit extremely interesting, have been challenged with respect to the clinical usefulness of cell kinetic information compared to or in association with other pathobiological information. Recently, in fact, the results became available of the first therapeutic clinical trials in which the determination of proliferation indices was planned *a priori*, with a sufficiently powered study design to define the role of prognostic/predictive markers. These provided preliminary information on the actual utility of a cell kinetic determination in the presence of a risk profile defined by other clinicopathological and biological factors.

LOE II studies *(50)*, companion to therapeutic clinical trials, provided evidence in favor of the following:

1. A contribution of cell proliferation evaluated as FCM-SPF to define, in association with patient age, PgR status and tumor size, a broad spectrum of clinicopathobiological categories with a different 10-yr risk of distant metastases within a subset of 800 node-negative ER$^+$ cancer patients given tamoxifen *(110)*. The risk probability ranged from 70%

(for patients under 35 yr of age with large, PgR-negative tumors and a very high FCM-SPF) to 20% (for patients older than 50 yr of age with PgR-positive, 1-cm tumors and a negligible proliferative activity), and, on an overall 1118 women with node-negative invasive breast cancer up to 5 cm in size, in which Ki67/MIB-1 was considered in addition to FCM-SPF;

2. A favorable prognosis for women with slowly proliferating tumors, with superimposable disease-free survival rates for patients who received only surgery or adjuvant tamoxifen or doxorubicin and cyclophosphamide *(111)*;

3. A survival advantage for patients with rapidly proliferating tumors who received postoperative adjuvant chemotherapy with doxorubicin and cyclophosphamide, with disease-free survival similar to that of patients with slowly proliferating tumors *(112)*.

Such information provides an accurate assessment of individual patient prognosis and suggests that an aggressive therapy is indicated for only some of the women with node-negative tumors, that is, for those presenting with rapidly proliferating cancers. In keeping with this line of evidence are the findings provided by the prospective randomized clinical trial (LOE I) conducted by the U.S. Intergroup, in which FCM-SPF was able to identify, within the "uncertain" risk subset (ER- or PgR-positive tumors ≤2 cm), patients at a low or high risk of relapse *(82)*.

The successive step of prospective translational studies was to investigate whether node-negative breast cancer patients defined at high risk on the basis of tumor cell proliferation could benefit from adjuvant polychemotherapy. One monoinstitutional and two multicenter phase III randomized trials using TLI *(7,8)* or MAI *(113)* were activated in Europe, in which the prognostic factor hypothesis was combined with a treatment hypothesis *(114)*. In these studies, patients with node-negative breast cancer were stratified into low- and high-risk groups based on the proliferation index of the primary tumor. Patients with slowly proliferating tumors were not treated with systemic therapy following radical or conservative surgery plus radiotherapy. Patients with rapidly proliferating tumors were randomized to receive or not adjuvant chemotherapy (CMF or FAC). Activation of these trials, as well as of similar studies involving the determination of proliferation indices, was paralleled by the promotion and maintenance of quality control programs for analytical and preanalytical phases of cell kinetic determinations *(6,12,23,24,115)*.

Results are available from the study by Amadori et al. *(7)* and Paradiso et al. *(8)*, in which 278 and 248 patients with histologically assessed node-negative tumors were randomized to receive or not to receive chemotherapy. Survival curves showed a disease-free survival benefit in CMF or FAC-treated compared to untreated patients (83% vs 72% *[7]* and 81% vs 69%

[8]), with a reduction in both locoregional and distant relapses. It was also observed *(7)* that the benefit from CMF treatment was evident mainly for cases at very high risk, that is, with the highest TLI values.

Overall, these results support the use of cell proliferation in the node-negative subset to identify patients at low or minimal risk of relapse and spare them from aggressive treatments, and to select those at high risk as candidates for systemic adjuvant therapy. The finding of a greater benefit from antimetabolite-based regimens in patients with tumors with the highest proliferative rate is in keeping with evidence of a relationship between cell kinetics and response to specific treatments, previously discussed in Subheading 2.3.3.3.

3. CONCLUSIONS

Proliferation indices can be considered markers of clinical utility. In fact, in node-negative breast cancers the usefulness of the different proliferation indices to identify subsets at very low risk of relapse has been assessed in large retrospective studies and validated in prospective studies *(82,111).* A benefit from antimetabolite-including chemotherapy regimens has been indicated from retrospective analyses performed in companion studies of randomized treatment protocols and assessed in phase III prospective confirmatory studies *(7,8).* All these findings have contributed to the ranking of mitotic figure count as a category I prognostic factor by the College of American Pathologists *(116),* that is, as a factor proven to be of prognostic importance and usefulness in clinical patient management. Mitotic figure count is the oldest measurement of cell proliferation, with a high degree of accuracy, and represents an integral part of histological grade. Furthermore, it is routinely assessable on histological sections/cytological smears, without the need for additional processing or staining procedures. These advantages over the other proliferation indices probably convinced panelists of the most recent NIH-NCI Consensus Development Conferences to support the use of mitotic figure count in clinical practice, alone or in association to the other components of grading systems *(116,117).* However, if mitotic figure count is used in clinical routine, the standardization of its measurement and the assessment of its intra- and interlaboratory reproducibility is mandatory. In fact, in addition to clinicobiological effectiveness and usefulness, defined as the ability to describe a biological process and its impact on clinical outcome when it influences the choice of therapy, laboratory effectiveness (in terms of the presence of quality assurance programs and methods comparison for any analyte) should also be considered to improve the diagnostic armamentarium in oncology.

Proliferative activity is an example of a biomarker that may be both prognostic and predictive. However, present data are insufficient to draw firm conclusions regarding its predictive role when choosing either endocrine or chemotherapy, but only suggestive of a relationship that should be investigated further in independent adjuvant settings and analyzed with techniques appropriately designed to determine the clinical utility of biomarkers.

ACKNOWLEDGMENTS

This work was supported in part by grants from the Italian Ministry of Health and the Italian National Research Council (CNR).

REFERENCES

1. Clurman BE, Roberts JM. Cell cycle and cancer. *J Natl Cancer Inst* 1995;87:1499–2005.
2. Gillett CE, Barnes DM. Demystified...cell cycle. *Mol Pathol* 1998;51:310–316.
3. Barnes DM, Gillett CE. Determination of cell proliferation. *J Clin Pathol Mol Pathol* 1995;48:M2–M5.
4. Amadori D, Silvestrini R. Prognostic and predictive value of thymidine labelling index in breast cancer. *Breast Cancer Res Treat* 1998;51:267–281.
5. Daidone MG, Silvestrini R. Prognostic and predictive role of proliferation indices in adjuvant therapy of breast cancer. *J Natl Cancer Inst* 2001;30:27–35.
6. Paradiso A, Volpe S, Iacobacci A, et al. Quality control for biomarker determination in oncology: the experience of the Italian Network for Quality Assessment of Tumour Biomarkers (INQAT). *Int J Biol Markers* 2002;17:201–214.
7. Amadori D, Nanni O, Marangolo M, et al. Disease-free survival advantage of adjuvant cyclophosphamide, methotrexate and fluorouracil in patients with node-negative rapidly proliferating breast cancer: a randomized multicenter study. *J Clin Oncol* 2000;18:3125–3134.
8. Paradiso A, Schittulli F, Cellamare G, et al. Randomized clinical trial of adjuvant fluorouracil, epirubicin, and cyclophosphamide chemotherapy for patients with fast-proliferating, node-negative breast cancer. *J Clin Oncol* 2001;19:3929–3937.
9. Silvestrini R. Cell kinetics: prognostic and therapeutic implications in human tumors. *Cell Prolif* 1994;27:579–596.
10. van Diest PJ, Brugal G, Baak JPA. Proliferation markers in tumours: interpretation and clinical value. *J Clin Pathol* 1998;51:716–724.
11. Quinn CM, Wright NA. The clinical assessment of proliferation and growth in human tumours: evaluation of methods and applications as prognostic variables. *J Pathol* 1990;160:93–102.
12. van Diest PJ, Baak JP, Matze-Cok P, et al. Reproducibility of mitosis counting in 2,469 breast cancer specimens: results from the Multi-Center Morphometric Mammary Carcinoma Project. *Hum Pathol* 1992;23:603–607.
13. Meyer JS, Connor RE. In vitro labeling of solid tissues with tritiated thymidine for autoradiographic detection of S-phase nuclei. *Stain Technol* 1977;52:185–195.
14. Hedley DW. Flow cytometry using paraffin-embedded tissue: five years on. *Cytometry* 1989;10:229–241.
15. Bagwell CB, Clark GM, Spyratos F, et al. Optimizing flow cytometric DNA ploidy and S-phase fraction as independent prognostic markers for node-negative breast cancer specimens. *Cytometry* 2001;46:121–135.
16. Cattoretti G, Becker MHG, Key G, et al. Monoclonal antibodies against recombinant parts of the Ki-67 antigen (MIB 1 and MIB 3) detect proliferating cells in

microwave-processed formalin-fixed paraffin sections. *J Pathol* 1992;168: 357–363.

17. Galand P, Degraef C. Cyclin/PCNA immunostaining as an alternative to tritiated thymidine pulse labeling for marking S phase cells in paraffin sections from animal and human tissues. *Cell Tissue Kinet* 1989;22:383–392.

18. Scholzen T, Gerdes J. The Ki-67 protein: from the known and the unknown. *J Cell Physiol* 2000;182:311–322.

19. Rudolph P, Alm P, Heidebrecht HJ, et al. Immunologic proliferation marker Ki-S2 as prognostic indicator for lymph node-negative breast cancer. *J Natl Cancer Inst* 1999;91:271–278.

20. Howell WM. Selective staining of nucleolar organizer regions (NORs) In: Bush H, Tothblum L, eds. *The Cell Nucleus.* Academic Press, New York, 1982:89–142.

21. He W, Meyer JS, Scrivner DL, Koehm S, Hughes J. Assessment of proliferating cell nuclear antigen (PCNA) in breast cancer using anti-PCNA and 19A2: correlation with 5-bromo-2´-deoxyuridine or tritiated thymidine labeling and flow cytometric analysis. *Biotechn Histochem* 1994;69:203–212.

22. Silvestrini R and the SICCAB Group for Quality Control of Cell Kinetic Determination. Feasibility and reproducibility of the ³H-dT labeling index in breast cancer. *Cell Prolif* 1991;24:437–445.

23. Collan YU, Kuopio T, Baak JP, et al. Standardized mitotic counts in breast cancer. Evaluation of the method. *Pathol Res Pract* 1996;192:931–941.

24. Baldetorp B, Bendahl PO, Ferno M, et al. Reproducibility in DNA flow cytometric analysis of breast cancer: comparison of 12 laboratories' results for 67 sample homogenates. *Cytometry* 1995;22:115–127.

25. Mengel M, von Wasielewski R, Wiese B, Rudiger T, Muller-Hermelin HK, Kreipe H. Inter-laboratory and inter-observer reproducibility of immunohistochemical assessment of the Ki-67 labelling index in a large multicentre trial. *J Pathol* 2002;198:292–299.

26. Silvestrini R, Daidone MG, Del Bino G, et al. Prognostic significance of proliferative activity and ploidy in node-negative breast cancers. *Ann Oncol* 1993;4: 213–219.

27. Rudas M, Gnant MFX, Mittlböck M, et al. Thymidine labeling index and Ki-67 growth fraction in breast cancer: comparison and correlation with prognosis. *Breast Cancer Res Treat* 1994;32:165–175.

28. Gaglia P, Bernardi A, Venesio T, et al. Cell proliferation of breast cancer evaluated by anti-BrdU and anti-Ki-67 antibodies: its prognostic value on short-term recurrences. *Eur J Cancer* 1993;29A:1509–1513.

29. Thor AD, Liu S, Moore II DH, Edgerton SM. Comparison of mitotic index, in vitro bromodeoxyuridine labeling, and MIB-1 assays to quantitate proliferation in breast cancer. *J Clin Oncol* 1999;17:470–477.

30. Meyer JS, Province MA. S-phase fraction and nuclear size in long-term prognosis of patients with breast cancer. *Cancer* 1994;74:2287–2299.

31. Peirò G, Lerma E, Climent MA, Seguf MA, Alonso MC, Prat J. Prognostic value of S-phase fraction in lymph-node-negative breast cancer by image and flow cytometric analysis. *Mod Pathol* 1997;10:216–222.

32. Winchester DJ, Duda RB, August CZ, et al. The importance of DNA flow cytometry in node-negative breast cancer. *Arch Surg* 1990;125:886–889.

33. Simpson JF, Gray R, Dressler LG, et al. Prognostic value of histological grade and proliferative activity in axillary node-positive breast cancer: results from the East-

ern Cooperative Oncology Group Companion Study, EST 4189. *J Clin Oncol* 2000;18:2059–2069.

34. Hatschek T, Gröntoft O, Fagerberg G, et al. Cytometric and histopathological features of tumors detected in a randomized mammography screening program: correlation and relative prognostic influence. *Breast Cancer Res Treat* 1990;15: 149–160.

35. Eskelinen M, Lipponen P, Papinaho S, et al. DNA flow cytometry, nuclear morphometry, mitotic indices and steroid receptors as independent prognostic factors in female breast cancer. *Int J Cancer* 1992;51:555–561.

36. Lipponen P, Papinaho S, Eskelinen M, et al. DNA ploidy, S-phase fraction and mitotic indices as prognostic predictors of female breast cancer. *Anticancer Res* 1992;12:1533–1538.

37. Joensuu H, Toikkanen S, Klemi PJ. DNA index and S-phase fraction and their combination as prognostic factors in operable ductal breast carcinoma. *Cancer* 1990;66:331–340.

38. Keshgegian AA, Cnaan A. Proliferation markers in breast carcinoma. Mitotic figure count, S-phase fraction, proliferation cell nuclear antigen, Ki-67 and MIB-1. *Anat Pathol* 1995;104:42–49.

39. Dettmar P, Harbeck N, Thomssen C, et al. Prognostic impact of proliferation-associated factors MIB (Ki-67) and S-phase in node-negative breast cancer. *Br J Cancer* 1997;75:1525–1533.

40. Harbeck N, Dettmar P, Thomssen C, et al. Prognostic impact of tumor biological factors on survival in node-negative breast cancer. *Anticancer Res* 1998;18:2187–2197.

41. Railo M, Lundin J, Haglund C, von Smitten K, von Boguslawsky K, Nordling S. Ki-67, p53, Er-receptors, ploidy and S-phase as prognostic factors in T1 node negative breast cancer. *Acta Oncol* 1997;36:369–374.

42. Brown WR, Allred DC, Clark GM, Osborne CK, Hilsenbeck SG. Prognostic value of Ki-67 compared to S-phase fraction in axillary node-negative breast cancer. *Clin Cancer Res* 1996;2:585–592.

43. Wiesener B, Hauser-Kronberger CE, Zipperer E, Dietze O, Menzel C, Hacker GW. p34cdc2 in invasive breast cancer: relationship to DNA content, Ki67 index and c-erbB-2 expression. *Histopathology* 1998;33:522–530.

44. Gasparini G, Boracchi P, Verderio P, Bevilacqua P. Cell kinetics in human breast cancer: comparison between the prognostic value of the cytofluorimetric S-phase fraction and that of the antibodies to Ki-67 and PCNA antigens detected by immunocytochemistry. *Int J Cancer* 1994;57:822–829.

45. Jansen RL, Hupperets PS, Arends JW, et al. MIB-1 labelling index is an independent prognostic marker in primary breast cancer. *Br J Cancer* 1998;78:460–465.

46. Leong AC, Hanby AM, Potts HW, et al. Cell cycle proteins do not predict outcome in grade I infiltrating ductal carcinoma of the breast. *Int J Cancer* 2000;89:26–31.

47. Clahsen PC, van de Velde CY, Duval C, et al. The utility of mitotic index, oestrogen receptor and Ki-67 measurements in the creation of novel prognostic indices for node-negative breast cancer. *Eur J Surg Oncol* 1999;25:356–363.

48. Jacquemier JD, Penault-Llorca FM, Bertucci F, et al. Angiogenesis as a prognostic marker in breast carcinoma with conventional adjuvant chemotherapy: a multi-parametric and immunohistochemical analysis. *J Pathol* 1998;184:130–135.

49. Pietilainen T, Lipponen P, Aaltomaa S, Eskelinen M, Kosma VM, Syrjanen K. The important prognostic value of Ki-67 expression as determined by image analysis in breast cancer. *J Cancer Res Clin Oncol* 1996;122:687–692.

50. Hayes DF, Trock B, Harris AL. Assessing the clinical impact of prognostic factors: when is "statistically significant" clinically useful? *Breast Cancer Res Treat* 1998;52:305–319.

51. Medri L, Nanni O, Volpi A, et al. Tumor microvessel density and prognosis in node-negative breast cancer. *Int J Cancer* 2000;89:74–80.

52. Paradiso A, Mangia A, Barletta A, et al. Heterogeneity of intratumour proliferative activity in primary breast cancer: biological and clinical aspects. *Eur J Cancer* 1995;31A:911–916.

53. Silvestrini R, Daidone MG, Di Fronzo G, Morabito A, Valagussa P, Bonadonna G. Prognostic implication of labelling index versus estrogen receptors and tumor size in node-negative breast cancer. *Breast Cancer Res Treat* 1986;7:161–169.

54. Courdi A, Hery M, Dahan E, et al. Factors affecting relapse in node-negative breast cancer. A multivariate analysis including the labeling index. *Eur J Cancer Clin Oncol* 1989;25:351–356.

55. Silvestrini R, Daidone MG, Luisi A, et al. Biologic and clinico-pathological factors as indicators of specific relapse types in node-negative breast cancer. *J Clin Oncol* 1995;13:697–704.

56. Cooke TG, Stanton PD, Winstanley J, et al. Long term prognostic significance of thymidine labeling index in primary breast cancer. *Eur J Cancer* 1992;28:424–426.

57. Tubiana M, Pejovic MH, Koscielny S, Chavaudra N, Malaise E. Growth rate, kinetics of tumor cell proliferation and long-term outcome in human breast cancer. *Int J Cancer* 1989;44:17–22.

58. Aubele M, Auer G, Falkmer U, et al. Identification of a low-risk group of stage I breast cancer patients by cytometrically assessed DNA and nuclear texture parameters. *J Pathol* 1995;177:377–384.

59. Sigurdsson H, Baldetorp B, Borg A, et al. Indicators of prognosis in node-negative breast cancer. *N Engl J Med* 1990;322:1045–1049.

60. O'Reilly SM, Camplejohn RS, Barnes DM, Millis RR, Rubens RD, Richards MA. Node-negative breast cancer: prognostic subgroups defined by tumor size and flow cytometry. *J Clin Oncol* 1990;8:2040–2045.

61. Harbeck N, Dettmar P, Thomssen C, et al. Risk-group discrimination in node-negative breast cancer using invasion and proliferation markers: 6-year median follow-up. *Br J Cancer* 1999;80:419–426.

62. Merkel DE, Winchester DJ, Goldschmidt RA, August CZ, Wruck DM, Rademaker AW. DNA flow cytometry and pathological grading as prognostic guides in axillary lymph node-negative breast cancer. *Cancer* 1993;72:1926–1932.

63. Balslev I, Christensen IJ, Bruun Rasmussen B, et al. Flow cytometric DNA ploidy defines patients with poor prognosis in node-negative breast cancer. *Int J Cancer* 1994;56:16–25.

64. Stal O, Dufmats M, Hatscheck T, et al. S-phase is a prognostic factor in stage I breast carcinoma. *J Clin Oncol* 1993;11:1717–1722.

65. Isola J, Visakorpi T, Holli K, Kallioniemi OP. Association of overexpression of tumor suppressor protein p53 with rapid cell proliferation and poor prognosis in node-negative breast cancer patients. *J Natl Cancer Inst* 1992;84:1109–1114.

66. Bosari S, Lee AK, Tahan SR, et al. DNA flow cytometric analysis and prognosis of axillary lymph node-negative breast carcinoma. *Cancer* 1992;70:1943–1950.

67. Johnson H Jr, Masood S, Belluco C, et al. Prognostic factors in node-negative breast cancer. *Arch Surg* 1992;127:1386–1391.

68. Witzig TE, Ingle JN, Cha SS, et al. DNA ploidy and the percentage of cells in S-phase as prognostic factors for women with lymph node-negative breast cancer. *Cancer* 1994;74:1752–1761.

69. Joensuu H, Toikkanem S. Identification of subgroups with favorable prognosis in breast cancer. *Acta Oncol* 1992;31:293–301.

70. Klintenberg C, Stal O, Nordenskjold B, Wallgren A, Arvidsson S, Skoog L. Proliferative index, cytosol estrogen receptor and axillary node status as prognostic predictors in human mammary carcinoma. *Breast Cancer Res Treat* 1986;7: S99–106.

71. Arnerlov C, Emdin SO, Lundgren B, et al. Mammographic growth rate, DNA ploidy, and S-phase fraction analysis in breast carcinoma. *Cancer* 1992;70:1935–1942.

72. Stanton PD, Cooke TG, Oakes SJ, et al. Lack of prognostic significance of DNA ploidy and S phase fraction in breast cancer. *Br J Cancer* 1992;66:925–929.

73. Fisher B, Gunduz N, Costantino J, et al. DNA flow cytometric analysis of primary operable breast cancer. *Cancer* 1991;68:1465–1469.

74. Toikkanen S, Joensuu H, Klemi P. The prognostic significance of nuclear DNA content in invasive breast cancer—a study with long-term-follow-up. *Br J Cancer* 1989;60:693–700.

75. Laderkarl M, Jensen V. Quantitative histopathology in lymph node-negative breast cancer. Prognostic significance of mitotic count. *Virchows Arch* 1995;427:265–270.

76. Kato T, Kimura T, Miyakawa R, et al. Clinicopathological study associated with long-term survival in Japanese patients with node-negative breast cancer. *Br J Cancer* 2000;82:404–411.

77. Aaltomaa S, Lipponen P, Eskelinen M, et al. Prognostic scores combining clinical, histological and morphometric variables in assessment of the disease outcome in female breast cancer. *Int J Cancer* 1991;49:886–892.

78. Clayton F. Pathologic correlates of survival in 378 lymph node-negative infiltrating ductal breast carcinomas. Mitotic count is the best single predictor. *Cancer* 1991;68:1309–1317.

79. Iacopetta B, Grieu F, Powell B, Soong R, McCaul K, Seshadri R. Analysis of p53 gene mutation by polymerase chain reaction-single strand conformational polymorphism provides independent prognostic information in node-negative breast cancer. *Clin Cancer Res* 1998;4:1597–1602.

80. Pinder SE, Wencyk P, Sibbering DM, et al. Assessment of the new proliferation marker MIB1 in breast carcinoma using image analysis: associations with other prognostic factors and survival. *Br J Cancer* 1995;71:146–149.

81. Goldhirsch A, Glick JH, Gelber RD, Senn HJ. Meeting highlights: international consensus panel on the treatment of primary breast cancer. *J Natl Cancer Inst* 1998;90:1601–1608.

82. Hutchins L, Green S, Ravdin P, Lew D, Martino S, Abeloff M. CMF versus CAF with and without tamoxifen in high-risk node-negative breast cancer patients and a natural history follow-up study in low-risk node-negative patients: first results of Intergroup trial INT 0102. In: Proceedings of the 34th Annual Meeting of the American Association of Cancer Research, 1998; Abstr 2.

83. Sulkes A, Livingstone RB, Murphy WK. Tritiated thymidine labeling index and response in human breast cancer. *J Natl Cancer Inst* 1979;62:513–515.

84. Amadori D, Volpi A, Maltoni R, et al. Cell proliferation as a predictor of response to chemotherapy in metastatic breast cancer: a prospective study. *Breast Cancer Res Treat* 1997;43:7–14.

85. Remvikos Y, Beuzeboc P, Zajdela A, Voillemot N, Magdelenat H, Pouillart P. Correlation of pretreatment proliferative activity of breast cancer with the response to cytotoxic chemotherapy. *J Natl Cancer Inst* 1989;81:1383–1387.

86. Hietanen P, Blomqvist C, Wasenius VM, Niskanen E, Franssila K, Nordling S. Do DNA ploidy and S-phase fraction in primary tumor predict the response to chemotherapy in metastatic breast cancer? *Br J Cancer* 1995;71:1029–1032.

87. Stål O, Skoog L, Rutqvist LE, et al. S-phase fraction and survival benefit from adjuvant chemotherapy or radiotherapy of breast cancer. *Br J Cancer* 1994;70: 1258–1272.

88. O'Reilly SM, Camplejohn RS, Millis RR, Rubens RD, Richards MA. Proliferative activity, histological grade and benefit from adjuvant chemotherapy in node-positive breast cancer. *Eur J Cancer* 1990;26:1035–1038.

89. Dressler LG, Eudey L, Gray R, et al. Prognostic potential of DNA flow cytometry measurements in node-negative breast cancer patients: preliminary analysis of an Intergroup study (INT 0076). *J Natl Cancer Inst Monogr* 1992;11:167–172.

90. Zambetti M, Valagussa P, Bonadonna G. Adjuvant cyclophosphamide, methotrexate and fluorouracil in node-negative and estrogen receptor-negative breast cancer. Updated results. *Ann Oncol* 1996;7:481–485.

91. Silvestrini R, Luisi A, Zambetti M, et al. Cell proliferation and outcome following doxorubicin plus CMF regimens in node-positive breast cancer. *Int J Cancer* 2000;87:405–411.

92. Daidone MG, Veneroni S, Benini E, et al. Biological markers and changes induced in their profiles following primary chemotherapy: relevance for short- and long-term clinical outcome. In: Howell A and Dowsett M, eds. ESO Scientific Updates, Vol. 4. Elsevier, Philadelphia, 1999:53–72.

93. Baldini E, Giannessi PG, Collecchi P, et al. Effects of primary chemotherapy on proliferative activity, IGF-1R and bcl2 expression in locally advanced breast cancer (Meeting abstract). *Proc Annu Meet Am Soc Clin Oncol* 1996;15:Abstr 139.

94. Briffod M, Tubiana-Hulin M, Spyratos F, et al. Fine-needle cytopunctures for early prediction of tumor response to preoperative chemotherapy in 94 operable breast carcinomas. *Proc Annu Meet Am Soc Clin Oncol* 1995;14:Abstr 261.

95. Chevillard S, Pouillart P, Beldjord C, et al. Sequential assessment of multidrug resistance phenotype and measurement of S-phase fraction as predictive markers of breast cancer response to neoadjuvant chemotherapy. *Cancer* 1996;77:292–300.

96. Collecchi P, Baldini E, Giannessi P, et al. Primary chemotherapy in locally advanced breast cancer (LABC): effects on tumour proliferative activity, bcl-2 expression and the relationship between tumour regression and biological markers. *Eur J Cancer* 1998;34:1701–1704.

97. Daidone MG, Silvestrini R, Luisi A, et al. Changes in biological markers after primary chemotherapy for breast cancers. *Int J Cancer* 1995;61:301–305.

98. Pierga JY, Lainé-Bidron C, Beuzeboc P, De Crémoux P, Pouillart P, Magdelénat H. Plasminogen activator inhibitor-1 (PAI-1) is not related to response to neoadjuvant chemotherapy in breast cancer. *Br J Cancer* 1997;76:537–540.

99. Rozan S, Vincent-Salomon A, Zafrani B, et al. No significant predictive value of c-erbB-2 or p53 expression regarding sensitivity to primary chemotherapy or radiotherapy in breast cancer. *Int J Cancer (Pred Oncol)* 1998;79:27–33.

100. Remvikos Y, Mosseri V, Asselain B, et al. S-phase fractions of breast cancer predict overall and post-relapse survival. *Eur J Cancer* 1997;33:581–586.

101. Dowsett M. Preoperative models to evaluate endocrine strategies for breast cancer. *Clin Cancer Res* 2003;9:502S–510S.

102. Decensi A, Robertson C, Viale G, et al. A randomized trial of low dose tamoxifen on breast cancer proliferation and blood estrogenic biomarkers. *J Natl Cancer Inst* 2003;95:779–790.

103. Meyer JS, Lee J. Relationships of S-phase fraction of breast carcinoma in relapse to duration of remission, estrogen receptor content, therapeutic responsiveness, and duration of survival. *Cancer Res* 1980;40:1890–1896.

104. Amadori D, Bonaguri C, Nanni O, et al. Cell kinetics and hormonal features in relation to pathological stage in breast cancer. *Breast Cancer Res Treat* 1991;18:19–25.

105. Paradiso A, Tommasi S, Mangia A, Lorusso V, Simone G, De Lena M. Tumor proliferative activity, progesterone receptor status, estrogen receptor level, and clinical outcome of estrogen receptor-positive advanced breast cancer. *Cancer Res* 1990;50:2958–2962.

106. Daidone MG, Luisi A, Martelli G, et al. Biomarkers and outcome after tamoxifen treatment in node-positive breast cancers from elderly women. *Br J Cancer* 2000;82:270–277.

107. Wenger CR, Clark GM. S-phase fraction and breast cancer—a decade of experience. *Breast Cancer Res Treat* 1998;51:255–265.

108. Volpi A, De Paola F, Nanni O, et al. Prognostic significance of biologic markers in node-negative breast cancer patients: a prospective study. *Breast Cancer Res Treat* 2000;63:181–192.

109. Ferno M, Stal O, Baldetorp B, et al. Results of two or five years of adjuvant tamoxifen correlated to steroid receptor and S-phase levels. *Breast Cancer Res Treat* 2000;59:69–76.

110. Bryant J, Fisher B, Gunduz N, Costantino JP, Emir B. S-phase fraction combined with other patient and tumor characteristics for the prognosis of node-negative, estrogen-receptor-positive breast cancer. *Breast Cancer Res Treat* 1998;51:239–253.

111. Jones S, Clark G, Koleszar S, et al. Low proliferative rate of invasive node-negative breast cancer predicts for a favorable outcome: a prospective evaluation of 669 patients. *Clin Breast Cancer* 2001;1:310–314.

112. Jones S, Clark G, Koleszar S, et al. Adjuvant chemotherapy with doxorubicn and cyclophosphamide in women with rapidly proliferating node-negative breast cancer. *Clin Breast Cancer* 2002;3:147–152.

113. Baak JP, van Diest PJ, Benraadt T, et al. The Multi-Center Morphometric Mammary Carcinoma Project (MMMCP) in The Netherlands; value of morphometrically assessed proliferation and differentiation. *J Cell Biochem Suppl* 1993;17G: 220–225.

114. Sargent D, Allegra C. Issues in clinical trial design for tumor marker studies. *Semin Oncol* 2002;29:222–230.

115. D'hautcourt JL, Spyratos F, Chassevent A. Quality control study by the French Cytometry Association on flow cytometric DNA content and S-phase fraction (S%). Assoc Francaise de Cytometrie. *Cytometry* 1996;26:32–39.

116. Fitzgibbons PL, Page DL, Weaver D, et al. Prognostic factors in breast cancer. College of American Pathologists Consensus Statement 1999. *Arch Pathol Lab Med* 2000;124:966–978.

117. NIH-NCI consensus development conference. *J Natl Cancer Inst* 2001;93: 979–989.

7

Urokinase-Type Plasminogen Activator and PAI-1

Validated Prognostic Factors for Breast Cancer

Michael J. Duffy, PHD, FRCPATH, FACB

CONTENTS

SUMMARY

Urokinase plasminogen activator (uPA) is a serine protease caus-ally involved in tumor progression. In vivo, uPA can be inhibited by the serpin inhibitor plasminogen activator inhibitor-1 (PAI-1). How-ever, PAI-1 is a multifunctional protein that can also play a role in cell migration, cell adhesion, angiogenesis, and apoptosis. Multiple single-institutional studies have shown that both uPA and PAI-1 are potent

Cancer Drug Discovery and Development: Biomarkers in Breast Cancer:
Molecular Diagnostics for Predicting and Monitoring Therapeutic Effect
Edited by: G. Gasparini and D. F. Hayes © Humana Press Inc., Totowa, NJ

and independent prognostic factors in breast cancer. Recently, this prognostic impact was validated in both a prospective randomized trial and a pooled analysis. As well as being prognostic, high levels of uPA/PAI-1 have been shown to predict for relative resistance to hormone therapy in patients with advanced breast cancer but are associated with an enhanced response to adjuvant chemotherapy in early breast cancer. As uPA and PAI-1 are both prognostic and predictive, assay of these factors has the potential to result in the enhanced management of patients with breast cancer. Measurement of these analytes should thus be now considered for use in the routine management of patients with breast cancer.

Key Words: Urokinase plasminogen activator; PAI-1; cancer; tumor marker; Level 1 evidence.

1. INTRODUCTION

The prognosis of a cancer is dependent primarily on its ability to invade locally and form distant metastasis. The formation of metastasis consists of a series of sequential steps involving processing or remodeling of the extracellular matrix (ECM), local invasion, angiogenesis, intravasation, survival of malignant cells in the circulation, extravasation, and finally growth at a secondary site (for review, *see* ref. *1*). To complete the metastatic cascade, malignant cells must also evade apoptosis and resist entering a dormant state. A key molecule causally involved in a number of these steps is the trypsin-like protease, urokinase plasminogen activator (uPA).

2. UPA: STRUCTURE, FUNCTION, AND MODE OF ACTION

The *uPA* gene, which in humans is located on chromosome 10q (10q22) *(2)*, encodes a 53-kDa protein. The protein is initially synthesized as a catalytically inactive single-chain peptide. Conversion to the active form can be brought about, at least in vitro, by a number of proteases such as plasmin, cathepsin B, and cathepsin L (for review, *see* ref. *3*). The active form of uPA consists of a two-chain molecule in which the amino terminal A-chain is linked to the B-chain by a single disulfide bond. The A-chain (amino acids 1–158) contains an epidermal growth factor (EGF)-like domain (amino acids 1–49) while the B-chain possesses the catalytic site *(3)*.

As a protease, uPA catalyzes conversion of the zymogen plasminogen to the active plasmin. Unlike uPA, plasmin is a broad-spectrum protease capable of hydrolyzing several different substrates. First, it can promote processing of diverse ECM substrates such as fibrin, fibronectin, and laminin *(3)*. Second, it can activate the precursor forms of specific matrix metalloproteses (MMPs) such as MMP-3, MMP-9, MMP-12, and MMM-13 *(4)*. The formation of the active MMPs allows further processing of the ECM, especially interstitial and type IV collagen. Third, plasmin can activate or release a number of growth factors such as fibroblast growth factor-2 (FGF-2), vascular endothelial growth factor (VEGF), and transforming growth factor-β (TGF-β) *(5)*. These pleiotrophic peptides have the potential to enhance tumour progression by stimulating angiogenesis, cell proliferation and migration.

In vivo, uPA-catalyzed proteolysis occurs while the protease is attached to a membrane-anchored receptor known as uPA receptor (uPAR). uPAR, which is a member of the Ly-6 family of molecules, is a 55–60-kDa glycoprotein *(3)*. It consists of three homologous domains—D1, D2, and D3—and is bound to the cell membrane by a glycosyl phosphatidylinositol (GPI) moiety. The primary binding region in uPA for uPAR resides in the growth factor domain, especially in the sequence containing amino acids 19–32 *(6)*. At least four distinct regions in uPAR attach directly to uPA. These sequences included amino acids 13–20 and amino acids 74–84 of domain 1 as well as regions in the putative loop of both domains 2 and 3 *(7)*.

Binding of uPA to its receptor has two main consequences. First, it leads to both enhanced and focused proteolysis. Second, ligand receptor interaction results in signal transduction that involves activation of mitogen-activated protein kinase (MAPK), extracellular regulated kinases (ERK) 1 and 2, and other signaling pathways *(8)*. These signaling pathways allow uPA to stimulate cell migration and mitogenesis, modulate cell adhesion, and prevent cell dormancy *(3,8)*.

3. ENDOGENOUS INHIBITORS OF UPA

uPA activity can be blocked by at least three naturally occurring inhibitors—plasminogen activator inhibitor-1 and -2 (PAI-1, PAI-2) and maspin. These are relatively nonhomologous proteins belonging to the serpin family of protease inhibitors (for review, *see* refs. *9,10*). Of the three inhibitors, PAI-1 is thought to be the primary endogenous inhibitor of uPA. The mature form of PAI-1 consists of 381 amino acids and has an apparent molecular mass of 50 kDa. PAI-1 can exist in different conformations *(9)*. The active conformation spontaneously converts into a latent inactive form that in vitro can be reactivated by protein-denaturing agents such as urea and sodium dodecyl sulfate. Alternatively, following inhibition of target proteases, the active conformation is transformed into a center-cleaved inactive form.

As well as binding to uPA, PAI-1 can also associate with a number of different proteins including fibrin, heparin, α_1 acid glycoprotein, and the ECM protein vitronectin. Binding to both vitronectin and α_1 acid glycoprotein stabilizes PAI-1 *(10)*. Furthermore, the interaction with vitronectin allows PAI-1 to modulate cell adhesion by competing with integrins and uPAR for binding to vitronectin *(11)*. By associating with fibrin, PAI-1 can control dissolution of blood clots *(12)* while binding to heparin enhances the inhibitory capacity of PAI-1 against thrombin *(13)*.

Recently, PAI-1 was shown to prevent both spontaneous and drug-induced apoptosis in a number of different cell lines *(14)*. In contrast to a stable variant of PAI-1, apoptosis was not blocked by a latent form of PAI-1, a stable variant inactivated by specific neutralizing antibodies or a stable variant in complex with uPA. These findings suggest that the inhibitory action of PAI-1 is required for its antiapoptotic effects but that uPAR was not involved *(14)*.

Clearly, PAI-1 can be regarded as a multifunctional protein with several activities in additional to its well-established role in the inhibition of uPA catalytic action. The particular action(s) may depend on factors such as its concentration, its cellular or extracellular localization, and its conformations state.

3. UPA AND PAI-1 IN BREAST CANCER

Multiple studies have shown increased expression of both uPA and PAI-1 in breast carcinomas vis-a vis nonmalignant breast tissue *(15–17)*. The mechanism(s) responsible for this enhanced expression in malignancy are unknown. In breast cell lines in culture, various hormones and growth factors have been shown to modulate uPA expression (Table 1). Other factors known to alter uPA expression in vitro include methylation of gene promoter regions *(28)* and specific transcription factors, especially members of the ets family *(29)*.

Several groups have related levels of both uPA and PAI-1 in breast cancers to tumor and patient characteristics. In a pooled analysis of 8175 primary breast cancers, uPA levels were not significantly associated with patient age, menopausal status, or lymph node status. Levels however, were positively correlated with tumor grade, negatively with hormone receptors and higher in pT2 and pT4 tumors than pT1 and pT3 samples *(30)*.

In contrast to uPA, PAI-1 levels were significantly related to patient age, were higher in postmenopausal than premenopausal women, and higher in lymph node–positive than lymph node–negative cancers. As with uPA, PAI-1 levels were also positively correlated with tumor grade, negatively with hormone receptors and higher in pT2 and pT4 tumors than pT1 and pT3 samples *(30)*.

Conflicting reports have been published on the cell type(s) expressing uPA and PAI-1 in breast cancer. Early work using immunohistochemistry suggested that uPA protein was mostly located in malignant cells *(15,31,32)*. Christensen et al. *(33)*, however, reported that uPA immunostaining was present in a number of different cell types, being most intense in macrophages and mast cells but showing moderate intensity in epithelial, fibro-

Table 1
Factors Shown to Regulate Expression of uPA Levels
in Cell Lines Derived from Breast Cancers

Factor	Cell line/type	↑ or ↓	Authors (ref.)
Estradiol	ZR-75-1	↑	Mangel et al. 1988 (18)
Estradiol	T47-D	↑	Mangel et al. 1988 (18)
Estradiol	MCF-7	↑	Pourreau-Schneider et al. 1989 (19)
EGF	SP1	↑	Korczak et al. 1991 (20)
EGF	A3a	↑	Korczak et al. 1991 (20)
EGF	MDA-MB-231	↑	Long et al. 1996 (21)
Estradiol	S30	↓	Levenson et al. (22)
FGF-1	Breast fibroblast	↑	Sieuwerts et al. 1999 (23)
FGF-2	Breast fibroblast	↑	Sieuwerts et al. 1999 (23)
IGF-1	Breast fibroblast	↓	Sieuwerts et al. 1999 (23)
IGF1	MDA-MB-231	↑	Dunn et al, 2000 (24)
Progesterone	MDA-MB-231[a]	↓	Lin et al. 2001 (25)
Amphiregulin	MCF-7	↑	Silvy et al. 2001 (26)
Heregulin	LM3	↓	Puricelli et al. 2002 (27)

↑, Increase expression; ↓, decreased expression.
[a]Transfected with progesterone receptor.

blasts, and endothelial cells. Kennedy et al. (34) also found uPA staining in both stromal and epithelial cells, although the predominant location was in stromal cells. Finally, Nielsen et al. (35) identified uPA immunoreactivity in myofibroblasts and macrophages in all 25 breast cancers examined. In 12 cases, endothelial cell staining was also seen. Only three cases exhibited cancer cell positivity and in each, only a small subpopulation of cells stained. These findings of Nielsen et al. (35) are consistent with previous in situ hybridization studies from the same group showing that mRNA for uPA was located almost exclusively in fibroblasts (36). The finding of uPA in stromal cells suggests that these cells synergize with cancer cells to promote metastasis.

Disagreement also exists on the location of PAI-1 in breast cancer. For example, Reilly et al. (16) detected PAI-1 protein in both endothelial and cancer cells. Similarly, Christensen et al. (33) found PAI-1 in endothelial and cancer cells, but also located it in stromal cells. In contrast, Jankum et al. (32) reported that PAI-1 was present mostly in malignant cells.

Possible reasons for these conflicting results on the location of uPA and PAI-1 in breast carcinomas include use of different methods of processing tissue (fresh vs formalin-fixed and paraffin-embedded tissue), different pretreatments of tissue, use of antibodies of different specificities, and possible failure in some studies to rigorously exclude nonspecific staining.

Table 2
Evidence Implicating uPA in Invasion and Metastasis

Positive correlations are found between levels of uPA in both cell lines and animal tumors and metastatic potential.

Inhibition of uPA activity (e.g., by inhibitors or antibodies) or uPA expression (e.g., by antisense oligonucleotides) suppresses metastasis in model systems.

Transfection of cell lines with cDNA for uPA enhances the metastatic phenotype of recipient cells.

Prevention of uPA from binding to uPAR decreases metastasis in model systems.

Tumors in uPA deficient mice undergo less progression than in control wild-type mice.

Data summarized from refs. *37,38.*

4. UPA AS A PROGNOSTIC MARKER IN BREAST CANCER

Studies with multiple model systems have shown that uPA is causally involved in metastasis *(37,38)* (Table 2). Originally, uPA was thought to play a role in these processes simplify by degrading the ECM, thus permitting local invasion and ultimately the formation of distant metastasis. The degradation of the ECM is now thought to be highly specific with limited substrate cleavage, that is, protein processing. However, in addition to protein processing, it is now clear that uPA has other actions allowing it mediate cancer cell dissemination *(3).* These activities include its ability to enhance angiogenesis, stimulate both cell proliferation and migration, and inhibit dormancy (for review, *see* refs. *3,8*).

Because the formation of distant metastasis is the principal cause of mortality in patients with cancer and uPA is a critical mediator of the process, the latter should be a good candidate for investigation as a prognostic marker *(39).* Furthermore, the positive correlations found between uPA levels and metastatic ability in both cell lines and animal cancers *(37)* might also be expected to apply to human cancers.

Duffy et al. *(40,41)* first reported that breast cancer patients with high levels of uPA activity in their primary cancer exhibited both a shorter disease-free interval and shorter overall survival than those with low activity levels. These preliminary results have now been confirmed by approx 20 independent groups, worldwide (Tables 3 and 4). These single-center studies showed that the prognostic value of uPA was:

- Independent of that provided by the traditional prognostic factors for this disease such as tumor size, tumor grade, or axillary node status.
- Stronger than that of other biological factors such as estrogen receptor, progesterone receptor, *HER2*, EGFR, p53, and Nottingham Index *(60,62,63).*

Table 3
Different Groups Showing a Prognostic Value for uPA in Breast Cancer

Authors (ref.)	No.	R or P study	Comments
Duffy et al. 1988 (40)	52	R	
Janicke et al. 1989 (42)	104	P	
Spyratos et al. 1992 (43)	319	R	
Cook et al. 1992 (44)	48	NS	
Foekens et al. 1992 (45)	671	R	
Grondahl-Hansen et al. 1993 (46)	119	NS	Only premenopausal patients
Bouchet et al. 1994 (47)	316	NS	
Sumiyoshi et al. 1995 (48)	80	NS	
Ferno et al. 1997 (49)	688	NS	
Shiba et al. 1997 (50)	226	P	
Umeda et al. 1997 (51)	73	R	
Koop et al. 1998 (52)	429	R	
Peyrat et al. 1998 (53)	634	NS	
Kim et al. 1998 (54)	130	P	
Tetu et al. 1998 (55)	575	R	
Eppenberger et al. 1998 (56)	305	NS	Only node-negative patients
Kute et al. 1998 (57)	116	NS	Only node-negative patients
Broet et al. 1999 (58)	1245	R	
Konecny et al. 2001 (59)	587	R	
Malmstrom et al. 2001 (60)	237	P	Only premenopausal node-negative patients
Meo et al. 2002 (61)	196	NS	Only node-negative patients

Many of the above-listed groups have published follow-up studies with greater numbers of patients and longer follow-up. Only the original study is cited above. P, Prospective study; R, Retrospective study; NS, not stated.

- Independent of the cutoff point used for separating patients with low and high levels of uPA, that is, whether the median, tertile, or quartile value was used (64). uPA was also predictive when used as continuous variable (64).
- Prognostic in axillary node-negative patients (Table 4), including node-negative patients who did not receive systemic adjuvant therapy (65).

Table 4
Different Groups Showing a Prognostic Value for uPA
in Axillary Node-Negative Breast Cancer Patients

Authors (ref.)	No.	R or P study
Janicke et al. 1990 (15)	50	P
Foekens et al. 1992 (45)	272	R
Duffy et al. 1994 (66)	75	R
Ferno et al. 1997 (49)	265	NS
Peyrat et al. 1998 (53)	634	NS
Kim et al. 1998 (54)	130	P
Eppenberger et al. 1998 (56)	305	NS
Malmstrom et al. 2001 (60)	237	P
Meo et al. 2002 (61)	196	NS

Some of the above-listed groups have published follow-up studies with greater numbers of patients and longer follow-up. Only the original study is cited above. P, Prospective study; R, retrospective study; NS, not stated.

5. PAI-1 AS A PROGNOSTIC MARKER IN BREAST CANCERS

Intuitively, it might be expected that high levels of an inhibitor of uPA in cancer tissue would correlate with a low probability of metastasis and thus with good outcome. Paradoxically, however, high levels of PAI-1 in breast cancer are also strongly and independently associated with poor outcome (Tables 5 and 6). Furthermore, the prognostic information available from PAI-1 is additional to that of uPA. Thus, the combined measurement of both proteins results in enhanced prognostic data over that available from either factor alone (65).

Why high levels of PAI-1 correlate with adverse prognosis is not clear. Possible explanations include:

- A critical concentration of PAI-1 is necessary to prevent excessive degradation of the ECM by uPA during cancer invasion. Excessive breakdown of the matrix could leave insufficient substrate for migration of cancer cells.
- PAI-1 is necessary for angiogenesis (72,73), which in turn is essential for malignant cells to gain access to the circulation and for progression at both primary and metastatic sites.
- PAI-1 can modulate both cell adhesion and migration (11) and as result may accelerate the metastatic process.
- PAI-1 can inhibit apoptosis (14). For malignant cells to complete the metastatic process, they must survive and evade apoptosis. Resistance

Table 5
Different Groups Showing a Prognostic Value for PAI-1 in Breast Cancer

Authors (ref.)	No.	R or P study	Comments
Janicke et al. 1991 (67)	102	P	
Grondahl-Hansen et al. 1993 (46)	72	NS	Only postmenopausal patients
Bouchet et al. 1994 (47)	314	NS	
Foekens et al. 1994 (68)	657		
Sumiyoshi et al. 1995 (48)	80	NS	
Duggan et al. 1997 (69)	148	R	
Eppenberger et al. 1998 (56)	305	NS	Only node-negative patients
Kute et al. 1998 (57)	135	NS	Only node-negative patients
Knoop et al. 1988 (52)	429	R	
Kim et al. 1988 (54)	130	P	Only node-negative patients
Billgren et al. 2000 (70)	1851	NS	
Konecny et al. 2001 (59)	587	R	
Meo et al. 2002 (61)	196	NS	Only node-negative patients

Many of the above-listed groups have published follow-up studies with greater numbers of patients and longer follow-up. Only the original study is cited above. P, Prospective study; R, retrospective study; NS, not stated.

Table 6
Different Groups Showing a Prognostic Value for PAI-1 in Axillary Node-Negative Breast Cancer Patients

Authors (ref.)	No.	R or P study
Janicke et al. 1993 (71)	101	P
Foekens et al. 1994 (68)	272	R
Bouchet et al. 1994 (47)	146	NS
Kim et al. 1998 (54)	130	P
Meo et al. 2002 (61)	96	NS

Many of the above-listed groups have published follow-up studies with greater numbers of patients and longer follow-up. Only the original study is cited above. P, Prospective study; R, retrospective study; NS, not stated.

to apoptosis might therefore be expected to increase the likelihood of forming a distant metastasis. Evasion of apoptosis could also confer resistance to specific therapies (74), which in turn could result in a more adverse outcome.

6. TRANSFER OF UPA AND PAI-1 TO THE CLINIC

Prior to entering routine clinical use, new markers should be rigorously evaluated with respect to both analytical and clinical performance. Several research and commercially available enzyme-linked immunosorbent assay (ELISA) kits have now been described for the measurement of uPA and PAI-1 concentration (75). A number of these have been subjected to detailed evaluation with the following conclusions (75,76).

- All the assays tested that were designed for the measurement of uPA in tissue extracts had adequate sensitivity for application in breast cancer extracts.
- Within assay precision for all the assays investigated was satisfactory.
- All assays investigated displayed an acceptable degree of parallelism following dilution of tissue extracts.
- Although the absolute level of uPA measured varied with the different methods, in general, good correlations were found between the different assays.
- Higher yields of uPA were obtained with a Triton X-100–containing buffer than with a detergent-free buffers.
- Some uPA and PAI-1 kits (American Diagnostica, Stamford, CT) were subsequently investigated in external quality assurance studies and shown to perform in a satisfactory manner (76). For example, in a German multicenter clinical trial in which six different laboratories all used these kits, the interlaboratory coefficient of variation (CV) varied between 6.2 and 8.2 for uPA and between 13.2 and 16.6 for PAI-1. Expressing results as nanograms per milligram of protein however, led to a substantial increase in the interlaboratory variation, that is, CVs of 10.8–20.4 for uPA and 15.5–23.6 for PAI-1.

Clinical validation of a new marker, requires validation in either a large randomized prospective trial in which evaluation of the marker is the primary objective of the study or a meta-analysis/pooled analysis of small-scale prospective or retrospective trials (77). Recently, the prognostic impact of uPA/PAI-1 in breast cancer patients was confirmed using both these types of Level 1 Evidence studies (30,78).

The prospective randomized investigation was a multicenter study containing almost 600 patients carried out in Germany (78). In this trial, node-negative breast cancer patients with low levels of uPA and PAI-1 were monitored but received no systemic adjuvant chemotherapy. On the other hand, patients with high levels of the protease and/or its inhibitor were randomized to receive adjuvant CMF treatment or to be observed. Following an interim analysis after 32 mo of follow-up, patients with low levels of both proteins had an estimated 3-yr recurrence rate of 6.7% whereas those with high concentrations of the protease and/or its inhibitor had a recurrence rate of 14.7% ($p = 0.006$).

Multivariate analysis showed that the prognostic impact of uPA/PAI-1 was independent of tumor grade, tumor size, surgical treatment of the primary cancer, and steroid receptor status. Although tumor grade was a stronger predictor of outcome than uPA/PAI-1, if grade was used to classify risk, only 10% of the node-negative patients would be regarded as having a low risk of recurrence, that is, those with grade 1 disease. In contrast, based on uPA/PAI-1, 56% would be considered at low risk of developing disease recurrence (78).

The second type of Level 1 Evidence study to have validated the prognostic significance of uPA and PAI-1 in breast cancer involved a pooled analysis of 18 different data sets containing a total of 8377 patients (30). Of these 18 studies, 11 were previously published while seven contained unpublished data. Raw data from all the 18 studies were used in the statistical analysis. Following a median follow-up of 79 mo, both uPA and PAI-1 were found to independent prognostic factors. Although less potent than axillary nodal status, both uPA and PAI-1 were stronger predictors of outcome than tumor size, tumor grade, hormone receptor status, or patient age. In the node-negative patients, uPA and PAI-1 were the strongest predictors of both disease-free interval and overall survival. Significantly, both uPA and PAI-1 were also prognostic in the subgroup of node-negative patients who did not receive systemic adjuvant therapy (30).

To the author's knowledge, uPA and PAI-1 are the first biological factors for which prognostic value was validated using either a prospective randomized trial or a pooled analysis. The results of the two studies clearly show that node-negative breast cancer patients have a low risk of disease relapse and consequently could avoid the side effects and financial costs of adjuvant chemotherapy. Assay of uPA and PAI-1 should therefore be now considered for routinely determining prognosis in axillary node-negative breast cancer patients.

7. PREDICTIVE VALUE OF UPA AND PAI-1

According to Clark (79), prognostic factors are necessary not only for predicting patient outcome but also to indicate which patients are likely to benefit from specific therapies. In a pilot study containing 235 patients with recurrent breast cancer, Foekens et al. (80) reported that women with uPA-negative tumors exhibited a better response to tamoxifen therapy than those with uPA-positive tumors. This predictive impact of uPA appeared to be independent of steroid receptor status. When patients were stratified by receptor concentration, however, the relationship between high levels of uPA and resistance to tamoxifen was observed only in the subgroup with intermediate levels of estrogen receptors (ERs) and progesterone receptors (PgRs) (i.e., >10 fmol/mg of protein for both receptors with at least 1 being not more than 75 fmol/mg). High levels of PAI-1 were also associated with reduced benefit from tamoxifen but the predictive effect of the inhibitor was less pronounced than that of the protease *(80)*.

While high levels of uPA/PAI-1 have been reported to predict for resistance to hormone therapy in patients with advanced breast cancer, recent data suggest that elevated levels of these proteins correlate with an enhanced response to adjuvant chemotherapy. In the German prospective randomized trial referred to in the preceding *(78)*, administration of chemotherapy to patients with high levels of uPA and/or PAI-1 reduced the relative risk of recurrence by approx 44% (relative risk = 0.56, p, NS). However, if patients who violated the study protocol were excluded from the analysis, the benefit of CMF became more pronounced ($p = 0.016$, relative risk = 0.27). This finding suggested that lymph node–negative breast cancer patients with high levels of uPA/PAI-1 benefit from adjuvant CMF.

Consistent with these findings, Harbeck et al. *(65)*, in a single-institution prospective study ($n = 761$), found that while uPA/PAI-1 predicted outcome in patients who did not receive systematic adjuvant therapy, the prognostic impact was lost in patients treated with either adjuvant chemotherapy or adjuvant hormone therapy. Again, this study suggested a benefit from adjuvant treatment in patients with high uPA/PAI-1 levels. More direct evidence of a predictive role for uPA/PAI-1 has come from a large two-center study ($n = 3424$), which showed that breast cancer patients with high levels of these proteins benefited more strongly from adjuvant chemotherapy than those with low levels *(81)*.

These preliminary findings suggest that in advanced breast cancer, high levels of uPA and PAI-1 predict for resistance to tamoxifen therapy. On the other hand, in early breast cancer, patient with high levels appear to derive an enhanced benefit from CMF-based chemotherapy. These promising results should now be confirmed in high-powered prospective randomized trials.

8. CONCLUSIONS

uPA and PAI-1 are among the few tumor markers whose clinical value has been validated using Level 1 Evidence data, and to the author's knowledge are the only markers to have been validated using two different types of such studies. Because assays for these markers have also been shown to perform satisfactorily in EQA trials, both should now be ready for routine clinical use. In the clinic, the immediate application of these markers is likely to be in selecting node-negative breast cancer patients who do not need or are unlikely to benefit from adjuvant chemotherapy, that is, patients with low levels of uPA and/or PAI-1.

In addition to being prognostic, uPA and PAI-1 have been reported to predict for likely response or resistance to therapy in patients with breast cancer. As mentioned earlier, emerging data suggests that high levels of these proteins are associated with resistance to hormone therapy in advanced breast cancer but correlate with enhanced benefit from adjuvant CMF therapy in early breast cancer.

As well as being able to predict for likely response to specific therapies, uPA can also be a direct target for new forms of anticancer therapies. Data from model systems show that either inhibition of uPA activity or blocking uPA from binding to its receptor reduces tumor growth and metastasis *(82)*. Recently, a serine protease inhibitor known as WX-UK1 (Wilex AG, Munich, Germany) and which is directed against uPA and plasmin, entered clinical trials. It might be expected that the tumors most likely to respond to uPA-directed therapy will be those expressing high levels of uPA. Thus, like ER and HER-2, uPA/PAI-1 has the potential to be both prognostic and predictive as well as a target for therapy.

In conclusion, clearly a knowledge of uPA and PAI-1 levels have the potential to result in the enhanced management of patients with breast cancer. Assay of these factors is therefore likely to be introduced into routine clinical practice in the near future. A limiting factor of the traditional assays for uPA and PAI-1 was the requirement for at least 100 mg of tumor tissue. Recently, however, a microassay for the detection of uPA/PAI-1 has been described *(83)*. This assay utilizes one or two breast tissue core biopsies or 5–10 of 90-μM-thick cryosections of a frozen tumor block. The availability of this new assay should allow the determination of uPA and PAI-1 in small breast cancers.

ACKNOWLEDGMENT

Our research was supported by grants from both the Irish Cancer Society and the Health Research Board of Ireland.

REFERENCES

1. Chambers AF, Groom AC, MacDonald IC. Dissemination and growth of cancer cells in metastatic sites. *Nat Rev Cancer* 2002;2:563–572.
2. Helenius, MA Saramaki, OR, Linja MJ, Tammela, TLJ, Visakorpi T. Amplification of urokinase gene in prostate cancer. *Cancer Res* 2001;61: 5340–5344.
3. Andreasen PA, Kjoller L, Christensen L, Duffy MJ. The urokinase-type plasminogen activator system in cancer metastasis: a review. *Int J Cancer* 1997;72:1–22.

4. Carmeliet P, Moons L, Lijnen R, et al. Urokinase-generated plasmin activates matrix metalloproteinase during aneurysm formation. *Nat Genet* 1997;17: 439–444.

5. Rifkin DB. Cross-talk among proteases and matrix in the control of growth factor action. *Fibrinol Proteol* 1997;11:3–9.

6. Magdolen V, Rettenberger P, Koppitz M, Goretzki L, Kessler H, Weidle U. Systematic mutational analysis of the receptor-binding region of the human urokinase-type plasminogen activator. *Eur J Biochem* 1996;237:743–751.

7. Liang OD, Chavakis T, Kanse SM, Preissner KT. Ligand binding region in the receptor for urokinase-type plasminogen activator. *J Biol Chem* 2001;276,28946–28953.

8. Ossowski L, Aguirre JA. Urokinase receptor and integrin partnership: coordination of signalling for cell adhesion, migration and growth. *Curr Opin Cell Biol* 2000;12:613–620.

9. Andreasen PA, Egelund R, Petersen HH. The plasminogen activation system in tumor growth, invasion and metastasis. *Cell Mol Life Sci* 2000;57:25–40.

10. Schroeck F, de Prada NA, Sperl S, et al. Interaction of plasminogen activator inhibitor type-1 (PAI-1) with vitronectin (Vn): mapping the binding sites on PAI-1 and Vn. *Biol Chem* 2002;383:1143–1149.

11. Loskutoff, DJ, Curriden SA, Hu G, Deng G. Regulation of cell adhesion by PAI-1, Review article. *APMIS* 1999;107:54–61.

12. Hoylaerts M, Rijken DC, Lijnen HR, Collen D. Kinetics of the activation of plasminogen by human tissue plasminogen activator. Role of fibrin. *J Biol Chem* 1982;257:2912–2919.

13. Ehrlich HJ, Keijer J, Preissner KT, et al. Functional interaction of PAI-1 and heparin. *Biochemistry* 1991;30:1021–1028.

14. Kwaan HC, Wang J, Svoboda K, Declerck PJ. Plasminogen activator inhibitor 1 may promote tumor growth through inhibition of apoptosis. *Br J Cancer* 2000;82:1702–1708.

15. Janicke F, Schmitt M, Hafter A. Urokinase-type plasminogen activator (upA) antigen is a predictor of early relapse in breast cancer. *Fibrinolysis* 1990;4:6978.

16. Reilly D, Christensen L, Duch M, et al. Type-1 plasminogen activator inhibitor in human breast carcinomas. *Int J Cancer* 1992;50:208–214.

17. Duggan C, Maguire T, McDermott E, et al. Urokinase plasminogen activator and urokinase plasminogen activator receptor in breast cancer. *Int J Cancer* 1995;61: 597–600.

18. Mangel WF, Toledo DL, Nardulli AM, et al. Plasminogen activator in human breast cancer cell lines: hormonal regulation and properties. *J Steroid Biochem* 1988;30:79–88.

19. Pourreau-Schneider N, Delori P, Boutiere B, et al. Modulation of plasminogen activator systems by matrix components in 2 breast cancer cell lines: MCF-7 and MDA-MB-231. *J Natl Cancer Inst* 1989;81:259–266.

20. Korczak B, Kerbel RS, Dennis JW. Autocrine and paracrine regulation of tissue inhibitor of metalloproteinases, transin and urokinase gene expression in metastatic and nonmetastatic mammary carcinoma cells. *Cell Growth Differ* 1991;2: 335–341.

21. Long BJ, Rose DP. Invasive capacity and regulation of urokinase-type plasminogen activator in estrogen receptor (ER)-negative MDA-MB-231 human breast cancer cells and a transfection (S30) stably expressing ER. *Cancer Lett* 1996;99:209–215.

22. Levenson AS, Kwaan HC, Svoboda KM, et al. Oestradiol regulation of the components of the plasminogen-plasmin system in MDA-MB-231 human breast cancer cells stably expressing the oestrogen receptor. *Br J Cancer* 1998;78:88–95.

23. Sieuwerts AM, Klijn JG, Henzen-Logmans SC, et al. Cytokine-regulated urokinase-type-plasminogen activator (uPA) production by human breast fibroblasts in vitro. *Breast Cancer Res Treat* 1999;55:9–20.

24. Dunn SE, Torres JV, Nihei N, Barrett JC. The insulin-like growth factor-1 elevates urokinase-type plasminogen activator in human breast cancer cells: a new avenue for breast cancer therapy. *Mol Carcinogen* 2000;27:10–17.

25. Lin VC, Eng AS, Hen NE, et al. Effect of progesterone on the invasive properties and tumor growth of progesterone receptor-transfected breast cancer cells MDA-MB-231. *Clin Cancer Res* 2001;7:2880–2886.

26. Silvy M, Giusti C, Martin PM, Berthois Y. Differential regulation of cell proliferation by epidermal growth and amphiregulin in tumoral versus normal breast epithelial cells. *Br J Cancer* 2001;84:936–945.

27. Puricelli L, Proiettii CJ, Labriola L, et al. Heregulin inhibits proliferation via ERKs and phosphatidylinositol 3-kinase activation but regulates urokinase plasminogen activator independently of these pathways in metastatic mammary tumor cells. *Int J Cancer* 2002;100:642–653.

28. Guo Y, Pakneshan P, Gladu J, et al. Regulation of DNA methylation in human breast cancer: effect on the urokinase-type plasminogen activator gene production and tumor invasion. *J Biol Chem* 2002;277:41571–41579.

29. Watabe, T, Yoshida K, Shindoh M, et al. The ets-1 and ets-2 transcription factors activate the promoters for invasion-associated urokinase and collagenase genes in response to epidermal growth factor. *Int J Cancer* 1998;77:128–137.

30. Look M P, van Putten WLJ, Duffy MJ, et al. Pooled analysis of prognostic impact of tumor biological factors uPA and PAI-1 in 8377 breast cancer patients. *J Natl Cancer Inst* 2002;94:116–128.

31. Del Vecchio S, Stoppelli MP, Carriero MV, et al. Human urokinase receptor concentration in malignant and benign breast tumors by in vitro quantitative autoradiography: comparison with urokinase levels. *Cancer Res* 1993;53:3198–3206.

32. Jankum J, Merrick HW, Goldblatt PJ. Expression and localisation of elements of the plasminogen activation system in benign breast disease and breast cancer. *J Cell Biochem* 1993;53:135–144.

33. Christensen L, Simonsen ACW, Heegaard CW, et al. Immunohistochemical localisation of urokinase-type plasminogen activator, type-1 plasminogen activator inhibitor, urokinase receptor and alpha-2-macroglobulin receptor in human breast carcinomas. *Int J Cancer* 1996;66:441–452.

34. Kennedy S, Duffy MJ, Duggan C, et al. Semi-quantitation of plasminogen activator and its receptor in breast carcinomas by immunocytochemistry. *Br J Cancer* 1998;77:1638–1641.

35. Nielsen BS, Sehested M, Duun S, et al. Urokinase plasminogen activator is localized in stromal cells in ductal breast cancer. *Lab Invest* 2001;81:1485–1501.

36. Nielsen BS, Sehested M, Timshel S, et al. Messenger mRNA for urokinase plasminogen activator (uPA) is expressed in myofibroblasts adjacent to cancer cells in human breast cancer. *Lab Invest* 1996;74:168–177.

37. Duffy MJ. Then role of proteolytic enzymes in cancer invasion and metastasis. *Clin Exp Med* 1992;10:145–155.

38. Duffy MJ. Urokinase-type plasminogen activator: a potent marker of metastatic potential in human cancer. *Biochem Soc Trans* 2002;30:207–210.
39. Duffy MJ: Do proteases play a role in cancer invasion and metastasis? *Eur J Cancer Clin Oncol* 1987;23:583–589.
40. Duffy MJ, O'Grady P, Devaney D, O'Siorain L, Fennelly JJ, Lijnen RJ. Urokinase-plasminogen activator, a marker for aggressive breast cancer. Preliminary report. *Cancer* 1988;62:531–533.
41. Duffy MJ, Reilly D, O'Sullivan C, O'Higgins N, Fennelly JJ. Urokinase plasminogen activator and prognosis in breast cancer. *Lancet* 1990;335:109.
42. Janicke F, Schmitt M, Ulm K, Gossner W, Graeff H. Urokinase-type plasminogen activator antigen and early relapse in breast cancer. *Lancet* 1989;ii:1049.
43. Spryatos F, Martin P-M, Hacene K, et al. Multiparametric prognostic evaluation of biological factors in primary breast cancer. *J Natl Cancer Inst* 1992;84:1266–1272.
44. Cook D, Mahmoud-Alexandroni N, Gaffney PJ, et al. Plasminogen activators are powerful indicators of prognosis in breast cancer. *Br J Surg* 1991;78:1495.
45. Foekens J, Schmitt M, Pache L, et al. Prognostic value of urokinase-type plasminogen activator in 671 primary breast cancer patients. *Cancer Res* 1992;52:6101–6105.
46. Grondahl-Hansen J, Christensen IJ, Rosenquist C, et al. High levels of urokinase-type plasminogen activator and its inhibitor PAI-1 in cytosolic extracts of breast carcinoma are associated with poor prognosis. *Cancer Res* 1993;53:2513–2521.
47. Bouchet C, Spyratos F, Martin P-M, et al. Prognostic role of urokinase-type plasminogen activator (uPA) and plasminogen activator inhibitors PAI-1 and PAI-2 in breast carcinomas. *Br J Cancer* 1994;69:398–405.
48. Sumiyoshi K, Urano T, Takada Y, Takada A. PAI-1 and PAI-2 levels as predictors in staging malignancy in breast cancer. In: Glas-Greenwalt P, ed. *Fibrinolysis in Disease*, CRC Press, Boca Raton, FL, 1995:26–30.
49. Ferno M, Bendahl PO, Borg A, et al. Urokinase plasminogen activator, a strong independent prognostic factor in breast cancer: analysed in steroid receptor cytosols with a luminometric immunoassay. *Eur J Cancer* 1996;32A:793–801.
50. Shiba E, Kim SJ, Taguchi T, et al. A prospective study on the prognostic significance of urokinase-type plasminogen activator levels in breast cancer tissue. *J Cancer Res Clin Oncol* 1997;123:555–559.
51. Umeda T, Eguchi Y, Okino K, et al. Cellular localisation of urokinase-type plasminogen activator, its inhibitors and their mRNA in breast cancer tissue. *J Pathol* 1997; 183:388–397.
52. Knoop A, Andreasen PA, Anderson JA, et al. Prognostic significance of urokinase-type plasminogen activator and plasminogen activator inhibitor-1 in primary breast cancer. *Br J Cancer* 1998;77:932–940.
53. Peyrat J-P, Vanlemmens L, Fournier J, et al. Prognostic value of p53 and urokinase-type plasminogen activator in node-negative human breast cancer. *Clin Cancer Res* 1998;4:189–196.
54. Kim SJ, Shiba E, Kobayashi T, et al. Prognostic impact of urokinase-type plasminogen activator (uPA), PA inhibitor type-1 and tissue-type PA antigen levels in node-negative breast cancer: a prospective study on multicenter basis. *Clin Cancer Res* 1998;4:177–182.
55. Tetu B, Brisson J, Lapointe H. Prognostic significance of stromelysin 3, gelatinase A and urokinase expression in breast cancer. *Hum Pathol* 1998;29:979–985.

56. Eppenberger U, Kueng W, Schlaeppi J-M, et al. Markers of tumor angiogenesis and proteolysis independently define high- and low-risk subsets of node-negative breast cancer patients. *J Clin Oncol* 1998;16:3129–3136.

57. Kute TE, Grondahl-Hansen J, Shao S-M, et al. Low cathepsin D and low plasminogen activator type 1 inhibitor in tumor cytosols define a group of node-negative breast cancer patients with low risk of recurrence. *Breast Cancer Res Treat* 1998;47:9–16.

58. Broet P, Spyratos F, Romain S, et al. Prognostic value of uPA and p53 accumulation measured by quantitative biochemical assays in 1245 primary breast cancer patients: a multicenter study. *Br J Cancer* 1999;80:536–545.

59. Konecny G, Untch M, Arboleda J, et al. HER-2 and urokinase-type plasminogen activator and its inhibitor in breast cancer. *Clin Cancer Res* 2001;7:2448–2457.

60. Malmstrom P, Bendahl P-O, Boiesen P, et al. S-phase fraction are urokinase plasminogen activator are better markers for distant recurrences that Nottingham Prognostic Index and histological grade in a prospective study of premenopausal lymph node-negative breast cancer. *J Clin Oncol* 2001;19:2010–2019.

61. Meo S, Dittadi R, Sweep CGJ, et al. Prognostic value of VEGF, uPA, PAI-1 in 196 node negative breast cancers. *Int J Biol Markers* 2002;17:S44.

62. Harbeck N, Dettmar C, Thomssen C, et al. Risk-group discrimination in node-negative breast cancer using invasion and proliferation markers: 6-year median follow-up. *Br J Cancer* 1999;80:419–426.

63. Le Goff JM, Lavayssiere L, Rouesse J, Spyratos F. Nonlinear discriminant analysis and prognostic factor classification in node-negative primary breast cancer using probabilistic neural networks. *Anticancer Res* 2000;20:2213–2218.

64. Duffy MJ, Duggan C, Maguire T, et al. Urokinase plasminogen activator as a predictor of aggressive disease in breast cancer. *Enzyme Protein* 1996;49:85–93.

65. Harbeck N, Kates RE, Schmitt M. Clinical relevance of invasion factors urokinase-type plasminogen activator and plasminogen activator inhibitor type 1 for individualized therapy in primary breast cancer is greatest when used in combination. *J Clin Oncol* 2002;20:1000–1007.

66. Duffy MJ, Reilly D, McDermott E, et al. Urokinase plasminogen activator as a prognostic marker in different subgroups of patients with breast cancer. *Cancer* 1994;74:2276–2280.

67. Janicke F, Schmitt M, Graeff H. Clinical relevance of the urokinase-type and tissue-type plasminogen activators and their type 1 inhibitor in breast cancer. *Semin Thromb Hemostas* 1991;17:303–312.

68. Foekens JA, Schmitt M, van Putten WLJ, et al. Plasminogen activator inhibitor-1 and prognosis in primary breast cancer. *J Clin Oncol* 1994;12:1648–1658.

69. Duggan C, Kennedy S, Kramer MD, et al. Plasminogen activator inhibitor type 2 in breast cancer. *Br J Cancer* 1997;76:622–627.

70. Billgren AM, Ritqvist LE, Johansson H, Hagerstrom T, Skoog L. The role of cathepsin D and PAI-1 in primary invasive breast cancer as prognosticators and predictors of treatment with adjuvant tamoxifen. *Eur J Cancer* 2000;36:1374–1380.

71. Janicke F, Schmitt M, Pache L, et al. Urokinase plasminogen activator (uPA) and its inhibitor PAI-1 are strong and independent prognostic factors in node-negative breast cancer. *Breast Cancer Res Treat* 1993;24:195–208.

72. Bajou K, Noel A, Gerard RD, et al. Absence of host plasminogen activator inhibitor 1 prevents cancer invasion and vascularization. *Nat Med* 1998;4:923–928.

73. Bajou K, Masson V, Gerard RD, et al. The plasminogen activator inhibitor PAI-1 controls in vivo vascularization by interaction with proteases, not vitronectin: implications for antioangiogenic strategies. *J Cell Biol* 2001;152:777–784.
74. Johnstone RW, Ruefli AA, Lowe SW. Apoptosis: a link between cancer genetics and chemotherapy. *Cell* 2002;108:153–164.
75. Benraad TH, Geurts-Moespot J, Grondahl-Hansen J, et al. Immunoassays (ELISA) of urokinase-type plasminogen activator (uPA): report of an EORTC/BIOMED-1 Workshop. *Eur J Cancer* 1996;32:1371–1381.
76. Sweep CGJ, Geurts-Moespot J, Grebenschikov N, et al. External quality assessment of trans-European multicenter antigen determination (enzyme-linked immunosorbent assay) of urokinase plasminogen activator (uPA) and its type-1 inhibitor (PAI-1) in human breast cancer extracts. *Br J Cancer* 1998;78:1434–1441.
77. Hayes D, Bast RC, Desch CE, et al. Tumor marker utility grading system: a framework to evaluate clinical utility of tumor markers. *J Natl Cancer Inst* 1996;88:1456–1466.
78. Janicke F, Prechtl A, Thomssen C, et al. For the German Chemo N_0 Study Group. Randomized adjuvant chemotherapy trial in high-risk node-negative breast cancer patients identified by urokinase-type plasminogen activator and plasminogen activator inhibitor type 1. *J Natl Cancer Inst* 2001;93:913–920.
79. Clark GM. Do we really need prognostic factors for breast cancer? *Breast Cancer Res Treat* 1994;30:117–126.
80. Foekens J, Look MP, Peters HA, et al. Urokinase-type plasminogen activator and its inhibitor PAI-1: predictors of poor response to tamoxifen therapy in recurrent breast cancer. *J Natl Cancer Inst* 1995;87:751–756.
81. Harbeck N, Kates RE, Look MP, et al. Enhanced benefit from adjuvant chemotherapy in breast cancer patients classified high-risk according to urokinase-type plasminogen activator (uPA) and plasminogen activator inhibitor type 1 (N = 3424). *Cancer Res* 2002;62:4617–4622.
82. Schmitt M, Magdolen V, Sperl S, et al. Interference with the urokinase plasminogen activator system: a promising therapy concept for solid tumors. *Expert Opinion Biol Ther* 2001;1:683–691.
83. Schmitt M, Eickler A, Welk A, et al. Procedure for the quantitative protein determination of urokinase (uPA) and its inhibitor PAI-1 in human breast cancer tissue extracts by ELISA. In: Harris A, Brooks S, eds., *Breast Cancer Protocols*, Humana Press, Totowa, NJ.

8   Predictive Value of c-*erb*-B2 for Endocrine Therapy and Chemotherapy in Breast Cancer

Vered Stearns, MD

CONTENTS

SUMMARY

c-*erb*-B2, also designated *HER-2/neu* or c-*neu*, is a tyrosine kinase proto-oncogene that may be overexpressed or amplified in 20–40% of breast tumors. Data reported to date suggest that the proto-oncogene may be a predictive factor of response to several therapies that are commonly used to treat breast cancer. Tumors that are both hormone receptors and c-*erb*-B2 positive may be associated with a relative resistance to tamoxifen. Preliminary data suggest that aromatase inhibitors may be more effective in such tumors. Available data suggest that women with c-*erb*-B2–positive tumors may have a

Cancer Drug Discovery and Development: Biomarkers in Breast Cancer:
Molecular Diagnostics for Predicting and Monitoring Therapeutic Effect
Edited by: G. Gasparini and D. F. Hayes © Humana Press Inc., Totowa, NJ

preferential response to anthracycline-containing regimens compared to cyclophosphamide, methotrexate, 5-fluorouracil (CMF)-like regimens. Anthracycline-based therapy should be recommended to women with c-*erb*-B2–positive breast cancer unless there is a contraindication to the administration of this group of agents. However, other regimens should not be withheld from women who cannot receive an anthracyline. Current clinical data also suggest a possible sensitivity to taxane-based therapy, especially when combined with an anthracycline. Trastuzumab-based therapy should be considered as first line therapy for women with metastatic breast cancer with c-*erb*-B2–positive disease who are hormone receptor negative, or those with hormone receptor–positive disease who have progressed on endocrine treatments. Adjuvant trastuzumab should be considered in women with high-risk primary breast cancer.

Key Words: c-*erb*-B2; *HER-2/neu*; predictive factor; hormone therapy; chemotherapy; trastuzumab.

1. INTRODUCTION

c-*erb*-B2, also designated *HER-2/neu* or c-*neu*, is a tyrosine kinase proto-oncogene that belongs to the epidermal growth factor receptor (EGFR) family. The EGFR family includes four members designated HER-1 (EGFR), HER-2, HER-3, and HER-4. The receptor consists of a transmembrane domain connected to an extracellular domain and an intracellular domain. When a ligand binds to the extracellular domain, the receptor homo- or heterodimerizes with another HER receptor and the intracellular tyrosine kinase domain is activated via phosphorylation. A cascade of protein-to-protein interactions is initiated, and a signal of growth and proliferation is transmitted to the nucleus. Of note, a ligand to c-*erb*-B2 has not been identified. Up to 20–40% of breast cancers overexpress or amplify c-*erb*-B2. Despite two decades of investigation and hundreds of publications, the role of c-*erb*-B2 as a prognostic and predictive factor in breast cancer is still in question. Indeed, members of the American Society of Clinical Oncology (ASCO) Tumor Marker Expert Panel, the NIH Consensus Panel, and the St. Gallen International Consensus Panel determined that c-*erb*-B2 status should not be used to alter treatment recommendations for individual patients *(1–3)*.

Prior to discussing individual studies that evaluated the predictive role of c-*erb*-B2, it is important to review some of the reasons for the controversial role of the marker. Difficulties assessing the true predictive role of a marker such as c-*erb*-B2 stem from heterogeneity in study design and patient population as well as variability in methods of marker evaluation (Table 1). Generally, anecdotal or preclinical data that suggest a marker may have a

Table 1
Reasons for the Controversial Role of c-*erb*-B2
as a Predictive Marker for Treatments of Breast Cancer

Heterogeneity in study design, patient population, and follow-up
   Retrospective analyses of archival tissue
   No distinction between prognostic and predictive role
   Include patients with many Tumor–Node–Metastasis (TNM) stages
   Include patients with many treatments
   Treatments may be suboptimal by today's standards
   Not all trial patients included in marker study
   Patients' outcomes not known
Heterogeneity of methods of marker detection
   Assays used detect different abnormal processes
      Gene amplification
      RNA amplification
      Protein overexpression
   Evaluated tissue or circulating marker levels
   Different specimen preparation
   Different reagents
   Different cutoff level

prognostic or predictive role in a specific cancer led to retrospective analyses of samples that may have been collected through previous clinical trials or simply from tissue banks. The patient population in a marker study may be heterogeneic and information regarding therapy, follow-up, specimen selection, or statistical analysis is not usually prospectively determined. Such studies are hypothesis-generating and designated level of evidence (LOE) III or IV studies *(4)*. Results of LOE III or IV studies must be further tested and validated before a marker is ready for clinical use. After establishing a possible role, LOE I evidence (i.e., evidence from a single high-powered prospective study that is specifically designed to test the marker or evidence from meta-analysis and/or overview of lower evidence studies) is required prior to accepting the marker for clinical use *(4)*. Unfortunately, most investigations that evaluated the role of c-*erb*-B2 in predicting response to breast cancer treatments include LOE III or IV studies. Several studies have evaluated c-*erb*-B2 in samples that have been collected through a prospective trial that was designed to test therapeutic hypothesis with a marker study as a secondary objective defined in the protocol (LOE II studies). Unfortunately, despite prospective collection of samples for the marker study, samples are often available only from a subgroup of patients who were included in the clinical trial.

Heterogeneity in study design also contributes to the confusion of whether a marker is prognostic, predictive, or both. A true prognostic marker reflects tumor biology and, in the absence of treatment, its presence may suggest improved long-term outcomes such as disease free and/or overall survival (positive prognostic marker) or worse outcomes (negative prognostic marker). To evaluate the true prognostic role of a marker, absence of systemic treatment is desired. In contrast, the presence or absence of a predictive marker is associated with sensitivity or resistance to specific therapy. To evaluate the predictive role of a marker, outcomes such as response rates, disease-free survival, and overall survival may be calculated for study participants with marker-positive vs marker-negative disease. The presence of the estrogen receptor (ER) is an example of a strong predictive marker for response to endocrine manipulations that is also a weak positive prognostic marker. Current data suggest that c-erb-B2 may be a weak negative prognostic factor and will not be reviewed in this chapter (5).

It is also difficult to compare results of individual marker studies owing to the heterogeneity in methods used to analyze the marker. While most early studies of c-erb-B2 used immunohistochemistry (IHC) to detect protein expression, others evaluated amplification of the oncogene. Even when the same method is used, different antibodies or cutoff levels may be utilized (Table 1). In this chapter, studies that assessed the predictive role of c-erb-B2 to endocrine therapies and to chemotherapies are discussed with an emphasis on studies with high LOE. In this review, c-erb-B2–positive tumors are referred to tumors that overexpress or amplify the oncogene using the cutoff levels and criteria defined in the individual study.

2. c-erb-B2 AS A PREDICTIVE FACTOR FOR RESPONSE TO ENDOCRINE MANIPULATIONS

Tumors from more than 50% of women diagnosed with breast cancer will express the ER and/or progesterone receptor (PgR). Most of hormone receptor-positive women will be offered endocrine manipulations at some point during the treatment course. The most common endocrine therapy administered to women with breast cancer is tamoxifen. Aromatase inhibitors are commonly administered as first- or second-line therapy for menopausal women with metastatic breast cancer. Based on the results from the Arimidex, Tamoxifen, Alone or in Combination (ATAC) Trial, the United States Food and Drug Administration recently approved the aromatase inhibitor anastrozole for adjuvant therapy for women with hormone receptor–positive breast cancer (6). Other studies support the use of the aromatase inhibitor letrozole following 5 yr of tamoxifen, or exemestane for 2–3 yr following 2–3 yr of tamoxifen for a total of 5 yr (7,8). Based on these recent reports, aromatase inhibitors are likely to have an increasing role in the adjuvant treatment of hormone receptors positive postmenopausal women (9). Ovarian ablation may be employed in premenopausal or perimenopausal women with hormone receptor–positive disease *(10)*. Initial reports from preclinical studies and retrospective clinical trials suggested that c-*erb*-B2–positive tumors may be associated with relative resistance to hormone therapies. However, the data are inconclusive. Reports from recent studies may also suggest that the presence of c-*erb*-B2 may not confer resistance to all endocrine therapies.

2.1. Preclinical Data

Breast cancer cell lines that overexpress c-*erb*-B2 or those that have been transfected with the oncogene are tamoxifen resistant *(11–13)*. Tamoxifen inhibits the growth of parental MCF-7 xenografts but not the growth of c-*erb*-B2–transfected MCF-7 xenografts *(11–13)*. One hypothesis that may explain tamoxifen resistance is that while tamoxifen inhibits ER-stimulated growth, the cells may be activated through the c-*erb*-B2 signal transduction pathway. Other data suggest that tamoxifen, unlike estrogen, may up-regulate the expression of c-*erb*-B2. Indeed, MCF-7 cells transfected with c-*erb*-B2 are associated with mitogen-activated protein (MAP) kinase hyperactivity and tamoxifen resistance. When c-*erb*-B2 and MAP kinase are blocked, tamoxifen sensitivity is restored *(14)*. It is also possible that hormone receptor–positive tumors that also overexpress c-*erb*-B2 have lower expression of the hormone receptors compared to similar tumors that are c-*erb*-B2 negative *(15)*. Thus, the c-*erb*-B2–positive tumors may be less responsive to the hormone therapies simply because of a lower hormone receptor content.

These preclinical studies suggest that there may be a "cross-talk" between the signal transduction associated with c-*erb*-B2 and that of the ER. Tumors that overexpress or amplify c-*erb*-B2 may be hormone independent and may indeed be relatively resistant to tamoxifen. However, these preclinical studies do not provide data regarding the predictive role of c-*erb*-B2 to hormonal manipulations that deprive the cells of estrogen without a direct association with the ER, such as aromatase inhibitors or ovarian suppression.

2.2. Studies of Hormone Therapies in Metastatic Breast Cancer

Several studies evaluated the predictive role of c-*erb*-B2 to hormonal therapies in metastatic breast cancer. Because women with metastatic breast cancer require effective therapy, randomized clinical trials with a control group are not available. However, one can assume that in the absence of treatment the response rate of the tumor will be nil. Then, with the use of any therapy, response rates and other outcomes can be compared between women with tumors that are c-*erb*-B2 positive vs those whose tumors are c-*erb*-B2 negative.

Most studies that investigated tissue c-*erb*-B2 status using IHC in patients with metastatic breast cancer reported that overexpression of the marker was associated with relative resistance to tamoxifen. In addition to differences in patient population and methods of c-*erb*-B2 detection, the studies are mostly small and may have included women with hormone receptor–positive and –negative tumors who may have received one of several hormone therapies. In one large study, women received first line tamoxifen ($n = 211$) or ovarian ablation ($n = 30$). Response rate and time to progression (TTP) were statistically significantly worse in women who overexpressed c-*erb*-B2 compared to women with c-*erb*-B2–negative disease *(16)*. When the analysis was restricted to the 189 women whose tumors were ER positive, TTP (5.5 vs 11.2 months, $p < 0.001$) and response rate (24% vs 64%, $p = 0.05$) were worse in c-*erb*-B2–positive patients. In a study of 104 women who received tamoxifen and 22 who received high-dose progestin or other hormone therapies, response rates were worse in c-*erb*-B2–positive women as was disease-free survival (DFS) *(17)*. A smaller study included samples from 65 women treated with tamoxifen or aminoglutetamide and hydrocortisone. Response rates were 7% for c-*erb*-B2–positive patients compared to 37% for c-*erb*-B2–negative patients *(18)*.

Studies that were restricted to ER-positive women who received tamoxifen only revealed no association between c-*erb*-B2 status and response to tamoxifen. In South West Oncology Group (SWOG) study 8228, evaluation of 205 samples of 349 study participants revealed no significant difference in response rate (54% and 57%), DFS (6 and 8 mo), or OS (29 and 31 mo) between women with c-*erb*-B2–positive and –negative disease *(19)*. In a smaller study that evaluated circulating extracellular domain (ECD) of c-*erb*-B2, significant difference in response to tamoxifen was not observed regardless of c-*erb*-B2 status *(20)*. Although both women with ER-positive or -negative disease were included in the initial analysis, the results remained insignificant even when the analysis was restricted to ER-positive patients.

Early reports suggested that c-*erb*-B2 positivity may also predict resistance to endocrine treatments other then tamoxifen. Response rates to treatments with megestrol acetate, fadrazole, and droloxifene were worse in women with elevated levels of ECD-c-*erb*-B2 compared to those who did not have elevated levels of the circulating marker *(21,22)*. These results supported the hypothesis that c-*erb*-B2 may confer a worse response to hormone therapies. However, while ECD shedding closely correlates with tumors that overexpress or amplify c-*erb*-B2 (high specificity), not all women whose tumors overexpress c-*erb*-B2 will have detectable circulating levels of the ECD of the marker *(23)*. At the same time, ECD–c-*erb*-B2 concentrations can be more precisely quantified compared to IHC, and the degree of marker elevation may be predictive of response.

Large studies correlating c-*erb*-B2 status and response to the aromatase inhibitor letrozole have demonstrated conflicting results. Colomer evaluated ECD–c-*erb*-B2 levels in 223 women with hormone receptor–positive metastatic breast cancer who received second-line hormone therapy with letrozole. Time to failure (TTF) was shorter for women with elevated concentrations of ECD–c-*erb*-B2 compared with those whose levels were below the cutoff value *(24)*. Similar results were observed in a study of 711 women who received megestol acetate, fadrazole, or letrozole. Women with elevated concentrations of ECD–c-*erb*-B2 had a worse response rate (23% vs 45%, $p < 0.0001$), TTP (3 vs 6 mo, $p < 0.0001$), and overall survival (17.2 vs 29.6 mo, $p < 0.0001$) compared to those whose concentrations were below the cutoff *(25)*.

Outcomes of women with c-*erb*-B2–positive or –negative breast cancer were evaluated in two randomized clinical trials of tamoxifen vs letrozole. In the first study, postmenopausal women with hormone receptor–positive locally advanced breast cancer received neoadjuvant therapy with letrozole or tamoxifen. Overall, response rate was greater for patients who received letrozole compared to those who received tamoxifen (60% and 41%, respectively, $p = 0.004$). In a post hoc analysis, the presence of c-*erb*-B2 (IHC) predicted for improved response to letrozole compared to tamoxifen (Table 2). Response rate to letrozole was 69% and 53% for women with c-*erb*-B2–positive and –negative disease (odds ratio [OR] for response 1.93, 95% CI 0.63–5.88, $p = 0.25$), compared to much lower response rates to tamoxifen of 17% and 40% for women with marker-positive and -negative disease, respectively (OR 0.31, 95% CI 0.10–0.97, $p = 0.045$). The odds ratio for response to letrozole vs tamoxifen for women whose tumors overexpressed *erb*-B1 or *erb*-B2 was 28 (response rate 88% vs 21%, respectively, $p = 0.0004$) compared to an odds ratio of 1.7 (response rate 54% vs 42%, $p = 0.078$) in c-*erb*-B1- or -2–negative patients *(26)*. Similar results were reported in a randomized trial comparing neoadjuvant anastrozole vs tamoxifen. Women with both ER and c-*erb*-B2 positive tumors were much more likely to respond to anastrozole compared to tamoxifen *(27)*. While intriguing, these data are a result of an unplanned analysis of a small number of patients whose tumors were c-*erb*-B2 positive and validation is required in larger studies. In addition, it is not known whether the greater response rates in the c-*erb*-B2-positive women will translate to improved DFS and/or OS. In another large study of tamoxifen vs letrozole as first line therapy for metastatic breast cancer, letrozole-treated women had improved outcomes compared to tamoxifen-treated women regardless of ECD–c-*erb*-B2 concentrations. Importantly, women without elevated ECD–c-*erb*-B2 who were treated with tamoxifen had substantially better outcomes compared to women with elevated ECD–c-*erb*-B2 who were treated with either tamoxifen or letrozole (Table 2). Thus, even if women with c-*erb*-B2–

Table 2
Randomized Clinical Trials of Endocrine Treatments

a. Advanced Breast Cancer

Author	Patient population and number in marker study (% c-erb-B2–positive)	Treatment arms (randomized, unless otherwise specified)	Response rate arm 1 vs arm 2 (p value)		Time to progression arm 1 vs arm 2 (p value)	
			c-erb-B2–positive	c-erb-B2–negative	c-erb-B2–positive	c-erb-B2–negative
Ellis (26)	LABC, first line, ER or PR+ 250 (14%)	1. Tamoxifen 20 mg 2. Letrozole 2.5 mg	17% vs 69%	40% vs 53%	NR	NR
Lipton (84)	LABC, metastatic, first line 562 (29%)	1. Tamoxifen 20 mg 2. Letrozole 2.5 mg	13% vs 17% (0.4507)	26% vs 39% (0.078)	3.3 vs 6.1 mo[a] (0.0596)	8.5 vs 12.2 mo[a] (0.0019)

b. Early Breast Cancer (Adjuvant)

Author	Patient population and number in marker study (% c-erb-B2-positive)	Treatment arms	HR disease-free survival (95% CI, p value) arm 1 vs arm 2		HR overall survival (95% CI, p value) arm 1 vs arm 2	
			c-erb-B2-positive	c-erb-B2-negative	c-erb-B2-positive	c-erb-B2-negative
Carlamango/ (GUN 1) (28)	N-, ER+/-, no CT 145 (30%)	1. Tamoxifen × 2 yr 2. No therapy	51% vs 63%[b] (0.3)	82% vs 54%[b] (0.003)	57% vs 82%[b] (0.03)	86% vs 68%[b] (0.09)
Muss, Berry (CALGB 8541) (30,58)	N+, 3 dose level CAF 650 (24%)	1. Tamoxifen × 5 yr 2. No tamoxifen (not randomized)	0.68 (0.42–1.1, 0.12)	0.61 (0.47–0.79, 0.0001)	0.70 (0.41–1.18, 0.18)	0.64 (0.47–0.87, 0.0037)
Stal (34)	ER+ 405 (11%)	1. Tamoxifen × 5 yr 2. Tamoxifen × 2 yr	2.0 (0.49–7.9)	0.58 (0.37–0.90)	NR	NR
Love (85)	N+/-, ER+, no CT 282 (26%)	1. Ovarian ablation and tamoxifen 2. No therapy	0.37 (0.26–0.89, 0.047)	0.48 (0.31–0.71, 0.019)	0.26 (0.07–0.92, 0.038)	0.68 (0.32–1.42, 0.30)

CAF, Cyclophosphamide, doxorubicin, 5-fluorouracil; CI, confidence interval; CT, chemotherapy; ER, estrogen receptor; HR, hazard ratio; LABC, locally advanced breast cancer; N, node; NR, data not reported; PgR, progesterone receptor.
[a]Median. [b]% DFS or OS per treatment arm.

positive disease may be more responsive to aromatase inhibitors compared to tamoxifen, their outcomes following letrozole treatment may still be worse than outcomes of women whose tumors are c-*erb*-B2 negative, reflecting the prognostic role of the marker.

Taken together, the results of studies in advanced breast cancer suggest that women whose tumors were c-*erb*-B2 positive may or may not be relatively resistant to tamoxifen. Whether c-*erb*-B2–positive women may derive greater benefit from aromatase inhibitors compared to tamoxifen is also not clear.

2.3. Studies of Hormone Manipulations in the Adjuvant Setting

Samples for c-*erb*-B2 analysis were available from only a handful of studies that compared adjuvant tamoxifen or other endocrine therapies to no treatment. The Gruppo Universitario Napoletano (GUN-1) was the first large randomized clinical trial that suggested that c-*erb*-B2 may be a negative predictive factor for response to tamoxifen. From 1978 to 1983, 433 women whose ER status was unknown were randomly assigned to 30 mg of tamoxifen daily for 2 yr or to no hormone therapy. Of those, 173 women were node negative and did not receive adjuvant chemotherapy, and tumors from 145 (84%) were available for c-*erb*-B2 analysis by IHC. Treatment with tamoxifen was associated with worse 10-yr overall survival (OS) in women whose tumors overexpressed c-*erb*-B2. In contrast, women with c-*erb*-B2–negative disease who received tamoxifen had improved OS (Table 2) *(28)*. In a recent update of this report, c-*erb*-B2 was one of eight markers that were retrospectively assayed in tissues from 83% of the patients enrolled in the original clinical trial (i.e., with or without chemotherapy). With a median follow-up of 15 yr, hazard ratio (HR) of death of tamoxifen over no-tamoxifen for c-*erb*-B2–positive subjects was 1.09 (95% confidence interval [CI]: 0.63–1.87, $p = 0.04$) compared to HR of 0.59 in women who did not overexpress c-*erb*-B2 (95% CI: 0.40–0.87) *(29)*. The presence of c-*erb*-B2 was predictive of response to tamoxifen in the subgroup of patients with hormone receptor–positive tumors. The results of this updated report suggest that women with tumors overexpressing c-*erb*-B2 have a worse outcome in the presence of 2 yr of tamoxifen; however, this update included premenopausal patients who received adjuvant systemic chemotherapy with the CMF regimen (cyclophosphamide, methotrexate, 5-fluorouracil) in both groups. HR for c-*erb*-B2–negative patients who received only tamoxifen vs no systemic therapy was 0.54 (0.47–1.14) compared to 2.23 (0.95–5.23) for c-*erb*-B2–positive patients. These results were not statistically significant. When comparing women who received CMF and tamoxifen to those who received CMF only, significant differences in HR of response to tamoxifen were not seen. The multiple subgroup analyses of the GUN-1 study reflect the many shortcomings that are associated with investigations of the predictive role of c-*erb*-B2 in breast cancer.

In the Cancer and Leukemia Group B (CALGB) study 8541, 1572 women with node-positive breast cancer were randomly assigned to one of three dose groups of the CAF combination (cyclophosphamide, doxorubicin, 5-fluorouracil). In an analysis of 650 women with ER-positive disease who received 5 yr of adjuvant tamoxifen vs not in a *nonrandomized* fashion after the completion of CAF, tamoxifen was associated with similar risk reduction in DFS in the c-*erb*-B2–positive and c-*erb*-B2–negative groups (Table 2) *(30)*. Although these results are from a nonrandomized assignment of tamoxifen, the number of samples available for the marker study was large, several methods assessing c-*erb*-B2 status were used, and the patient population was relatively homogeneous (node-positive, hormone receptor-positive). However, all the patients included in the analysis received doxorubicin-based therapy, albeit one of three-dose levels, prior to tamoxifen. Given the clinical data suggesting that c-*erb*-B2–positive tumors may be associated with relative sensitivity to anthracyclines (reviewed below), it can be hypothesized that doxorubicin may reverse relative resistance to tamoxifen. Other reports from nonrandomized investigations suggested a relative resistance to tamoxifen for the subgroups of patients with c-*erb*-B2–positive breast cancer vs those with marker-negative disease *(31–33)*.

Others suggested that the optimal treatment duration of tamoxifen might differ for women with c-*erb*-B2–positive vs –negative disease. c-*erb*-B2 status was assessed either by DNA amplification assay ($n = 181$) or by flow cytometry of the protein ($n = 396$) in women who received 2 or 5 yr of adjuvant tamoxifen in a randomized clinical trial. Patients with c-*erb*-B2–negative disease had a significant benefit from 5 yr of tamoxifen treatment (relative risk [RR] = 0.62, 95% CI: 0.42–0.93), while no added benefit was seen for c-*erb*-B2–positive patients (RR = 1.1, 95% CI: 0.41–3.2) *(34)*. However, when the analysis was restricted to ER-positive patients, the difference in relative hazard was not statistically significant ($p = 0.065$).

Recently, results were reported from a large clinical trial of adjuvant oophorectomy and tamoxifen (20 mg/day for 5 yr) or observation. From 1993 to 1999, 709 premenopausal women with operable breast cancer were recruited to this trial. Hormone receptor status, which was not available at the time of recruitment, was subsequently evaluated in 66% of the participants, of those 62% were ER positive (i.e., 288 women or 41% of the study participants). With a median follow-up of 3.6 yr, 5-yr DFS and OS were improved for the women in the treatment group with hormone receptor-positive disease *(35)*. Overall, 282 samples were available for IHC analysis. The HR for DFS in c-*erb*-B2–positive patients with adjuvant endocrine therapy was 0.37 (95% confidence interval [CI], 0.26–0.89) compared to 0.48 (95% CI, 0.31–0.71) for c-*erb*-B2–negative patients, suggesting that both marker groups benefited from the treatment equally. Likewise, the HR for OS was similar for c-*erb*-B2–positive and –negative patients. When analyses were restricted to patients with ER-positive tumors, c-*erb*-B2 positivity was associated with worse DFS and OS compared to women with c-*erb*-B2–negative tumors. These results suggest that women with c-*erb*-B2–positive and –negative disease derive similar proportional benefit from a combination of oophorectomy and tamoxifen, however, it is possible that the c-*erb*-B2–positive tumors may be associated with a more aggressive biology (negative prognostic factor) and the outcomes, although improved with the treatment, may still be inferior to outcomes of women with c-*erb*-B2–negative disease.

2.4. c-erb-B2 as a Predictive Factor
for Response to Endocrine Therapies: Conclusions

The results outlined above demonstrate the multiple limitations of the studies reported to date that evaluated the predictive role of c-*erb*-B2 to endocrine therapies. Most studies are very small, with patients who may or may not have received a uniform treatment, and may or may not have been enrolled in a single clinical trial. The assays used to determine c-*erb*-B2 status vary among different investigations, as do the antibodies used, cutoff levels, and scoring algorithms. While initial reports supported preclinical studies that suggested that c-*erb*-B2 may indeed be associated with a worse response to endocrine manipulations, recent reports indicate that women with either c-*erb*-B2–positive or –negative disease derive similar proportional benefit from endocrine treatments, and/or that not all endocrine treatments are alike.

Given the deficiencies of most marker studies and inconsistent results from larger randomized studies, it is difficult to conclude whether c-*erb*-B2 is predictive of response to all or to specific hormone therapies. Based on the available data, hormone therapies should not be withheld from women simply because their tumors overexpress or amplify c-*erb*-B2. Hormone treatment recommendations should be based on hormone receptor status, risk of relapse, menopausal status, and comorbidities. Until further data are available, it may be reasonable to offer adjuvant anthracycline-based chemotherapy in addition to tamoxifen to women with primary breast cancer with expression of hormone receptors and overexpression/amplification of c-*erb*-B2. Whether the addition of ovarian ablation to tamoxifen in pre- or perimenopausal women with small hormone receptor–positive c-*erb*-B2–positive disease will reverse possible tamoxifen resistance is simply not known. Likewise, conclusive data to support the use of aromatase inhibitors instead of tamoxifen in postmenopausal women with c-*erb*-B2–positive disease are not available.

3. c-*erb*-B2 AS A PREDICTIVE FACTOR FOR RESPONSE TO CHEMOTHERAPY

3.1. Preclinical Data

Results from preclinical experiments suggested that breast cancer cell lines that overexpress or amplify the c-*erb*-B2 receptor have not provided conclusive evidence regarding c-*erb*-B2 status and relative sensitivity or resistance to chemotherapy. In breast cancer cell lines that were transfected with c-*erb*-B2, significant difference in the response to seven different chemotherapy agents was not observed between the wild-type or transfected cells *(36)*. Similarly, normal human mammary epithelial cells that were designed to overexpress c-*erb*-B2 did not demonstrate resistance to single-agent doxorubicin, paclitaxel, cisplatin, 5-fluorouracil, or methotrexate *(37)*. It is possible that overexpression of the oncogene by itself may not be sufficient to confer relative sensitivity or resistance to common chemotherapies. In human cancers c-*erb*-B2 positivity may be associated with several additional subcellular changes. For example, breast cancer specimens commonly coamplify c-*erb*-B2 and the enzyme topoisomerase II, the target of anthracyclines *(38)*. Investigators thus evaluated c-*erb*-B2 status in 40 cell lines that were primarily derived from tissue of chemotherapy-naïve patients at the time of surgery. The tumors were then exposed to six different concentrations of CEF (cyclophosphamide, epirubicin, 5-fluorouracil) or CMF (cyclophosphamide, methotrexate, 5-fluorouracil) combination. Tumors with an intermediate or strong overexpression of the marker were more sensitive to either CMF or CEF compared to tumors with low or no c-*erb*-B2 expression. Of note, the results were statistically significant when the antibodies TAB250 and AO485 were used (p values 0.044 and 0.032, respectively) but not with the CB11 antibody ($p = 0.8$) *(39)*.

Other studies focused on response to taxanes. Breast cancer cell lines transfected with c-*erb*-B2 blocked paclitaxel- or docetaxel-induced apoptosis *(40,41)*. Furthermore, infection of the taxane-resistant cells with adenovirus type 5 *EIA* led to down-regulation of c-*erb*-B2 and subsequent restoration of paclitaxel sensitivity *(42)*.

3.2. CMF and Other Alkylating Agent-Based Therapy

Several uncontrolled clinical trials have demonstrated that patients who were treated with adjuvant CMF or CMF-containing regimens and whose tumors were c-*erb*-B2 positive had worse outcomes compared to patients with c-*erb*-B2–negative disease *(31,43–45)*. In contrast, in the metastatic setting, patients with c-*erb*-B2–positive cancers were more likely to respond to CMF compared to those with c-*erb*-B2–negative tumors *(17,46)*. Because of heterogeneity in patient population, small sample size and variability in methods of c-*erb*-B2 detection, a conclusive correlation between c-*erb*-B2 status and CMF cannot be made. Results from controlled studies demonstrated no correlation, relative resistance, or relative sensitivity to the CMF regimen (Table 3).

The first two controlled studies were reported more than a decade ago, and both suggested that c-*erb*-B2 may be a negative predictive factor for response to CMF-like regimens. Blocks were available from 306 node-negative women enrolled in U.S. Intergroup 0011. The women received cyclophosphamide, methotrexate, 5-fluorouracil, and prednisone (CMFP) or no systemic therapy. DFS was improved for c-*erb*-B2–negative women who were on the treatment group compared to control (80% vs 58%, *p* = 0.0003). However, c-*erb*-B2–positive women had similar DFS regardless of the treatment assignment (78% vs 68%, *p* = not significant) *(47)*. In International Breast Cancer Study Group (Ludwig) Trial V, node-positive women received six cycles of CMF vs one preoperative cycle of CMF. Node-negative women received one perioperative cycle of CMF vs no therapy. Postmenopausal women also received tamoxifen. Marker analysis was performed in 60% of the clinical trial participants. In c-*erb*-B2–negative patients, six cycles of CMF were superior to one cycle of therapy. However, outcomes were similar for women with c-*erb*-B2–positive disease who received six cycles or one cycle of CMF (Table 3) *(48)*.

More recently, British investigators compared outcomes of 274 node-positive women who received six cycles of CMF vs no adjuvant systemic therapy. For women with c-*erb*-B2–negative tumors, median survival was improved with CMF compared to the control group (12.7 vs 7.3 yr, *p* = 0.0014) *(49)*. Women whose tumors were c-*erb*-B2 positive had a worse survival compared to c-*erb*-B2–negative patients regardless of treatment assignment. However, CMF therapy was associated with an almost 2-yr survival benefit for c-*erb*-B2–positive patients (median survival 6.1 and 4.4 yr for CMF-treated and control patients, respectively, *p* = 0.08). In a multivariate analysis, c-*erb*-B2 positivity was marginally associated with worse survival (*p* = 0.03); however, the c-*erb*-B2–positive patients were also more likely to have ER-negative tumors and four or more involved nodes.

In another large study, 386 node-positive women were randomly assigned to 12 cycles of CMF vs no adjuvant chemotherapy, and 337 samples were available for IHC of c-*erb*-B2 *(50)*. HR for DFS for women treated with CMF vs not was 0.484 for c-*erb*-B2–positive patients, compared to 0.641 for c-*erb*-B2–negative patients (Table 3). HR for cause specific survival for c-*erb*-B2–positive patients was 0.495 compared to 0.73 in c-*erb*-B2–negative patients, suggesting that women benefited equally from CMF regardless of c-*erb*-B2 status.

Other small studies evaluated c-*erb*-B2 status and response to cyclophosphamide-based high-dose chemotherapy. In aggregate, the results suggest a worse DFS for women with tissue c-*erb*-B2 overexpression or high concentration of ECD–c-*erb*-B2. The patients included in these studies may have received a variety of different regimens prior to the high-dose therapy and the results may also be confounded by prior use of arthracyclines.

Taken together, results from large prospective clinical trials of CMF vs no therapy suggest that women with c-*erb*-B2–positive or –negative tumors derive benefit from the CMF regimen. However, women with c-*erb*-B2–positive disease may have a worse prognosis at baseline and thus even if the proportional benefit from CMF is equivalent in marker-positive or -negative patients, the marker-positive patients may still suffer worse outcome following CMF chemotherapy compared to women with c-*erb*-B2–negative tumors.

3.3. Anthracycline-Based Regimens

While several studies evaluated c-*erb*-B2 status and response to CMF vs no chemotherapy, most studies that correlated the role of the marker and response to anthracycline-based therapy included comparisons either to non-anthracyline–containing regimens or between different schedules and doses of the anthracycline (Table 3).

In SWOG Trial 9445 (Intergroup 0100), 1470 node-positive, ER-positive, postmenopausal women were randomly assigned to CAF combination with tamoxifen administered sequentially or concurrently (designated CAFT) vs tamoxifen alone. c-*erb*-B2 analysis was performed on 595 samples (41%) using IHC. CAFT was marginally superior to tamoxifen for the entire study population; however, women whose tumors overexpressed the c-*erb*-B2 receptor had substantial benefit form the addition of CAF to tamoxifen. Women whose tumors did not over express c-*erb*-B2 did not gain benefit from the addition of CAF to tamoxifen *(51)*.

In National Surgical Adjuvant Breast and Bowel Project (NSABP) study B-11, node-positive women were randomly assigned to melphalan and 5-fluorouracil with or without doxorubicin (PF or PAF). With a 13.5-yr median follow-up, outcomes were improved for women who received the doxorubicin-based regimen. For c-*erb*-B2–positive patients, RR for DFS was 0.6 (0.44–0.83, $p = 0.001$), and for OS it was 0.66 (0.47–0.92, $p = 0.01$). For c-*erb*-B2–negative patients DFS and OS were not significantly different between the two treatment groups *(52)*.

3.3.1. ANTHRACYCLINE-BASED VS CMF-LIKE REGIMENS

Based on early studies that suggested that women overexpressing c-*erb*-B2 may be relatively resistant to CMF-like regimens and sensitive to anthracyclines, studies that compared response to either of these regimens were of great interest (Table 3). In one study comparing CMF vs CAF, the 5-yr OS of the CMF-treated group was 84% for c-*erb*-B2–negative patients

Table 3
Randomized Clinical Trials of Adjuvant CMF-Based and Anthracycline-Based Regimens

Author and study	Number of patients in marker study (% c-erb-B2-positive)	Treatment arms	HR disease-free survival (95% CI, p value) arm 1 vs arm 2		HR overall survival (95% CI, p value) arm 1 vs arm 2	
			c-erb-B2-positive	c-erb-B2-negative	c-erb-B2-positive	c-erb-B2-negative
CMF-like						
Intergroup 0011 (47)	406 (14%)	1. CMFP 2. No therapy	78% vs 68%[a] (NS)	80% vs 58%[a] (0.0003)	NR	NR
Ludwig V (node positive group) (48)	746 (19%)	1. CMF × 6 2. CMF × 1	0.77 (0.51–1.16)	0.57 (0.46–0.72)	46% vs 40% (0.93)	71% vs 61% (0.01)
Miles (Guy's Hospital) (49)	274 (30%)	1. CMF × 6 2. No therapy	NR	NR	6.1 vs 4.4 yr (0.08)	12.7 vs 7.3 yr (0.0014)
Menrad (Milan) (50)	337 (16%)	1. CMF × 12 2. No therapy	0.484 (0.284–0.827, 0.004)	0.641 (0.481–0.853, 0.001)	0.495 (0.287–0.853, 0.006)	0.73 (0.537–0.991, 0.22)
Anthracycline-based therapy						
Anthracycline-based vs not						
SWOG 9445 (51)	595 (16%)	1. CAFT 2. Tamoxifen	74% vs 41%[a] (0.01)	84% vs 81%[a] (0.39)	NR	NR
NSABP B-11 (52)	638 (37%)	1. PAF 2. PF	0.6 (0.44–0.83, 0.001)	0.96 (0.75–1.23, 0.74)	0.66 (0.47–0.92, 0.01)	0.9 (0.69–1.19, 0.47)
Anthracycline vs CMF						
NSABP B-15 (86)	1355 (30%)	1. AC 2. CMF	0.84 (0.65–1.07, 0.15)	1.02 (0.86–1.2, 0.84)	0.82 (0.63–1.06, 0.14)	1.07 (0.88–1.3, 0.51)
Vera (53)	141 (13%)	1. CAF 2. CMF	NR NR		72% vs 42% (0.3)	82% vs 84% (NS)

DiLeo (54)	354 (21%)	1. HEC 2. EC 3. CMF	3 vs 1:1.42 (0.54–3.76, 0.48) 3 vs 2:1.65 (0.66–4.13, 0.29)	3 vs 1:0.84 (0.49–1.44, 0.53) 3 vs 2:0.66 (0.39–1.1, 0.11)	NR	NR
NCI-C MA.5 (56)	602 (24%)	1. CEF 2. CMF	1.54 (0.06)	1.07 (0.61)	1.29 (0.28)	0.90 (0.53)
Moliterni (57)	506 (19%)	1. CMF × 8 6 A × 4 2. CMF × 12	0.83 (0.46–1.49)	1.22 (0.91–1.64)	0.61 (0.32–1.16)	1.26 (0.89–1.79)
Anthracycline dose						
CALGB 8541 (58,59)	992 (24%)	1. High-dose CAF 2. Moderate-dose CAF 3. Low-dose CAF	71%, 52%, 51%[a] (<0.01)	65%, 66%, 60%[a] (0.058)	87%, 66%, 63%[a] (<0.01)	77%, 82%, 78%[a] (0.048)
DiLeo (54)	354 (21%)	1. HEC 2. EC	2 vs 1:0.93 (0.31–2.77, 0.9)	2 vs 1:1.33 (0.82–2.14, 0.25)	NR	NR

CAF, Cyclophosphamide, doxorubicin, 5-fluorouracil; CI, confidence interval; EC, epirubicin, cyclophosphamide; HEC, high-dose epirubicin, cyclophosphamide; HR, hazard ratio; NR, not reported; NS, not significant.
[a] % DFS or OS per treatment arm.

compared to 42% in those who overexpressed the marker ($p = 0.006$) *(53)*. In contrast, women who were treated with CAF had similar 5-yr OS regardless of c-*erb*-B2 status. These results were consistent with the hypothesis that women with c-*erb*-B2–positive disease were more likely to benefit from CAF while those with c-*erb*-B2–negative disease derived equal benefit from CMF or CAF.

European investigators evaluated c-*erb*-B2 status in 354 samples from 777 node-positive patients who were randomly assigned to six cycles of CMF vs eight cycles of either moderate dose epirubicin and cyclophosphamide combination (EC) or high-dose epirubicin and cyclophosphamide (HEC). Overall, HEC was associated with improved outcomes compared to EC, while the CMF and EC groups had equivalent outcomes. However, when outcomes were analyzed by c-*erb*-B2 status and treatment, marker-positive women were more likely to benefit from HEC or EC compared to CMF (Table 3) *(54)*. A significant difference was not seen between EC and HEC in either c-*erb*-B2–positive or –negative patients. However, the sample size of each group was small, and all comparisons were not significant with wide and overlapping confidence intervals. In another study, 348 women received adjuvant CMF or weekly epirubicin and 266 samples were available for marker analysis. OS was worse for women with c-*erb*-B2–positive disease in both groups ($p = 0.02$), but a significant difference in OS was not observed between the arms ($p = 0.12$) *(55)*.

In National Cancer Institute of Canada (NCI-C) study MA .5, 710 premenopausal node-positive women were randomly assigned CEF or CMF, and tissue for c-*erb*-B2 analysis was available from a large proportion (85%) of the study participants. DFS was statistically significantly worse for the patients whose tumors overexpressed or amplified c-*erb*-B2 *(56)*. These results suggested that women with marker-positive disease may have preferential sensitivity to CEF; however, data were not conclusive owing to a small sample size and a short follow-up. In another recent report, specimens from 506 patients who were included in a prospective study of 12 cycles of CMF vs 8 cycles of CMF followed by 4 cycles of doxorubicin were analyzed for c-*erb*-B2 status. With a 15-yr median follow-up, recurrence-free survival and OS were improved for patients who overexpressed c-*erb*-B2 who received sequential CMF followed by doxorubicin compared to the CMF-only group *(57)*.

3.3.2. ANTHRACYCLINE DOSE

Results from CLAGB study 8541 suggested that c-*erb*-B2 overexpression or amplification may be predictive for response to higher dose levels of doxorubicin. In this study, women received one of three dose levels of CAF, designated low, moderate, and high dose. DFS and OS were improved for women with c-*erb*-B2–positive tumors who received high-dose CAF ($p <$

0.01) *(58)*. The results were confirmed with a larger data set and with other methods including fluorescence *in situ* hybridization (FISH) and polymerase chain reaction (PCR) (Table 4) *(59,60)*. However, the regimen designated "high-dose" is now considered standard while the moderate- and low-dose regimens may be suboptimal alternatives. Whether a higher than standard dose of doxorubicin will be associated with even further benefit for c-*erb*-B2–positive women is not known. The European study comparing CMF to EC or HEC outlined earlier, did not demonstrate a preferential outcome with HEC compared to EC *(54)*. Marker analysis from patients included in CALGB study 9344 who received one of three escalating doses of doxorubicin (60, 75, or 90 mg/m^2) may provide additional information *(61)*.

Although the studies described in the preceding are very heterogeneic, the data overall suggest that while both CMF and anthracyclines are effective treatments for c-*erb*-B2–positive or –negative breast cancer, it is possible that c-*erb*-B2–positive patients derive greater benefit from anthracycline-based therapy compared to CMF-like regimens. At the same time, c-*erb*-B2–negative patients may benefit equally from either type of therapy. While clinicians may choose anthracyclines preferentially for c-*erb*-B2–positive patients, CMF should be offered to women for whom anthracycline-based therapy is not appropriate regardless of c-*erb*-B2 status.

3.4. Taxane-Based Regimens

Preclinical studies suggested that c-*erb*-B2 overexpression may result in relative resistance to taxanes; however, reports from clinical trials are mixed. Taxanes have been available for more than a decade and only a handful of clinical studies evaluated the role of c-*erb*-B2 in predicting response to taxanes. Most studies were in the metastatic setting and included combination of taxanes and anthracyclines. In a study of women with metastatic breast cancer who received single agent paclitaxel ($n = 106$) or docetaxel ($n = 20$), the odds of responding to the taxane for c-*erb*-B2–positive patients were greater compared to the c-*erb*-B2–negative group. Women with c-*erb*-B2–positive disease had a response rate of 47% compared to a 39% response rate in the c-*erb*-B2–negative group ($p = 0.027$) *(62,63)*. c-*erb*-B2 was associated with a relative sensitivity to either taxane.

Colomer and colleagues evaluated the predictive role of tissue (IHC) or circulating ECD–c-*erb*-B2 and response to a combination of doxorubicin and paclitaxel administered as first-line chemotherapy to women with metastatic breast cancer. With a 23-mo follow-up, the authors reported that elevated circulating ECD–c-*erb*-B2 correlated with worse response rate (complete response 0% vs 26% for c-*erb*-B2–positive and –negative patients, respectively, $p = 0.35$) *(64)*. However, response to the therapy was similar for patients with tissue c-*erb*-B2–positive or –negative disease. Importantly, circulating ECD–c-*erb*-B2 correlated with bulk of disease and

Table 4
Randomized Clinical Trials of Taxane-Containing Regimens vs Not

Author	Patient population and number in marker study (% c-erb-B2-positive)	Treatment arms	Response rate (p value) c-erb-B2-positive	c-erb-B2-negative	Median time to progression (p value) arm 1 vs arm 2 c-erb-B2-positive	c-erb-B2-negative	Median overall survival (p value) arm 1 vs arm 2 c-erb-B2-positive	c-erb-B2-negative
Konecny (87)	Metastatic 256 (38%)	1. ET 2. EC	76% vs 46% (0.04)	50% vs 33% (0.02)	10.5 vs 7.1 mo (0.116)	9.6 vs 10.4 mo (0.35)	21.4 vs 16.4 mo (0.319)	27.5 vs 33.1 mo = (0.292)
Di Leo (66)	Metastatic 176 (20%)	1. Docetaxel 2. Doxorubicin	67% vs 27% (0.04)	40% vs 35% (0.70)	7 vs 4.7 mo (0.73)	5 vs 5.9 mo (0.21)	14.4 vs 10.8 (0.32)	12.6 vs 16.9 (0.07)
Nabholtz (68)	Adjuvant 1491 (20%)	1. TAC 2. FAC	NA	NA	HR: 0.59 (95% CI 0.38–0.91, 0.02)	HR: 0.74 (95% CI 0.54–1.01, 0.06)	NR	NR

CI, Confidence interval; EC, epirubicin and cyclophosphamide; ET, epirubicin and cyclophosphamide; FAC, 5-fluorouracil, doxorubicin, cyclophosphamide; HR, hazard ratio; NA, not applicable; NR, not reported; TAC, docetaxel, doxorubicin, cyclophosphamide.

may be a more quantitative assay compared to IHC. In a similar study of 49 patients who received combination doxorubicin and paclitaxel, overall response was equivalent in women with c-*erb*-B2–positive or –negative disease (90% and 93%, respectively). However, the percentage of women free from progression at 20 mo was greater in the c-*erb*-B2–positive group (63% and 48%, respectively) *(65)*.

In the Eastern Cooperative Oncology Group Study (ECOG) 1193, 107 women with metastatic breast cancer received combination of doxorubicin and paclitaxel, paclitaxel alone (*n* = 109), or doxorubicin alone (*n* = 64). The group who received doxorubicin alone was then allowed to cross over to paclitaxel. The authors correlated response to taxane (alone or in combination) with c-*erb*-B2 status. A difference in response was not observed among the c-*erb*-B2–positive and –negative patients ($p = 0.51$). However, women with c-*erb*-B2–positive disease had a worse survival compared to the c-*erb*-B2–negative group ($p = 0.0008$).

In a study of 326 women with metastatic disease were randomly assigned to single-agent doxorubicin or docetaxel, samples for c-*erb*-B2 analysis by FISH were available from 176 participants. Objective response, TTP, and OS were similar for women in either treatment group. However, when analyzed by c-*erb*-B2 status, docetaxel provided greater benefit compared to doxorubicin in the marker-positive group (Table 4) *(66)*. Marker-negative women had similar outcomes with either treatment.

Two other studies compared anthracycline-containing regimens with or without docetaxel. Konecny compared outcomes of women with metastatic breast cancer who were treated with combination epirubicin and cyclophosphamide (EC) or epirubicin and docetaxel (ET). ET-treated women with c-*erb*-B2–amplified tumors had improved response rate, DFS and OS as compared to those who received EC (Table 4) *(67)*. However, women whose tumors did not amplify the oncogene had similar response to either regimen. Others compared adjuvant combination FAC and TAC in women with node-positive breast cancer. While TAC was superior to FAC in all women, c-*erb*-B2–positive women derived substantial benefit from TAC (HR 0.59, $p = 0.02$), while the benefit for marker-negative patients was approaching but not statistically significant (HR 0.74, $p = 0.06$) *(68)*.

3.5. c-erb-B2 as a Predictive Factor for Response to Chemotherapy: Conclusions

Review of randomized clinical trials suggests that c-*erb*-B2 may indeed be predictive of response to specific chemotherapies. It is also possible that c-*erb*-B2 is a surrogate marker that reflects a more aggressive tumor biology and correlates with other factors that may predict for response to chemotherapy (e.g., lack of hormone receptors and worse grade). Based on the available data, systemic chemotherapy recommendations should be made based on the patient's risk of recurrence using accepted markers such as stage, nodal status, tumor size, grade, and hormone receptor status. The data overall suggest that women with c-*erb*-B2–positive disease may be more sensitive to anthracyclines and if a contraindication does not exist may be the combination of choice for those women. However, CMF should be considered for women who cannot tolerate anthracyclines. Sufficient evidence to preferentially recommend combination of anthracycline and taxane to women with c-*erb*-B2–positive disease is not available. Likewise, there is not sufficient evidence to recommend escalation of standard dose of anthracyclines to women with c-*erb*-B2–positive tumors.

4. c-*erb*-B2 AS A PREDICTIVE FACTOR FOR RESPONSE TO TRASTUZUMAB

Trastuzumab (Herceptin) is a humanized monoclonal antibody that targets the extracellular domain of c-*erb*-B2. In preclinical trials, trastuzumab suppressed tumor growth in breast cancer xenografts. Combination of trastuzumab with several chemotherapy agents such as doxorubicin, paclitaxel, and cisplatin provided synergistic tumor suppression *(69)*.

The efficacy of trastuzumab has been examined in several clinical trials in metastatic breast cancer. In women with metastatic breast cancer whose tumors overexpressed c-*erb*-B2, single-agent trastuzumab was associated with a response rate of 12–15% in heavily pretreated women and 26% as first-line therapy *(70–72)*. The initial clinical trials of single-agent trastuzumab have included patients with 2+ or 3+ overexpression of c-*erb*-B2 using IHC. In a study that evaluated response to single-agent trastuzumab in 111 women, response rate was 35% in those with a 3+ expression and 0% in women with a 2+ expression. When the same patients were evaluated using FISH, response rate in patients who amplified the oncogene was similar to those with the 3+ expression *(72)*.

Based on the encouraging results of studies of single-agent trastuzumab, several uncontrolled and controlled studies evaluated combination of this agent and chemotherapy. In the largest randomized clinical trial, 469 women received first-line chemotherapy with or without trastuzumab. Women who received prior anthracyclines received paclitaxel with or without trastuzumab, while women who had not received anthracyclines previously were treated with combination doxorubicin and cyclophosphamide with or without trastuzumab. Objective response (50% vs 32%, $p < 0.001$) and TTP (7.4 vs 4.6, $p < 0.001$) were improved in women who received chemotherapy and trastuzumab compared to chemotherapy alone *(73)*. More importantly, 1-yr survival was significantly improved for women who received trastuzumab (79% vs 68%, $p < 0.01$). Owing to the high rate of cardiac toxicity seen on the trastuzumab and doxorubicin/cyclophosphamide arm, the combination was not recommended for clinical use.

In other studies, combination trastuzumab and chemotherapy agents such as cisplatin, docetaxel, gemcitabine, paclitaxel, vinrelbine, or combination carboplatin and paclitaxel provides a higher response rates than expected with either agent alone *(74–79)*. Most studies included only patients with overexpression or amplification of c-*erb*-B2. In one study that enrolled patients regardless of c-*erb*-B2 status, combination of paclitaxel and trastuzumab provided improved response rates compared to paclitaxel alone in women who overexpressed c-*erb*-B2 (81% and 67%), while no difference in response was observed in women without c-*erb*-B2 expressing tumors (46% and 41%) *(77)*. Indeed, this study demonstrated that c-*erb*-B2 is the target of trastuzumab and c-*erb*-B2 status should be used for patient selection.

Studies of trastuzumab in the preoperative setting with paclitaxel or docetaxel demonstrated high response rates of 75% *(78,80)*. MD Anderson Cancer Center investigators have recently demonstrated that the addition of trastuzumab to preoperative anthracycline and taxane-based chemotherapy was associated with a marked increase in pathological complete response *(81)*. The role of adjuvant trastuzumab with or following systemic chemotherapy is under extensive investigation. Recent results from large cooperative group clinical trials designed to evaluate the efficacy and toxicity of trastuzumab in the adjuvant setting were recently presented in abstract form. The addition of trastuzumab to standard adjuvant systemic therapy provided a substantial improvement in DFS and OS. Importantly, investigators have found discrepancies in evaluation of c-*erb*-B2 testing of patients enrolled in adjuvant randomized clinical trials of chemotherapy with or without trastuzumab compared to a central laboratory *(82,83)*. Based on these evaluations, most centers and laboratories accept 3+ as overexpression but 2+ or 1+ is referred for further FISH testing. Other studies are evaluating the role of trastuzumab with other novel agents. Finally, several studies focus on newer agents and vaccines that target the c-*erb*-B2.

5. CONCLUSIONS

c-*erb*-B2 is clearly an important oncogene in breast cancer. However, after two decades of investigations, the predictive role of c-*erb*-B2 to specific treatments is still uncertain. With the exception of trastuzumab, c-*erb*-B2 status cannot be used to determine systemic treatment recommendations for breast cancer. Although some evidence suggests that women with c-*erb*-B2–positive disease may be less likely to benefit from a tamoxifen and CMF-like regimen, the data are mixed. Most controlled studies suggest that women with c-*erb*-B2–positive disease may have a preferential response to anthracycline-containing regimens. Thus, anthracycline-based therapy should be recommended to women with c-*erb*-B2–positive breast cancer unless there is a contraindication to the administration of this group of agents (such as cardiac disease or prior anthracycline use). Current clinical data also suggest a possible sensitivity to taxane-based therapy, especially when combined with an anthracycline. Finally, trastuzumab-based therapy should be clearly considered as first-line therapy for women with c-*erb*-B2 disease who are hormone receptor negative, or those with hormone receptor–positive disease who have progressed on endocrine treatments. In the adjuvant setting, the addition of trastuzumab should be considered for women with high-risk disease.

REFERENCES

1. 1997 update of recommendations for the use of tumor markers in breast and colorectal cancer. Adopted on November 7, 1997 by the American Society of Clinical Oncology. *J Clin Oncol* 1998;16:793–795.
2. National Institutes of Health Consensus Development Conference statement: adjuvant therapy for breast cancer, November 1–3, 2000. *J Natl Cancer Inst Monogr* 2001:5–15.
3. Goldhirsch A, Wood WC, Gelber RD, Coates AS, Thurlimann B, Senn HJ. Meeting highlights: Updated International Expert Consensus on the Primary Therapy of Early Breast Cancer. *J Clin Oncol* 2003;21:3357–3365.
4. Hayes DF, Bast R, Desch CE, et al. A tumor marker utility grading system (TMUGS): a framework to evaluate clinical utility of tumor markers. *J Natl Cancer Inst* 1996;88:1456–1466.
5. Trock BJ, Yamauchi H, Brotzman M, Stearns V, Hayes DF. c-erbB-2 as a prognostic factor in breast cancer: a meta-analysis. *Proc Am Soc Clin Oncol* 2000;19:97a.
6. Baum M, Budzar AU, Cuzick J, et al. Anastrozole alone or in combination with tamoxifen versus tamoxifen alone for adjuvant treatment of postmenopausal women with early breast cancer: first results of the ATAC randomised trial. *Lancet* 2002;359:2131–2139.
7. Goss PE, Ingle JN, Martino S, et al. A Randomized trial of letrozole in postmenopausal women after five years of tamoxifen therapy for early-stage breast cancer. *N Engl J Med* 2003;349:1793–1802.
8. Coombes RC, Hall E, Gibson LJ, et al. A randomized trial of exemestane after two to three years of tamoxifen therapy in postmenopausal women with primary breast cancer. *N Engl J Med* 2004;350:1081–1092.
9. Winer EP, Hudis C, Burstein HJ, et al. American Society of Clinical Oncology technology assessment on the use of aromatase inhibitors as adjuvant therapy for postmenopausal women with hormone receptor-positive breast cancer: status report 2004. *J Clin Oncol* 2005;23:619–629.
10. Emens LA, Davidson NE. Adjuvant hormonal therapy for premenopausal women with breast cancer. *Clin Cancer Res* 2003;9:486S–94S.
11. Benz CC, Scott GK, Sarup JC, et al. Estrogen-dependent, tamoxifen-resistant tumorigenic growth of MCF-7 cells transfected with HER2/*neu*. *Breast Cancer Res Treat* 1992;24:85–95.
12. Liu Y, el-Ashry D, Chen D, Ding IY, Kern FG. MCF-7 breast cancer cells overexpressing transfected c-erbB-2 have an in vitro growth advantage in estrogen-depleted conditions and reduced estrogen-dependence and tamoxifen-sensitivity in vivo. *Breast Cancer Res Treat* 1995;34:97–117.

13. Pietras R, Arboleda J, Reese D, et al. HER-2 tyrosine kinase pathway targets estrogen receptor and promotes hormone-independent growth in human breast cancer cells. *Oncogene* 1995;10:2435–2446.

14. Kurokawa H, Lenferink AE, Simpson JF, et al. Inhibition of HER2/neu (erbB-2) and mitogen-activated protein kinases enhances tamoxifen action against HER2-overexpressing, tamoxifen-resistant breast cancer cells. *Cancer Res* 2000;60: 5887–5894.

15. Konecny G, Pauletti G, Pegram M, et al. Quantitative association between HER-2/neu and steroid hormone receptors in hormone receptor-positive primary breast cancer. *J Natl Cancer Inst* 2003;95:142–153.

16. Houston SJ, Plunkett TA, Barnes DM, Smith P, Rubens RD, Miles DW. Overexpression of c-erbB2 is an independent marker of resistance to endocrine therapy in advanced breast cancer. *Br J Cancer* 1999;79:1220–1226.

17. Berns EMJJ, Foekens JA, van Staveren IL, et al. Oncogene amplification and prognosis in breast cancer: relationship with systemic treatment. *Gene* 1995;159: 11–18.

18. Wright C, Nicholson S, Angus B, et al. Relationship between c-*erb*B-2 protein product expression and response to endocrine therapy in advanced breast cancer. *Br J Cancer* 1992;65:118–121.

19. Elledge RM, Green S, Ciocca D, et al. HER-2 expression and response to tamoxifen in estrogen receptor-positive breast cancer: a Southwest Oncology Group Study. *Clin Cancer Res* 1998;4:7–12.

20. Willsher PC, Beaver J, Pinder S, et al. Prognostic significance of serum c-erbB-2 protein in breast cancer patients. *Breast Cancer Res Treat* 1996;40:251–255.

21. Leitzel K, Teramoto Y, Konrad K, et al. Elevated serum c-erbB-2 antigen levels and decreased response to hormone therapy of breast cancer. *J Clin Oncol* 1995;13:1129–1135.

22. Yamauchi H, O'Neill A, Gelman R, Carney W, Hosch S, Hayes DF. Prediction of response to antiestrogen therapy in advanced breast cancer patients by pretreatment circulating levels of extracellular domain of the HER-2/c-neu protein. *J Clin Oncol* 1997;15:2518–2525.

23. Nunes RA, Harris LN. The HER2 extracellular domain as a prognostic and predictive factor in breast cancer. *Clin Breast Cancer* 2002;3:125–135; discussion 136–137.

24. Colomer R, Llombart A, Ramos M, et al. Serum HER-2 ECD and the efficacy of letrozole in ER+/PR+ metastatic breast cancer: preliminary results of a prospective study. *Breast Cancer Res Treat* 2001:223a.

25. Lipton A, Ali SM, Leitzel K, et al. Elevated serum Her-2/neu level predicts decreased response to hormone therapy in metastatic breast cancer. *J Clin Oncol* 2002;20:1467–1472.

26. Ellis MJ, Coop A, Singh B, et al. Letrozole is more effective neoadjuvant endocrine therapy than tamoxifen for ErbB-1- and/or ErbB-2-positive, estrogen receptor-positive primary breast cancer: evidence from a phase III randomized trial. *J Clin Oncol* 2001;19:3808–3816.

27. Smith I, Dowsett M. Comparison of anastrozole vs tamoxifen alone and in combination as neoadjuvant treatment of estrogen receptor-positive (ER+) operable breast cancer in postmenopausal women: the IMPACT trial. *Breast Cancer Res Treat* 2003;82 (Suppl 1):1a.

28. Carlomagno C, Perrone F, Gallo C, et al. c-erbB2 overexpression decreases the benefit of adjuvant tamoxifen in early-stage breast cancer without axillary lymph node metastases. *J Clin Oncol* 1996;14:2702–2708.

29. De Placido S, De Laurentiis M, Carlomagno C, et al. Twenty-year results of the Naples GUN Randomized Trial: predictive factors of adjuvant tamoxifen efficacy in early breast cancer. *Clin Cancer Res* 2003;9:1039–1046.

30. Berry DA, Muss HB, Thor AD, et al. HER-2/neu and p53 expression versus tamoxifen resistance in estrogen receptor-positive, node-positive breast cancer [in process citation]. *J Clin Oncol* 2000;18:3471–3479.

31. Tetu B, Brisson J. Prognostic significance of HER-2/neu oncoprotein expression in node-positive breast cancer. The influence of the pattern of immunostaining and adjuvant therapy. *Cancer* 1994;73:2359–2365.

32. Borg A, Baldetrop B, Ferno M, et al. ERBB2 amplification is associated with tamoxifen resistance in steroid-receptor positive breast cancer. *Cancer Lett* 1994;81:137–144.

33. Sjögren S, Inganas M, Lindgren A, Holmberg L, Bergh J. Prognostic and predictive value of c-erbB-2 overexpression in primary breast cancer, alone and in combination with other prognostic markers. *J Clin Oncol* 1998;16:462–469.

34. Stal O, Borg A, Ferno M, Kallstrom AC, Malmstrom P, Nordenskjold B. ErbB2 status and the benefit from two or five years of adjuvant tamoxifen in postmenopausal early stage breast cancer. *Ann Oncol* 2000;11:1545–1550.

35. Love RR, Duc NB, Allred DC, et al. Oophorectomy and tamoxifen adjuvant therapy in premenopausal Vietnamese and Chinese women with operable breast cancer. *J Clin Oncol* 2002;20:2559–2566.

36. Pegram MD, Finn RS, Arzoo K, Beryt M, Pietras RJ, Slamon DJ. The effect of HER-2/neu overexpression on chemotherapeutic drug sensitivity in human breast and ovarian cancer cells. *Oncogene* 1997;15:537–547.

37. Orr MS, O'Connor PM, Kohn KW. Effects of c-erbB2 overexpression on the drug sensitivities of normal human mammary epithelial cells [in process citation]. *J Natl Cancer Inst* 2000;92:987–994.

38. Jarvinen TA, Liu ET. HER-2/neu and topoisomerase IIalpha in breast cancer. *Breast Cancer Res Treat* 2003;78:299–311.

39. Konecny G, Fritz M, Untch M, et al. HER-2/neu overexpression and in vitro chemosensitivity to CMF and FEC in primary breast cancer. *Breast Cancer Res Treat* 2001;69:53–63.

40. Yu D, Liu B, Tan M, Li J, Wang SS, Hung MC. Overexpression of c-erbB-2/neu in breast cancer cells confers increased resistance to Taxol via mdr-1-independent mechanisms. *Oncogene* 1996;13:1359–1365.

41. Yu D, Jing T, Liu B, et al. Overexpression of ErbB2 blocks Taxol-induced apoptosis by upregulation of p21Cip1, which inhibits p34Cdc2 kinase. *Mol Cell* 1998;2:581–591.

42. Ueno NT, Bartholomeusz C, Herrmann JL, et al. E1A-mediated paclitaxel sensitization in HER-2/neu-overexpressing ovarian cancer SKOV3.ip1 through apoptosis involving the caspase-3 pathway. *Clin Cancer Res* 2000;6:250–259.

43. Giai M, Roagna R, Ponzone R, De Bortoli M, Dati C, Sismondi P. Prognostic and predictive relevance of c-erbB-2 and ras expression in node positive and negative breast cancer. *Anticancer Res* 1994;14:1441–1450.

44. Stal O, Sullivan S, Wingren S, et al. c-erbB-2 expression and benefit from adjuvant chemotherapy and radiotherapy of breast cancer. *Eur J Cancer* 1995;31A:2185–2190.

45. Mehta R, McDermott J, Hieken T, et al. Plasma c-erbB-2 levels in breast cancer patients: prognostic significance in predicting response to chemotherapy. *J Clin Oncol* 1998;16:2409–2416.

46. Klijn J. Cell biological factors associated with the response of breast cancer to systemic treatment. *Cancer Treat Rev* 1993;19SB:45–63.

47. Allred DC, Clark G, Tandon A, et al. HER-2/neu in node-negative breast cancer: prognostic significance of overexpression influenced by the presence of *in situ* carcinoma. *J Clin Oncol* 1992;10:599–605.

48. Gusterson BA, Gelber RD, Goldhirsch A, et al. Prognostic importance of c-*erb*B-2 expression in breast cancer. *J Clin Oncol* 1992;10:1049–1056.

49. Miles DW, Harris WH, Gillett CE, Smith P, Barnes DM. Effect of c-erbB(2) and estrogen receptor status on survival of women with primary breast cancer treated with adjuvant cyclophosphamide/methotrexate/fluorouracil. *Int J Cancer* 1999;84:354–359.

50. Menard S, Valagussa P, Pilotti S, et al. Response to cyclophosphamide, methotrexate, and fluorouracil in lymph node-positive breast cancer according to HER2 overexpression and other tumor biologic variables. *J Clin Oncol* 2001; 19:329–335.

51. Ravdin P, Green S, Albain K, et al. Initial report of the SWOG biological correlative study of c-erbB-2 expression as a predictor of outcome in a trial comparing adjuvant CAF T with tamoxifen alone. *Proc Am Soc Clin Oncol* 1998;17:97a.

52. Paik S, Bryant J, Park C, et al. Erbb-2 and response to doxorubicin in patients with axillary lymph node-positive, hormone receptor-negative breast cancer. *J Natl Cancer Inst* 1998;90:1361–1370.

53. Vera R, Albanell J, Lirola J, Bermejo B, Sole L, Baselga J. HER2 overexpression as a predictor of survival in a trial comparing adjuvant FAC and CMF in breast cancer. *Proc Am Soc Clin Oncol* 1999;18:71a.

54. Di Leo A, Gancberg D, Larsimont D, et al. HER-2 amplification and topoisomerase IIalpha gene aberrations as predictive markers in node-positive breast cancer patients randomly treated either with an anthracycline-based therapy or with cyclophosphamide, methotrexate, and 5-fluorouracil. *Clin Cancer Res* 2002;8: 1107–1116.

55. Colozza M, Gori S, Mosconi A, et al. c-erbB-2 expression as a predictor of outcome in a randomized trial comparing adjuvant CMF vs. single agent epirubicin in stage I-II breast cancer patients. *Proc Am Soc Clin Oncol* 1999;18:70a.

56. Pritchard KI, O'Malley F, Andrulis I, et al. Prognostic and predictive value of HER2/neu in a randomized trial comparing CMF to CEF in premenopausal women with axillary lymph node positive breast cancer (NCIC CTG MA.5). *Proc Am Soc Clin Oncol* 2002;21:165a.

57. Moliterni A, Menard S, Valagussa P, et al. HER2 overexpression and doxorubicin in adjuvant chemotherapy for resectable breast cancer. *J Clin Oncol* 2003;21: 458–462.

58. Muss HB, Thor A, Berry DA, et al. c-*erb*B-2 expression and S-phase activity predict response to adjuvant therapy in women with node-positive early breast cancer. *N Engl J Med* 1994;330:1260–1266.

59. Thor A, Berry D, Budman D, et al. erbB2, p53, and adjuvant therapy interactions in node positive breast cancer. *J Natl Cancer Inst* 1998;90:1346–1360.

60. Dressler L, Berry D, Liu E, et al. Amplification of erbB-2 by fluorescent in situ hybridization (FISH): an alternate method to predict outcome following dose-escalated CAF in Stage II, node positive breast cancer patients. A Cancer and Leukemia Group B (CALGB) study. *Proc Am Soc Clin Oncol* 1999;18:75a.

61. Henderson IC, Berry DA, Demetri GD, et al. Improved outcomes from adding sequential paclitaxel but not from escalating doxorubicin dose in an adjuvant

chemotherapy regimen for patients with node-positive primary breast cancer. *J Clin Oncol* 2003;21:976–983.

62. Seidman A, Baselga J, Yao T-J, Gilewski T, Rosen PP, Norton L. HER-2/neu over-expression and clinical taxane sensitivity: a multivariate analysis in patients with metastatic breast cancer. *Proc Am Soc Clin Oncol* 1996;15:104a.

63. Baselga J, Seidman AD, Rosen PP, Norton L. HER2 overexpression and paclitaxel sensitivity in breast cancer: therapeutic implications. *Oncology (Huntingt)* 1997;11:43–48.

64. Colomer R, Montero S, Lluch A, et al. Circulating HER2 extracellular domain and resistance to chemotherapy in advanced breast cancer. *Clin Cancer Res* 2000;6: 2356–2362.

65. Gianni L, Capri G, Mezzelani A, et al. HER-2/neu amplification and response to doxorubicin/paclitaxel (AT) in women with metastatic breast cancer. *Proc Am Soc Clin Oncol* 1997;16:139a.

66. Di Leo A, Chan S, Paesmans M, et al. HER-2/neu as a predictive marker in a population of advanced breast cancer patients randomly treated either with single-agent doxorubicin or single-agent docetaxel. *Breast Cancer Res Treat* 2004;86: 197–206.

67. Konecny GE, Thomssen C, Luck HJ, et al. Her-2/neu gene amplification and response to paclitaxel in patients with metastatic breast cancer. *J Natl Cancer Inst* 2004;96:1141–1151.

68. Nabholtz JM, Pienkowski T, Mackey J, et al. Phase III trial comparing TAC (docetaxel, doxorubicin, cyclophosphamide) with FAC (5-fluorouracil, doxorubi-cin, cyclophosphamide) in the adjuvant treatment of node positive breast cancer (BC) patients: interim analysis of the BCIRG 001 study. *Proc Am Soc Clin Oncol* 2002;21:141a.

69. Pegram M, Hsu S, Lewis G, et al. Inhibitory effects of combinations of HER-2/neu antibody and chemotherapeutic agents used for treatment of human breast cancers. *Oncogene* 1999;18:2241–2251.

70. Baselga J, Norton L, Albanell J, Kim YM, Mendelsohn J. Recombinant humanized anti-HER2 antibody (Herceptin) enhances the antitumor activity of paclitaxel and doxorubicin against HER2/neu overexpressing human breast cancer xenografts. *Cancer Res* 1998;58:2825–2831.

71. Cobleigh MA, Vogel CL, Tripathy D, et al. Multinational study of the efficacy and safety of humanized anti-HER2 monoclonal antibody in women who have HER2-overexpressing metastatic breast cancer that has progressed after chemotherapy for metastatic disease. *J Clin Oncol* 1999;17:2639–2648.

72. Vogel CL, Cobleigh MA, Tripathy D, et al. Efficacy and safety of Trastuzumab as a single agent in first-line treatment of HER2-overexpressing metastatic breast cancer. *J Clin Oncol* 2002;20:719–726.

73. Slamon DJ, Leyland-Jones B, Shak S, et al. Use of chemotherapy plus a mono-clonal antibody against HER2 for metastatic breast cancer that overexpresses HER2. *N Engl J Med* 2001;344:783–792.

74. Pegram M, Lipton A, Hayes DF, et al. Phase II study of receptor-enhanced chemosensitivity using recombinant humanized anti-p185HER2/neu monoclonal antibody plus cisplatin in patients with HER2/neu-overexpressing metastatic breast cancer refractory to chemotherapy treatment. *J Clin Oncol* 1998;16:2659–2671.

75. Esteva FJ, Valero V, Booser D, et al. Phase II study of weekly docetaxel and trastuzumab for patients with HER-2-overexpressing metastatic breast cancer. *J Clin Oncol* 2002;20:1800–1808.

76. O'Shaughnessy J. Gemcitabine and trastuzumab in metastatic breast cancer. *Semin Oncol* 2003;30:22–26.

77. Seidman AD, Fornier MN, Esteva FJ, et al. Weekly trastuzumab and paclitaxel therapy for metastatic breast cancer with analysis of efficacy by HER2 immuno-phenotype and gene amplification. *J Clin Oncol* 2001;19:2587–2595.

78. Burstein HJ, Harris LN, Marcom PK, et al. Trastuzumab and vinorelbine as first-line therapy for HER2-overexpressing metastatic breast cancer: multicenter phase II trial with clinical outcomes, analysis of serum tumor markers as predictive factors, and cardiac surveillance algorithm. *J Clin Oncol* 2003;21:2889–2895.

79. Robert N, Leyland-Jones B, Asmar L, et al. Phase III comparative study of trastuzumab and paclitaxel with and without carboplatin in patients with HER-2/neu positive advanced breast cancer. *Breast Cancer Res Treat* 2002;76:35a.

80. Van Pelt AE, Elledge RM, Allred DC, Mohsin SK, Gutierrez MC, Chang JC. Phase II study of neoadjuvant trastuzumab plus docetaxel for locally advanced and metastatic breast cancer that overexpresses HER2/neu: a preliminary report. *Breast Cancer Res Treat* 2002;76:441a.

81. Buzdar AU, Ibrahim NK, Francis D, et al. Significantly higher pathologic complete remission rate after neoadjuvant therapy with trastuzumab, paclitaxel, and epirubicin chemotherapy: results of a randomized trial in human epidermal growth factor receptor 2–positive operable breast cancer. *J Clin Oncol* 2005;23:3676–3685.

82. Paik S, Bryant J, Tan-Chiu E, et al. Real-world performance of HER2 testing—National Surgical Adjuvant Breast and Bowel Project experience. *J Natl Cancer Inst* 2002;94:852–854.

83. Roche PC, Suman VJ, Jenkins RB, et al. Concordance between local and central laboratory HER2 testing in the breast intergroup trial N9831. *J Natl Cancer Inst* 2002;94:855–857.

84. Lipton A, Ali SM, Leitzel K, et al. Serum HER-2/neu and response to the aromatase inhibitor letrozole versus tamoxifen. *J Clin Oncol* 2003;21:1967–1972.

85. Love RR, Duc NB, Havighurst TC, et al. Her-2/neu overexpression and response to oophorectomy plus tamoxifen adjuvant therapy in estrogen receptor-positive premenopausal women with operable breast cancer. *J Clin Oncol* 2003;21:453–457.

86. Paik S, Bryant J, Tan-Chiu E, et al. HER2 and choice of adjuvant chemotherapy for invasive breast cancer: National Surgical Adjuvant Breast and Bowel Project Protocol B-15. *J Natl Cancer Inst* 2000;92:1991–1998.

87. Konecny G, Thomssen M, Pegram M, et al. HEr-2/neu gene amplification and response to paclitaxel in patients with metastatic breast cancer. *Proc Am Soc Clin Oncol* 2001;20:23a.

9   *erb*-B2 as a Therapeutic Target

Robert Mass, MD

CONTENTS

SUMMARY

Trastuzumab is a humanized monoclonal antibody that targets the type 1 tyrosine kinase receptor erb-B2 and has demonstrated survival benefit when used in combination with chemotherapy in the treatment of metastatic, HER2 overexpressing breast cancer. This chapter reviews the history of the development of trastuzumab including the biology of HER signaling, the technical issues of antibody "humanization," the diagnostic challenges in developing "targeted" therapeutic agents, and the clinical data that led to the approval of this agent for patients with HER2 overexpressing breast cancer.

Key Words: Breast cancer; HER2; erb-B2; trastuzumab; monoclonal antibody; targeted therapy.

1. INTRODUCTION

The human epidermal growth factor receptor 2 (HER2, c-erb-B2, HER2/*neu*) is one of four known members of the type 1 family of tyrosine kinase

Cancer Drug Discovery and Development: Biomarkers in Breast Cancer:
Molecular Diagnostics for Predicting and Monitoring Therapeutic Effect
Edited by: G. Gasparini and D. F. Hayes © Humana Press Inc., Totowa, NJ

receptors present in human epithelial cells. These receptors all share significant homology, structurally consisting of an extracellular (ligand binding)
domain, a transmembrane region, and an intracellular domain containing a
tyrosine kinase region *(1)*. In addition to the 4 known receptors, 12 ligands
have been described within this signaling pathway, each exhibiting highly
specific binding to the extracellular domain of one or more of the receptors.
More primitive species have a less diverse and robust HER signaling network. *C. elegans* contains a single receptor and ligand while *Drosophila*
contains four ligands and a single receptor. This evolutionary richness and
diversity is directly related to the critical role this signaling pathway plays
in regulating multiple cellular functions including proliferation, differentiation, adhesion, migration, and survival.

During the past 25 yr much has been learned regarding the precise mechanism by which these various receptors and their ligands associate to initiate
intracellular signal transduction pathways. Two of the receptors have peculiar characteristics. HER2 lacks any known ligand while HER3 has a "dead"
kinase domain. Neither of these receptors can signal without associating or
dimerizing with another member of the HER receptor family. Although
weak signaling may occur with ligand binding to a single receptor (HER1
or HER4), receptor aggregation forming homo- or heterodimeric pairs or
larger oligomeric structures result in sustained and potent signaling. In a
series of elegant experiments, Yarden and colleagues demonstrated that
heterodimers provide a significant increase in signaling potency over
homodimers. In addition, they showed that heterodimers containing HER2
were the most potent signaling complexes, suggesting a central, pivotal role
for HER2 in this pathway *(2)*.

Recently the crystalline structures of HER1, in both its unbound and
ligand bound conformations, HER2 and HER3 have been described *(3–5)*.
These structural observations show that receptor association occurs via a
short hairpin loop within the extracellular domain II region of the receptors.
HER1, in its non-ligand–bound state, assumes a "closed" conformation
with this hairpin loop "buried" within a pocket of domain IV, When ligand
binding occurs at a point between domains I and III there is a substantial
structural change with pivoting of the receptor complex, disruption of the
domain II–IV interaction, and exposure of the hairpin loop to form an "open"
conformation available for receptor interactions. The structure of HER2
demonstrated that this critical hairpin loop is constitutively exposed,
explaining the lack of need for a HER2 ligand. By adopting this fixed,
"open" conformation, HER2 is always "ready to partner" with other receptor members and serves to explain the pivotal role that HER2 plays in this
signaling pathway.

2. THE DEVELOPMENT OF HERCEPTIN®

Although these reports were published well after the development of Herceptin, earlier observations suggested that HER2 was an attractive target for therapeutic cancer drug development. Human *HER2* was initially cloned by Ullrich and colleagues at Genentech in the mid-1980s and soon thereafter shown to be an oncogene *(6)*. When *HER2* was transfected into normal cells they became transformed and displayed all the characteristics of malignant cells when grown in soft agar (Fig. 1) *(7,8)*. At the same time, the initial reports were published suggesting that 25–30% of human breast cancers demonstrated an abnormality of *HER2*, specifically high-level amplification of a nonmutated copy of the gene *(9)*. In this seminal observation, *HER2* was found to be amplified in a subset of breast cancers and that amplification was shown to be a significant negative prognostic indicator, implying an integral role for *HER2* in the biology of these cancers. This finding has been confirmed in many subsequent studies and there is considerable evidence that amplified *HER2* is an early and stable molecular abnormality in breast cancer and an adverse prognostic indicator in both node-positive and node-negative disease *(10–13)*. Because amplification is not associated with mutations or splice variants, corresponding increases in mRNA and protein expression by Southern, Northern, and Western blotting and immunohistochemistry were also seen *(14)*. The observation that *HER2* amplification was associated with high-level overexpression of its protein product, p185[HER2], provided a framework to consider strategies to antagonize or suppress this abnormal biologic phenotype in human breast cancer.

One strategic approach to suppress the function of a surface expressed protein product of an oncogene is the use of targeted monoclonal antibodies. In the late 1980s, a large (>100) library of murine antihuman HER2 antibodies was generated by immunizing mice with homogenates of human HER2 overexpressing cell lines *(15,16)*. These antibodies were then screened to determine their specificity and binding affinity to HER2. A short list of antibodies with the highest K_d is shown in Table 1.

Following this initial screen, the most promising antibodies were evaluated for antitumor activity in both in vitro and in vivo model systems across a range of tumor cell lines. The antibody that was selected from this screening process for clinical development was known as 4D5. These preclinical studies also provided a critical observation that guided the overall clinical development plan for Herceptin.

From the data shown in Fig. 2, it was apparent that the antitumor activity of 4D5 was confined to cell lines that expressed moderate to high levels of HER2 *(17)*. Although not unexpected, it did suggest that optimal clinical development of this antibody would require the parallel development of an assay to detect amplification or protein overexpression of HER2 in clinical

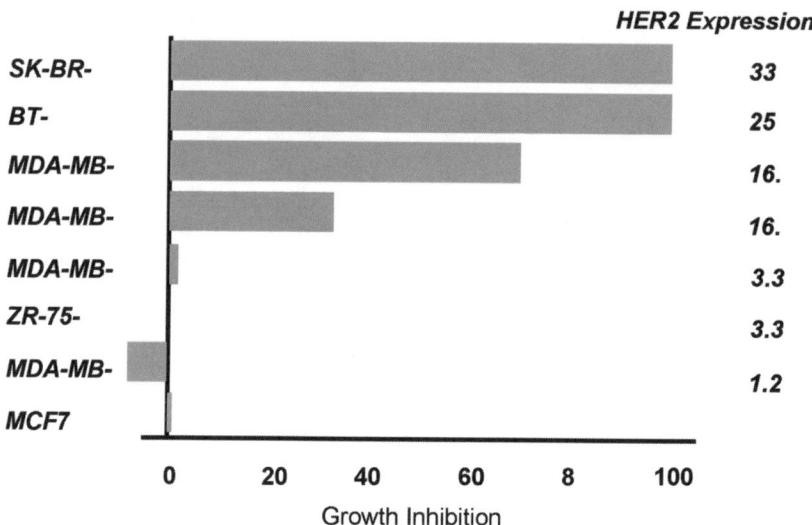

Fig. 1. Antibody inhibition of anchorage-independent growth is related to HER2 expression level.

Table 1
Binding Affinity and Internal Characteristics
of Several Monoclonal Antibodies Against HER2

Monoclonal antibody	Kd® (nm)	Internalization in SK-BR-3
4D5	9.3	243
2H11	2.6	24
7C2	5.0	236
7D3	8.4	133
2C4	8.6	313
7F3	63	1801

tumor material and then restrict enrollment in clinical trials to only those patients whose tumor demonstrated high levels of expressed HER2.

To standardize and validate an immunohistochemistry (IHC) assay to detect expressed p185^{HER2}, three breast cell lines were obtained from the American Type Culture Collection (ATCC); MDA-231, MDA-175, and SK-BR-3. The *HER2* gene copy number, using DNA slot blots (and subsequently by FISH to correct for chromosome 17 ploidy) and quantification of expressed HER2 receptors by Scatchard analysis, was determined as shown in Table 2. These cell lines served as performance controls for the development of a semiquantitative IHC assay, known as the Clinical Trials

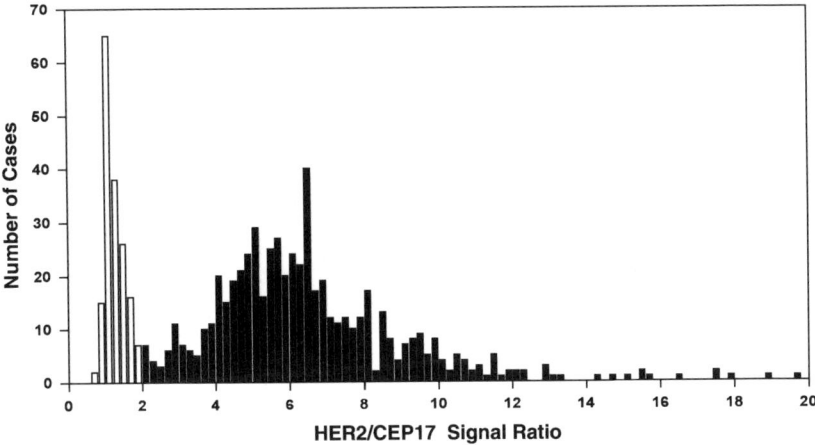

Fig. 2. Distribution of HER2/CEP17 signal ratios ($n = 765$).

Table 2
HER Expression Is Related to *HER2* Amplification
in Cultured Human Breast Cancer Cell Lines

Cell line	HER2 receptors/cell	HER2/neu/CEP17 ratio
MDA-231	21,600	~1.1
MDA-175	92,400	~1.3
SK-BR-3	2,390,000	~4.5

Table 3
Immunohistochemistry Staining of Cultured
Human Breast Cancer Cell Lines to Develop IHC Score for HER2

Cell line	IHC score	Description
MDA-231	0	No discernible membrane staining
MDA-175	1+	Faint/barely perceptible, incomplete membrane staining
SK-BR-3	3+	Moderate/strong complete membrane staining

Assay (CTA) subsequently utilized to select patients for the Herceptin development trials.

4D5 was the antibody selected for the assay with a standard antimouse antibody and an avidin–biotin horseradish peroxidase complex. The antigen retrieval consisted of limited protease treatment. The conditions for the assay were standardized to obtain a reliable and characteristic membrane-staining pattern from each of the performance control cell lines as shown in Table 3.

After the development and validation of this assay, human clinical trials using antibody 4D5 (murine) were initiated. Only patients whose tumor scored 2+ or 3+ using the CTA were enrolled in all subsequent clinical trials. A total of 26 women with advanced metastatic breast cancer, known to be HER2 positive, were treated in a single dose and a multiple dose phase I trial with this murine antibody. Infusion reactions were common and both trials demonstrated the rapid and frequent development of neutralizing human antimouse antibodies (HAMA). Despite these findings, several patients in these trials demonstrated clear, but transient, objective tumor regression, establishing the "proof of concept" that antibodies to HER2 could result in antitumor effects in humans.

Advances in protein and antibody engineering in the late 1980s made it possible to conceptualize the idea of "grafting" the backbone of a human immunoglobulin molecule onto the consensus determining regions (CDRs) or binding domains of a specific murine monoclonal antibody; essentially "humanizing" the antibody. This concept would theoretically enable chronic, long-term dosing by avoiding the development of HAMAs and, with an intact and functional human F_c domain, could provide for additional antitumor activity by initiating targeted antibody-dependent cellular cyto-toxicity (ADCC). Through a series of landmark technical achievements, a human IgG$_1$ molecule was successfully grafted onto antibody 4D5 (18). Hundreds of clones were created in this process to determine the precise sequence location where binding affinity began to degrade. The optimal clone was composed of 95% human and 5% murine sequences and was determined to have higher binding affinity to human HER2 and better antitumor activity in human xenograft model systems when compared with the native murine antibody, 4D5. This humanized antibody is now known as trastuzumab or Herceptin.

A small phase I program to establish the safety and pharmacokinetics of Herceptin was initiated in 1992. Infusion reactions continued to be seen with the humanized antibody in 30–40% of patients; however, they were rarely severe and typically confined only to the first infusion. The half-life was estimated to be 5–6 d and, most importantly, no HAMAs were detected with the humanized antibody. During the phase I period, additional preclinical studies were conducted to assess the interaction between Herceptin and several chemotherapeutic agents. Striking synergy was noted when HER2 overexpressing cells were exposed to the combination of Herceptin and the DNA damaging agent cisplatin (19). These observations led to the development of two phase II trials with Herceptin. The first trial (H0551g) evaluated single-agent Herceptin at the target dose of 4 mg/kg as a loading dose and then 2 mg/kg/wk until disease progression in highly refractory HER2-positive metastatic breast cancer. This trial showed that the drug was well tolerated and demonstrated an objective response rate of 11% (20). The second

Table 4
Trastuzumab and Chemotherapy:
In Vitro Cytotoxicity Against HER2-Positive Breast Cancer Cell Lines[a]

Synergistic (CI <1)		Additive (CI = 1)		Subadditive (CI >1)	
Vinorelbine	0.34	Doxorubicin	0.82–1.16	Fluorouracil	2.87
Docetaxel/carboplatin	0.34	Paclitaxel	0.91		
Docetaxel	0.41	Epirubicin	0.99		
Etoposide	0.54	Vinblastine	1.09		
Cyclophosphamide	0.57	Methotrexate	1.36		
Paclitaxel/carboplatin	0.64				
Thiotepa	0.67				
Cisplatin	0.67				
Liposomal doxorubicin	0.7				
Gemcitabine	1.25–5.34 (variable, dose-dependent)				

[a]Based on a Combination Index (CI) score from multiple drug-effect analysis at fixed molar ratios. Pegram et al. *Oncogene* 1999;18:2241; Pegram et al. *Semin Oncol* 2000;27(Suppl 11):21; Slamon and Pegram. *Semin Oncol* 2001;28(Suppl 3):13.

trial (H0552g) attempted to exploit the preclinical observations of synergy by utilizing the novel combination of Herceptin and cisplatin. The eligibility for this trial required patients to have particularly aggressive disease, demonstrating progressive disease *during* treatment with prior chemotherapy. Despite selecting for this very poor prognostic feature, the trial demonstrated an overall response rate of 24% with an additional 24% of patients achieving either a minor response or stable disease *(21)*. Subsequently a larger panel of agents was tested, in multiple HER2 overexpressing models, to guide the optimal combination of Herceptin with chemotherapeutic drugs *(22)*. Table 4 shows the results of those experiments. Many agents demonstrate additive or synergistic activity, with vinorelbine, the platinum salts cisplatin and carboplatin, docetaxel, and the antiestrogen tamoxifen showing the greatest synergistic interactions. Doxorubicin, cyclophosphamide, and paclitaxel all showed additive interactions and 5-fluorouracil (5-FU) was the only agent tested that demonstrated less than an additive interaction.

The pivotal development program for Herceptin included two large clinical trials: one phase II trial evaluating the agent as monotherapy in relapsed breast cancer following one or two prior regimens for metastatic disease and a second phase III trial evaluating doxorubicin and cyclophosphamide (AC) with or without Herceptin in first-line therapy of metastatic disease. Patients in both trials were required to have HER2 overexpression with a score of 2+ or 3+ using the CTA performed at a single reference laboratory. Because of the increasing use of doxorubicin in the adjuvant setting and the approval of paclitaxel for the treatment of metastatic breast cancer, the phase III trial was amended approximately halfway through recruitment to provide for two different chemotherapy strata. Patients naïve to anthracyclines in the adjuvant setting continued to be treated with AC ± Herceptin while patients who had received anthracyclines in the adjuvant setting were assigned to paclitaxel ± Herceptin. This second strata had more unfavorable baseline prognostic characteristics consisting of larger size tumors, higher lymph node burden, and a shorter disease-free interval following adjuvant chemotherapy. The phase III trial specified a minimum of six cycles of chemotherapy (AC or paclitaxel) with further chemotherapy at the discretion of the investigator. Few patients received more than six cycles of cytotoxic chemotherapy. Herceptin was given as a weekly dose concomitantly with chemotherapy and then continued until the point of disease progression, which was the primary end point of the clinical trial. At progression, patients in the control arm were eligible to receive Herceptin as part of a separate protocol and approx 65% went on to receive the drug from this treatment arm. Patients in the experimental arm were also permitted to continue to receive Herceptin after initial disease progression and approx 50% continued treatment in this arm. This aspect of the study design is important when assessing the results, given the possibility that this prespecified "crossover" design may have reduced some of the treatment effect from Herceptin on end points occurring after progression (i.e., overall survival).

The phase III trial (study H0648g) reached the predefined number of events in late 1997 and was unblinded, revealing a highly significant improvement in the primary end point, time to disease progression. The addition of Herceptin to standard chemotherapy for HER2 overexpressing metastatic breast cancer improved the time to disease progression from 4.6 to 7.4 mo ($p = 0.0001$; see Table 5). This treatment effect was seen in both chemotherapy strata (AC and paclitaxel), and secondary efficacy end points of response rate, duration of response, and time to treatment failure were also significantly improved with the addition of Herceptin to standard chemotherapy.

Although the trial was unblinded 9 mo after the last patient was enrolled, patients continued to be followed for survival until the final study analysis was completed 30 mo after the last patient was enrolled. This ensured that all patients were followed beyond the median survival time point. Despite the fact that 65% of the control patients crossed over and received Herceptin at the time of disease progression, median survival improved from 20.3 mo to 25.1 mo ($p = 0.046$) (23).

The large phase II trial (study H0649g) of single-agent Herceptin in HER2 overexpressing metastatic breast cancer following one or two prior chemotherapy regimens for metastatic disease also confirmed the clinical activity of Herceptin. A total of 222 patients were treated with Herceptin as a weekly dose and an overall response rate of 14% was confirmed by a blinded, external response evaluation committee (24). A subsequent clini-

Table 5
Trastuzumab Efficacy in Prospective Randomized Clinical Trial of Patients with Metastatic Breast Cancer

	Either chemotherapy		Efficacy (all enrolled patients) doxorubicin and cyclophosphamide		Paclitaxel	
	+ traztuzumab (n = 235)	Alone (n = 234)	+ traztuzumab (n = 143)	Alone (n = 138)	+ traztuzumab (n = 92)	Alone (n = 96)
Complete response (CR)	18/235 (8)	11/234 (5)	12/143 (8)	9/143 (7)	6/92 (7)	2/96 (2)
Partial response (PR)	96/235 (41)	66/234 (28)	63/143 (44)	50/138 (36)	33/92 (36)	13/96 (14)
Overall CR + PR 95%	114/235 (49)	74/234 (32)	75/143 (52)	59/138 (43)	39/92 (42)	15/96 (16)
	$p < 0.001$		$p = 0.10$		$p = <0.001$	
Median response duration (mo)	9.3	5.9	9.1	6.5	11.0	4.4
	$p < 0.001$		$p = 0.0025$		$p < 0.001$	
Median time to disease progression (mo)	7.4	4.6	8.1	6.1	6.9	3.0
Relative risk (95% CI)	0.51 (0.41, 0.63)		0.62 (0.47, 0.81)		0.38 (0.27, 0.53)	
	$p < 0.001$		$p < 0.001$		$p < 0.001$	
Median time to treatment failure (mo)	6.9	4.5	7.2	5.6	5.8	2.9
Relative risk (95% CI)	0.58 (0.47, 0.70)		0.67 (0.52, 0.86)		0.46 (0.33, 0.63)	
	$p < 0.001$		$p = 0.001$		$p < 0.001$	
Median survival (mo)	25.1	20.3	26.8	21.4	22.1	18.4
Relative risk (95% CI)	0.80 (0.64, 1.00)		0.82 (.61, 1.09)		0.80 (.56, 1.11)	
	$p = 0.046$		$p = 0.16$		$p = 0.18$	

Duration of response was defined as the time from first response to disease progression or death. Time to treatment failure was defined as the time from randomization to disease progression, study discontinuation for any reason, use of additional anti-tumor therapy, or death.

The final analysis of the primary end point was performed 9 mo after enrollment of the last patient. The most recent survival data were obtained 30 mo after enrollment of the last patient, with a median follow-up of 35 mo (range: 30–51 mo). As of the data cutoff date of December 31, 1997, 388 of 469 (83%) of patients had discontinued the study, including 173 of 235 (74%) of patients receiving rhuMAb HER2 plus chemotherapy and 215 of 234 (92%) of patients receiving chemotherapy alone. From ref. 23 with permission.

cal trial of single-agent Herceptin in previously untreated patients with HER2 overexpressing metastatic breast cancer (study H0650g) demonstrated an objective response rate of 26% *(25)*. The three single-agent Herceptin trials (H0551g, H0649g, and H0650g) treated patients with highly refractory metastatic disease, refractory metastatic disease, and untreated metastatic disease, respectively, and demonstrated response rates of 11%, 14%, and 26%, suggesting that Herceptin is most effective when used early in the treatment of HER2-positive breast cancer.

3. HER2 TESTING AND THE IMPACT ON TREATMENT EFFECT FROM HERCEPTIN

All of the pivotal trials described in the previous section utilized an IHC assay known as the Clinical Trials Assay (CTA) to define eligible patients. Scores of 2+ or 3+ were defined as "positive," rendering the patient eligible for enrollment while scores of 0 or 1+ were defined as "negative." Although the pivotal trials were not adequately powered to evaluate definitively the impact of IHC score (2+ vs 3+) on treatment effect, the retrospective analysis did suggest that the treatment effect was seen predominantly in the patients whose tumors had the highest (3+) expression of HER2. In the single-agent trial, H0649g, the response rate was 6% in the 2+ group and 18% in the 3+ group. In the pivotal chemotherapy trial, H0648g, median time to disease progression in the 2+ group went from 5.6 to 6.6 mo while in the 3+ group the improvement was from 4.6 to 8.5 mo.

Further confusion around the definition of HER2 overexpression in the Herceptin pivotal trials was introduced with the development of the HercepTest™ assay. Although the CTA was used to select patients during clinical development, this assay was complicated and not well suited to commercialization. The HercepTest is a different IHC assay that was designed and developed to provide "similar" results to those provided by the CTA. In a large concordance study performed on more than 600 clinical specimens, the HercepTest assay was found to provide the same result as the CTA in 82% of individual samples. Although HercepTest was approved by the US Food and Drug Administration (FDA) to aid in the selection of patients for Herceptin therapy, there were no prospective or retrospective analyses of the predictive value of a score of 2+ or 3+ on the treatment effect of Herceptin. Unfortunately, tissue blocks were not archived from any of the pivotal Herceptin studies. Only tissue sections, 4–6 μm thick and mounted on glass slides, were retained from the patients' original tumor specimens. These type of specimens are subject to oxidation and other factors, resulting in significant antigen degradation over time and an unacceptable rate of "false-negative" IHC assay results. A small, pilot study of the HercepTest assay on archived material from the pivotal trials confirmed this high rate of false-negative results and served to highlight the need to archive tissue blocks or tissue microarrays from patients enrolled in clinical trials of targeted agents such that retrospective analyses of various diagnostic assays can be performed and correlated with clinical results.

Since the introduction of the HercepTest assay for the selection of patients for Herceptin therapy, there has been increasing concern over the reliability of IHC assays to assess HER2 status accurately in routine (formalin-fixed and paraffin-embedded, or FFPE) clinical specimens. IHC assays for HER2 are subject to a number of potential shortcomings, including variability in fixation techniques, reagents, antigen retrieval methods, and subjectivity of staining interpretation. These shortcomings can result in both false-positive and false-negative results (26–30). Because the primary molecular abnormality resulting in HER2 overexpression in 25–30% of human breast cancer is amplification of a nonmutated copy of the gene, alternative diagnostic strategies to directly assess gene copy number were evaluated in the belief that these technologies might provide more consistent and precise information as compared to IHC. Fluorescence in situ hybridization (FISH) is a technique in which a highly specific complementary DNA sequence (probe) is developed to the gene of interest and then labeled (either directly or indirectly) with a florescent tag for eventual visualization/detection (31,32). Clinical tumor samples are subjected to mild protease digestion to disrupt histones and DNA crosslinking to allow the probe access to the gene of interest. Probe is applied to the digested samples, allowed to bind or "anneal" to the genetic sequence, and the gene copy number is simply quantitated by counting the number of fluorescent signals in each cell. Many FISH systems also include a "control" probe to a centromeric gene sequence to correct for chromosomal gain or loss and to differentiate ploidy from true amplification. When this approach is used, FISH status is expressed as the ratio of the number of copies of the gene of interest to the number of control genes. In a normal situation there would be two target genes and two control genes for a ratio of 1. Because of technical issues, ratios between 1 and 2 are typically consider a "gray zone" result, with ratios ≥ 2 clearly indicating gene amplification. FISH represents a huge technical advance over older methods of gene quantification, such as Southern or DNA slot-blotting, in that FISH assays can be performed on routinely processed, FFPE clinical material as opposed to fresh or frozen clinical material. In addition, the resilience of DNA makes this assay far more robust than IHC and avoids many of the problems of specimen processing and age effects that hamper protein detection assays such as IHC.

This technical advantage enabled the retrospective evaluation of FISH status as a predictor of clinical benefit in three large, pivotal Herceptin clinical trials; H0648g, H0649g, and H0650g. A total of 799 patients were enrolled in these trials, all patients tested positive at the 2+ or 3+ level using

Table 6
Objective Response Rates by HER2 Amplification Status
in Patients Treated with Trastuzumab Alone

Study	HER2 amplification	Evaluable patients (No.)	Objective responses No.	%
Study H0649g	FISH-positive	173	33	19
	FISH-negative	36	0	0
Study H0650g	FISH-positive	79	27	34
	FISH-negative	29	2	7

Table 7
Objective Response Rates by HER2 Amplification Status
for Patients Treated with Trastuzumab
and Chemotherapy vs Chemotherapy Alone—Study H0648g

HER2 amplification	Trastuzumab and chemotherapy			Chemotherapy alone			p
	Evaluable patients No.	Objective responses No.	%	Evaluable patients No.	Objective responses No.	%	
FISH-positive	176	95	54	168	51	30	<.0001
FISH-negative	50	19	38	57	22	39	NS

the CTA. Archival tissue sections were available from 784 (98%) and FISH results were generated from 765 (96%). This high rate of technical success confirmed the robust characteristics of FISH and served to minimize some of the risk associated with retrospective analyses where missing data points can hamper the generalization of results. The first interesting finding from this analysis was that only 78% of the tumors were found to be amplified, suggesting significant discordance between an IHC score of 2+ or 3+ and the presence of HER2 gene amplification. The distribution of FISH scores shown in Fig. 2 demonstrates a bimodal distribution, with a median ratio of 6.1 in the FISH positive group and 1.2 in the FISH-negative group. This distribution is similar to other reported data and supports the cutpoint of 2 in separating amplified and nonamplified tumors *(33,34)*.

The next series of tables and K–M graphs outline the clinical activity of Herceptin in these three trials, in both the FISH-positive and FISH-negative subgroups. Table 6 shows the single-agent response rates in studies H0649g and H0650g. Of the 65 FISH-negative patients in these two studies, objective responses were seen in only two patients and, on further testing, one

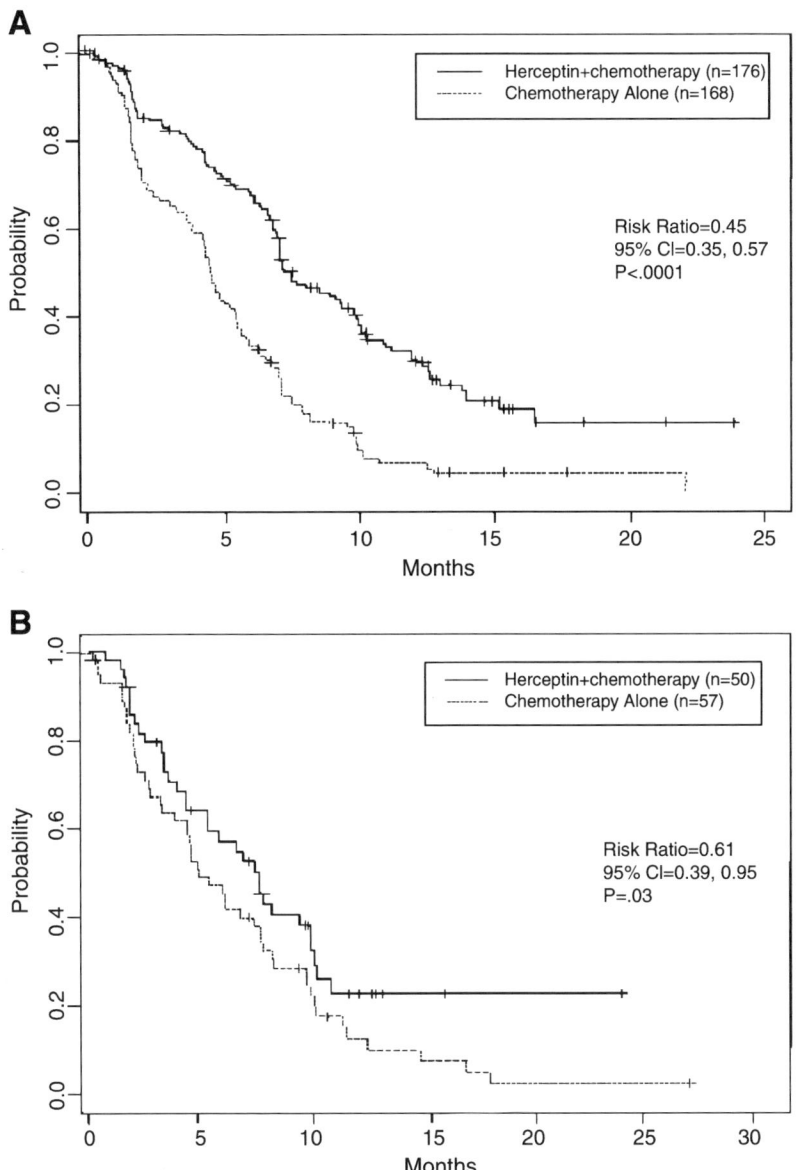

Fig. 3. Time to disease progression by HER2 amplification status for patients receiving chemotherapy + trastuzumab vs chemotherapy alone (study H0648g). (**A**) FISH-positive. (**B**) FISH-negative.

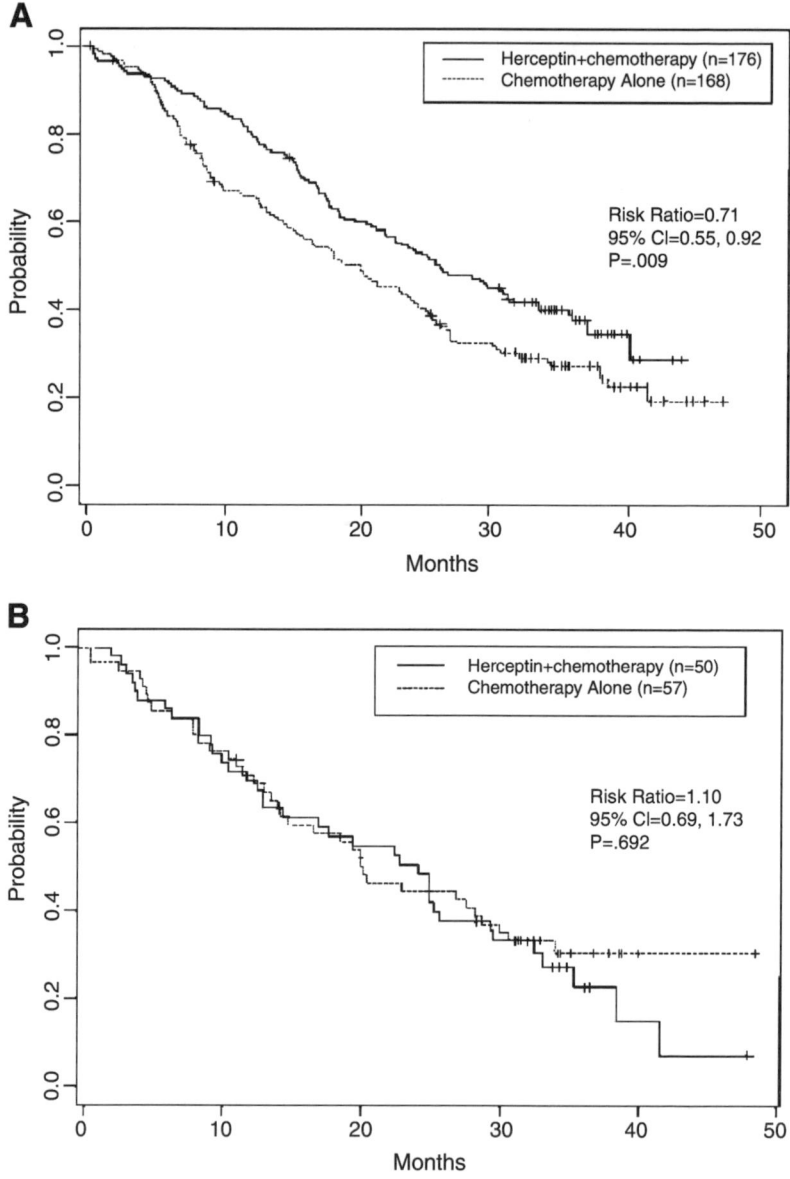

Fig. 4. Overall survival time by HER2 amplification status for patients receiving chemotherapy + trastuzumab vs chemotherapy alone (study H0648g). (**A**) FISH-positive. (**B**) FISH-negative.

of these two patients was found to have gene amplification. The same association was seen in study H0648g (*see* Table 7). In the FISH-negative group, response went from 39% to 38% with the addition of Herceptin while in the FISH-positive group response rate went from 30% to 54%.

The time to disease progression in study H0648g was strikingly improved in the FISH-positive group with a risk ratio of 0.45 ($p < 0.0001$); however, there was also borderline improvement for the FISH-negative group with a risk ratio of 0.61 ($p = 0.03$) (Fig. 3).

Finally, in evaluating the critical end point of survival there was clearly significant improvement from the addition of Herceptin in the FISH-positive population (risk ratio = 0.71, $p = 0.009$) that was not apparent in the FISH-negative group (risk ratio = 1.10, $p = 0.692$) (Fig. 4).

All the efficacy analysis in these three trials suggested that the treatment effect from Herceptin was limited to the FISH-positive population with the exception of the time to progression analysis in study H0648g. It is not clear whether this is a "real" treatment effect or whether this is a statistical anomaly, an inherent risk in the conduct of multiple retrospective subset analyses. The preponderance of the data from the other efficacy analyses, however, suggests the latter as the most reasonable conclusion.

4. CONCLUSIONS

Herceptin represents one of a few but growing class of "targeted" anticancer agents: agents that are specifically designed to precisely antagonize, or suppress, the abnormal biologic phenotype responsible for the malignant characteristics of a particular tumor. In some malignant conditions, the target biologic abnormality occurs with high frequency within the affected population, rendering screening prior to the therapeutic application of targeted therapy unnecessary. This situation is best exemplified by the abnormal *bcr–abl* tyrosine kinase in chronic myelogenous leukemia and the targeted therapeutic agent imatinib (Gleevec®). Unfortunately, this situation of "high prevalence" appears to be uncommon, with most solid tumors demonstrating significant phenotypic and/or genotypic heterogeneity. As new agents are developed targeting molecular abnormalities that affect a minority of patients with a specific tumor type, detection of the underlying abnormality and the specific methodology to detect that target will assume increasing importance when assessing therapeutic benefit. Important work to date suggests that the use of FISH to detect the primary biologic alteration, amplification of HER2, is the preferred methodology to select breast cancer patients for Herceptin therapy as compared to IHC. Diagnostic methods are inevitably destined to evolve along with remarkable advances in technology, however. This observation reinforces the vital need to prospectively incorporate tissue acquisition and archiving into ongoing clinical development plans for the new generation of targeted anticancer agents.

REFERENCES

1. Yarden Y, Sliwkowski MX. Untangling the ErbB signalling network. *Nat Rev Mol Cell Biol* 2001;2:127–137.
2. Pinkas-Kramarski R, et al. Diversification of *neu* differentiation factor and epidermal growth factor signaling by combinatorial receptor interactions. *EMBO J* 1996;15:2452–2467.
3. Ogiso H, et al. Crystal structure of the complex of human epidermal growth factor and receptor extracellular domains. *Cell* 2002;110:775–787.
4. Cho HS, Leahy DJ. Structure of the extracellular region of HER3 reveals an interdomain tether. *Science* 2002;297:1330–1333.
5. Cho HS, Mason K, Ramyar KX, et al. Structure of the extracellular region of HER2 alone and in complex with the Herceptin Fab. *Nature* 2003;421:756–760.
6. DiFiore PP, et al. ErbB-2 is a potent oncogene when overexpressed in NIH/3T3 cells. *Science* 1987;237:178–182.
7. Hudziak RM, Schlessinger J, Ullrich A. Increased expression of the putative growth factor receptor p185HER2 causes transformation and tumorigenesis of HIB3T3 cells. *PNAS* 1987;84:7159–7163.
8. Coussens L, Yang-Feng TL, Liao YC, et al. Tyrosine kinase receptor with extensive homology to EGF receptor shares chromosomal location with neu oncogene. *Science* 1985;230:1132–1139.
9. Slamon DJ, Clark G, Wong SG, Levin WJ, Ullrich A, McGuire WL. Human breast cancer: correlation of relapse and survival with amplification of the HER-2/*neu* oncogene. *Science* 1987;235:177–182.
10. Gusterson BA, Gelber RD, Goldhirsch A, et al. Prognostic importance of c-*erb*B-2 expression in breast cancer. *J Clin Oncol* 1992;7:1049–1056.
11. Andrulis IL, Bull SB, Blackstein ME, et al. *neu/erbB-2* amplification identifies a poor-prognosis group of women with node-negative breast cancer. *J Clin Oncol* 1998;16:1340–1349.
12. Press MF, Pike MC, Chazin VR, et al. Her-2/neu expression in node-negative breast cancer: direct tissue quantitation by computerized image analysis and association of overexpression with increased risk of recurrent disease. *Cancer Res* 1993;53:4960–4970.
13. Press MF, Bernstein L, Thomas PA, et al. HER-2/neu amplification characterized by fluorescence in situ hybridization: poor prognosis in node-negative breast carcinomas. *J Clin Oncol* 1997;15:2894–2904.
14. Slamon DJ, Godolphin W, Jones LA, et al. Studies of the HER-2/*neu* proto-oncogene in human breast and ovarian cancer. *Science* 1989;244:707–712.
15. Fendly BM, Winget M, Hudziak RM, Lipari MT, Napier MA, Ullrich A. Characterization of murine monoclonal antibodies reactive to either the human epidermal growth factor receptor or HER2/neu gene product. *Cancer Res* 1990;50:1550–1558.
16. Shepard HM, Lewis GD, Sarup JC, et al. Monoclonal antibody therapy of human cancer: taking the HER2 protooncogene to the clinic. *J Clin Immunol* 1991;11:117–127.
17. Lewis GD, Figari I, Fendly B, et al. Differential responses of human tumor cell lines to anti-p185HER2 monoclonal antibodies. *Cancer Immunol Immunother* 1993;37:255–263.
18. Carter P, Presta L, et al. Humanization of an anti-p185 antibody for human cancer therapy. *PNAS* 1992;89:4285–4289.

19. Pietras RJ, Fendly BM, Chazin VR, Pegram MD, Howell SB, Slamon DJ. Antibody to HER-2/neu receptor blocks DNA repair after cisplatin in human breast and ovarian cancer cells. *Oncogene* 1994;9:1829–1838.

20. Baselga J, Tripathy D, Mendelsohn J, et al. Phase II study of weekly intravenous recombinant humanized anti-p185HER2 monoclonal antibody in patients with HER2/neu-overexpressing metastatic breast cancer. *J Clin Oncol* 1996; 14:737–744.

21. Pegram MD, Lipton A, Hayes DF, et al. Phase II study of receptor-enhanced chemosensitivity using recombinant humanized anti-p185HER2/neu monoclonal antibody plus cisplatin in patients with HER2/neu-overexpressing metastatic breast cancer refractory to chemotherapy treatment. *J Clin Oncol* 1998;16:2659–2671.

22. Pegram M, Hsu S, Lewis G, et al. Inhibitory effects of combinations of HER-2/neu antibody and chemotherapeutic agents used for treatment of human breast cancers. *Oncogene* 1999;18:2241–2251.

23. Slamon DJ, Leyland-Jones B, Shak S, et al. Use of chemotherapy plus a monoclonal antibody against HER2 for metastatic breast cancer that overexpresses HER2. *N Engl J Med* 2001;344:783–792.

24. Cobleigh MA, Vogel CL, Tripathy D, et al. Multinational study of the efficacy and safety of humanized anti-HER2 monoclonal antibody in women who have HER2-overexpressing metastatic breast cancer that has progressed after chemotherapy for metastatic disease. *J Clin Oncol* 1999;17:2639–2648.

25. Vogel CL, Cobleigh MA, Tripathy D, et al. Efficacy and safety of trastuzumab (Herceptin) as a single agent in first-line treatment of HER2-overexpressing metastatic breast cancer. *J Clin Oncol* 2002;20:719–726.

26. Press MF, Hung G, Godolphin W, et al. Sensitivity of HER-2/new antibodies in archival tissue samples: potential source of error in immunohistochemical studies of oncogene expression. *Cancer Res* 1994;54:2771–2777.

27. Pauletti G, Godolphin W, Press MF, et al. Detection and quantitation of HER-2/ *neu* gene amplification in human breast cancer archival material using fluorescence *in situ* hybridization. *Oncogene* 1996;13:63–72.

28. Pauletti G, Dandekar S, Rong H, et al. Assessment of methods for tissue-based detection of the HER-2/Nneu alteration in human breast cancer: a direct comparison of fluorescence in situ hybridization and immunohistochemistry. *J Clin Oncol* 2000;18:3651–3664.

29. Tubbs RR, Pettay JD, Roche PC, et al. Discrepancies in clinical laboratory testing of eligibility for trastuzumab therapy: apparent immunohistochemical false-positives do not get the message. *J Clin Oncol* 2001;19:2714–2721.

30. Lebeau A, Deimling D, Kaltz C, et al. HER-2/neu analysis in archival tissue samples of human breast cancer: comparison of immunohistochemistry and fluorescence in situ hybridization. *J Clin Oncol* 2001;19:354–363.

31. Pinkel D, Straume T, Gray JW. Cytogenetic analysis using quantitative, high-sensitivity, fluorescence hybridization. *Proc Natl Acad Sci USA* 1986;83:2934–2938.

32. Kallioniemi OP, Kallioniemi A, Kurisu W, et al. ERBB2 amplification in breast cancer analyzed by fluorescence *in situ* hybridization. *Proc Natl Acad Sci USA* 1992;89:5321–5325.

33. Berry D, Muss H, Thor A, et al. HER-2/*neu* and p53 expression versus tamoxifen. Resistance in estrogen receptor-positive, node-positive breast cancer. *J Clin Oncol* 2000;18:3471–3479.

34. "PathVysion" HER-2 DNA Probe Kit package instructions. Vysis Inc., Downers Grove, IL, 2000.

10 The Epidermal Growth Factor Receptor Pathway as a Selective Molecular-Targeted Treatment in Human Breast Cancer

Fortunato Ciardiello, MD, Teresa Troiani, MD, and Giampaolo Tortora, MD

CONTENTS

Cancer Drug Discovery and Development: Biomarkers in Breast Cancer:
Molecular Diagnostics for Predicting and Monitoring Therapeutic Effect
Edited by: G. Gasparini and D. F. Hayes © Humana Press Inc., Totowa, NJ

SUMMARY

The regulation of normal breast development is dependent on several hormones. Among these hormones, estrogens play an essential role in the control of normal mammary development and in the etiology and progression of breast cancer.

Key Words: Breast cancer; EGF; EGFR.

1. INTRODUCTION

The regulation of normal breast development is dependent on several hormones. Among these hormones, estrogens play an essential role in the control of normal mammary development and in the etiology and progression of breast cancer. More recently, it has been recognized that normal and malignant mammary epithelial are also able to synthesize a number of different locally acting peptide growth factors that function through autocrine, juxtacrine, and paracrine pathways. Several studies have demonstrated that estrogens influence mammary epithelial cell growth both directly and indirectly by modulating growth factor production and growth factor receptor expression *(1)*. Among these, the epidermal growth factor (EGF) family of peptides, in combination with their specific cognate receptors, is involved in the regulation of mammary gland development, morphogenesis, and lactation, and also play a pivotal role in the pathogeneses of human breast cancer *(2)*. The purpose of this chapter is to describe the role of EGF-related growth factors and their receptors in the control of proliferation and differentiation of human mammary epithelial cells and in the pathogenesis of human breast cancer and to discuss the possibility of using drugs that selectively block the activation of the EGFR as anticancer therapy in human breast cancer.

2. EXPRESSION OF THE EGF FAMILY IN BREAST CANCER

EGF is a 6-kDa polypeptide of 53 amino acids. The human EGF gene is located on chromosome 4 *(3)*. It was originally isolated from the male mouse submaxillary gland as a factor that caused eyelid opening *(4)* and later from human urine as urogastrone *(5)*. EGF is a transmembrane glycosylated protein that is biologically active as it can bind to and activate EGF receptors in adjacent cell through a juxtacrine mode of action *(6)*. It has been found to stimulate the growth of both normal and transformed human mammary epithelial cells. Breast cancer cells are also able to synthesize EGF. In fact, EGF mRNA has been detected in a majority of human breast cancer cell lines, with the estrogen-receptor (ER)-positive breast cancer cell lines T47-D and ZR-75-1 showing higher levels of expression as compared to the ER-negative breast cancer cell lines *(7)*. Progestins were found to specifically increase the levels of EGF mRNA in T47-D cells, while 17β-estradiol had no effect on EGF mRNA levels in this cell line *(8,9)*. EGF mRNA was also detected in 83% of human breast tumors and in addition EGF protein has been detected in 15–30% of human primary invasive breast carcinomas *(8,9)*. EGF is a crucial regulator of growth and differentiation in the mouse mammary gland, especially during pregnancy and lactation and during the spontaneous formation of mammary tumors *(8,9)*.

Transforming growth factor-α (TGF-α) was first identified in the culture media of virus-transformed cells and of human tumors cell. It shares 42% homology with human EGF. Its tertiary structure is identical to EGF and is able to bind to the EGF receptor with the same affinity. Several clinical and experimental studies have demonstrated that TGF-α is an important modulator of the malignant progression of mammary epithelial cells in breast cancer *(8,9)*. In particular, TGF-α is a potent mitogen for normal and malignant mammary epithelial cell in vitro and, similar to EGF, is able to stimulate lobuloalveolar development of the mouse mammary gland in vivo *(8,9)*. The basal levels of TGF-α are higher in ER-positive estrogen-responsive, breast cancer cell lines. TGF-α mRNA and protein are induced by physiological concentration of 17β-estradiol. The mechanism of induction seems to be transcriptional because several imperfect estrogen response elements (EREs) that are located in the promoter region of the TGF-α gene are thought to be active, as determined by an increase in CAT activity of transiently transfected breast cancer cells. This induction can be blocked with the antiestrogen tamoxifen, suggesting that this effect is mediated through the ER. In this regard, it has been demonstrated that tamoxifen can reduce the production of TGF-α by 30–70% in primary human breast tumors that are ER positive *(8,9)*. In addition, in one study tamoxifen treatment of breast cancer patients resulted in a 10-fold reduction in TGF-α tumor levels. These data demonstrate that TGF-α can act as an autocrine growth factor and can function as a mediator in part for the growth-promoting effects of oestrogen in human breast cancer cells. The majority of the tumors that express higher levels of TGF-α also express higher levels of the EGF receptor (EGFR), suggesting that an autocrine loop may be operative. TGF-α mRNA and protein levels have been detected in 40–70% of human breast tumors. RNA *in situ* hybridization has shown that TGF-α mRNA is expressed mainly in breast cancer cells and not in the surrounding stromal cells or in infiltrating lymphoid cells *(8,9)*. TGF-α has also been detected in premalignant atypical ductal hyperplasias, ductal hyperplasias, ductal carcinoma *in situ*, and in 30–50% of primary and metastatic human breast carcinomas at levels that are generally two to threefold higher than the levels found in benign breast lesions or in normal mammary tissues *(8,9)*. TGF-α has also been found in the pleural effusions and in the urine samples from metastatic breast cancer patients. Higher levels of TGF-α in pleural effusions correlate with poor prognosis and performance status and with tumor burden. TGF-α mRNA has been detected during the proliferative, lobular development of both the rat and human mammary gland and its expression is enhanced during pregnancy and lactation, suggesting some form of hormonal control of TGF-α production in vivo *(8,9)*.

Amphiregulin (AR) is a glycoprotein that is structurally related to EGF, but it has lower affinity for the EGFR than TGF-α and EGF. Expression of high levels of endogenous AR mRNA and protein has also been found in several normal human mammary epithelial cell strains in culture and in nontransformed human mammary epithelial cell lines. Furthermore, AR and TGF-α can function as autocrine growth factor in these cells. AR has a bifunctional mode of action. Depending on the concentration, the presence of other growth factors and the target cells, it can either stimulate or inhibit cell proliferation. Although AR has been reported to inhibit the growth of some breast cancer cell lines, there is also evidence to suggest that AR can function as autocrine growth factor in human breast cancer cells. In fact, AR is expressed in a number of human ER-positive and ER-negative breast cancer cell lines *(8,9)*. ER-positive breast cancer cell lines generally express higher levels of AR when compared to ER-negative cell lines, and estrogen treatment induces the expression of AR mRNA in MCF-7 breast cancer cells. A significant correlation between AR and ER expression was found in a subset of human primary breast carcinomas that were examined for AR mRNA expression by Northern blot analysis. AR mRNA expression was found in approx 60% of these tumors, and all the tumors that were positive for AR expression were also found to be ER positive.

The possible role of heregulins (HRGs) in regulating the proliferation and the differentiation of human breast cancer cells has not yet been clarified, as HRGs have been demonstrated to either stimulate or inhibit the growth breast cancer cells in vitro and to induce the differentiation of breast cancer cells at least with respect to facilitating the expression of milk protein. HRG mRNA has been detected in both normal and malignant breast tissues and in a small number of human breast cancer cell lines *(8,9)*. Its distribution is more restricted than that of TGF-α or AR, because generally ER-negative, estrogen-independent cell line express HRG, whereas only one ER-negative breast cancer cell line was found to express low levels of HGR mRNA *(8,9)*. However, HRG seems to inhibit the effect of estrogen in ER-positive estrogen-responsive breast cancer cells *(8,9)*. It has been show that HRG can stimulate lobular–alveolar development and the production of milk proteins in the mouse mammary gland and that antisense oligonucleotides against HRG can abolish branching morphogenesis and lobular alveolar differentiation of the mammary gland *(8,9)*.

3. EXPRESSION OF THE EGFR FAMILY IN BREAST CANCER

The EGFR family consists of four closely related genes: c-*erb*-B1 or EGFR, c-*erb*-B2 or *HER2*, c-*erb*-B3 or *HER3*, and c-*erb*-B4 or *HER4*. These receptor proteins are glycosylated and share a similar primary structure consisting of an extracellular, ligand-binding domain (which has two cysteine-rich regions), a single transmembrane region, a short juxtamembrane sequence, and an intracellular domain that contains a tyrosine-kinase domain flanked by a large hydrophilic carboxyl tail. The carboxyl tail displays sequence heterogeneity and carries several tyrosine autophosphorylation sites. The four members of the EGFR family have a high degree of homology in the tyrosine kinase domain, while the extracellular domains are less conserved, which is indicative of different specificity in ligand binding. Different classes of ligands that bind to and activate distinct sets of individual receptors can be distinguished within the EGF-like growth factors. The first group, that includes EGF, TGF-α, and AR, can exclusively bind to EGFR. Heparin binding EGF (HB-EGF) and betacellulin (BTC) can efficiently interact with both the EGFR and c-*erb*-B4, whereas epiregulin is a broad-spectrum receptor ligand. Finally, HRGs can bind to *erb*-B3 and *erb*-B4. Following ligand binding, these receptors dimerize, which may result in either homodimerization or heterodimerization. Dimerization results in tyrosine kinase autophosphorylation, which then activates a number of different intracellular signaling pathways *(10,11)*. The signaling pathway involves activation of ras and mitogen-activated protein kinase (MAPK), which activates several nuclear proteins required for cell cycle progression from the G_1 to the S phase. This activation is critical not only for cell proliferation. Several studies have demonstrated that EGFR-mediated signals also contribute to other processes that are crucial to cancer progression, including angiogenesis, invasion, metastasis, and inhibition of apoptosis *(12)*. In cells that express EGFR and c-*erb*-B2, any of EGF agonists will induce formation of EGFR/c-*erb*-B2 heterodimers, as well as EGFR/EGFR homodimers. This cross-activation extends to most of the receptor combinations, so that activation of one receptor will generally lead to some activation of other coexpressed EGF family receptors *(13,14)*. Heteromerization with other *erbB* family receptors is required for the activation of c-*erb*-B3, which is devoid of intrinsic catalytic activity *(15)*. c-*erb*-B2 is an orphan receptor, because none of the known ligands bind to c-*erb*-B2. c-*erb*-B2 is activated as heterodimers through interactions with other EGF family receptors following ligand binding and as homodimers in cancer cells with an amplified and overexpressed c-*erb*-B2 gene *(16)*. The EGFR family is involved in the regulation of mammary growth and differentiation. The female mammary gland undergoes extensive postnatal development under the influence of systemic hormones, including EGF family ligands and their cognate receptors. All four *erb*-B family receptors are expressed in mammary glands of adult females, but the EGFR and c-*erb*-B2 are preferentially expressed in young females *(17–19)*. The first postnatal episode of mammary development occurs at puberty, and leads to elongation and branching of the mammary ducts to extend throughout the fatty mesenchyme. EGFR and c-*erb*-B2 are present both in the stroma and the epithelium and are tyrosine phosphorylated, which is indicative of signaling activity *(18,19)*. The EGFR is important at puberty, because expression of dominant-negative EGFR impairs ductal morphogenesis *(20)*. The second wave of activation of *erbB* family receptors occurs in pregnancy *(18,19)*. Dominant-negative c-*erb*-B2 and c-*erb*-B4 transgenes interfere with lobuloalveolar expansion and milk protein production early and late in the postpartum period, respectively, which is consistent with the ability of neuregulin-activated c-*erb*-B2 to drive mammary differentiation *(17,21–23)*. All four receptors have been reported to be expressed to some extent also in breast tumors. EGFR expression is generally found between 30% and 50%, although it can range from 14% to 91%, depending on the method of assessment *(24,25)*. EGFR positivity is also common in ductal carcinoma *in situ* (DCIS) *(26)*. In breast tumors, EGFR overexpression is almost never caused by gene amplification; rather, it is a result of increased receptor synthesis *(27)*. Overexpression of c-*erb*-B2 is reported in approx 30% of breast tumors *(28)* and it is generally associated with gene amplification *(29,30)*. Amplification and/or overexpression of c-*erb*-B2 occurs more frequently (in up to 60% of cases) in DCIS *(31,32)*. c-*erb*-B3 is overexpressed in approx 20% of infiltrating breast cancers. As gene amplification has not been observed, overexpresion is most likely to be a result of increased transcription *(33)*. Overexpression of c-*erb*-B4 is relatively uncommon in breast cancer, and *erb*-B4 expression may be suppressed in carcinoma *(34–37)*.

4. INTRACELLULAR SIGNALING THROUGH THE EGFR FAMILY IN BREAST CANCER DEVELOPMENT AND PROGRESSION AND ROLE AS POTENTIAL MOLECULAR TARGETS FOR THERAPY

Because activation of the TGF-α/EGFR autocrine growth pathway is a common mechanism for autonomous, dysregulated cancer cell growth in the most common types of human epithelial cancers, the EGFR-driven autocrine pathway is a rational target for cancer therapy. The design of anticancer therapies using a selective EGFR inhibitor was proposed by Mendelshon in the early 1980s as one the first approaches for interfering with a specific cancer cell molecular target *(38)*. In the past 20 yr, a large body of experimental and clinical studies have supported this hypothesis. In this respect, the identification of selective and potent inhibitors of EGFR and of c-*erb*-B2 that can be developed as anticancer drugs has been one of the most successful examples of translation research in cancer. Trastuzumab (Herceptin®), a humanized monoclonal antibody generated against the c-*erb*-B2 protein, has shown activity in c-*erb*-B2 overexpressing metastatic breast cancer *(39,40)*, and enhances survival when given in combination with chemotherapy *(41)*. Two anti-EGFR therapeutic approaches have been shown potentially effective in clinical trials: monoclonal antibodies (MAbs) and small molecule inhibitors of the EGFR tyrosine kinase enzymatic activity. MAbs are raised against the extracellular domain of the EGFR to block ligand binding and receptor activation. Tyrosine kinase inhibitors (TKIs) prevent the autophosphorylation of the EGFR intracellular tyrosine kinase domain. The molecules are generally reversible competitors of ATP for binding to the intracellular catalytic domain of the EGFR tyrosine kinase. The most promising small molecule selective EGFR-TKIs belong to three series of compounds: 4-anilinoquinazolines, 4-ar(alk)ylaminopyrido-pyrimidines, and 4-phenylaminopyrrolopyrimidines. Both anti-EGFR MAbs and EGFR-TKIs have shown efficacy in relevant preclinical models, such as human cancer cell lines in vitro and in vivo. The blockade of EGFR signaling in cancer cells determines not only inhibition of cell proliferation but also other effects by inhibition of cell proliferation that could be relevant in the clinical setting, such as antiangiogenetic effects by inhibition of tumor cell production of proangiogenetic growth factors and possibly by direct cytotoxicity on endothelial cells in tumor vessels such as antiinvasive and antimetastatic effects.

DCIS is a preinvasive breast lesion that accounts for 30% of screening-detected breast cancer *(42)*. Untreated DCIS progresses to invasive breast cancer in 25–30% of patients *(43–45)*. DCIS express both EGFR and c-*erb*-B2 which might play an important role in proliferation and progression of DCIS. Chan et al. *(46)* have investigated the effects of an anti-c-*erb*-B2 monoclonal antibody (trastuzmab, Herceptin) and of an anti-EGFR selective TKI (Gefitinib, Iressa) on in vivo growth of ER-negative DCIS. These authors have detected no significant effects on epithelial proliferation by trastuzmab treatment, while gefitinib decreases proliferation and activates apoptosis in DCIS. These data show that gefitinib may have potential as an adjuvant therapy for the treatment and chemoprevention of DCIS.

EGFR and c-*erb*-B2 overexpression has been also associated with cancer cell resistance to antineoplastic agents *(47–51)*. In this respect, the transfection of human breast cancer cells with an EGFR expression vector results in the development of resistance to several chemotherapeutic agents *(52)*. Moreover, human breast cancer cell lines that become resistant to various cytotoxic agents overexpress EGFR, c-*erb*-B2 and various ligands, including TGF-α *(53)*. Signaling from EGFR, via the mitogen-activated protein kinase (MAPK) pathway, is believed to protect breast cancer cells against ionizing radiation and to be involved in rapid repopulation following radiotherapy *(47,48,54)*. Consequently, disrupting EGFR signaling with selective anti-EGFR drugs should result in cellular radiosensitization and enhanced sensitivity to chemotherapeutic agents. In addition, it could slow repopulation after radiotherapy or chemotherapy *(54)*. It is conceivable that the cellular damage induced by chemotherapy or by ionizing radiation can convert EGFR ligands from growth factors into survival factors for cancer cells that express functional EGFR. In this situation, the blockade of EGFR signaling in combination with cytotoxic drugs or with radiotherapy could cause irreparable cancer cell damage leading to increased programmed cell death. The enhancement of anticancer activity of conventional cytotoxic treatments, by interfering with EGFR activation, may have relevant clinical implications. In this respect, treatment with conventional doses of cytotoxic drugs or of radiotherapy in combination with signal transduction inhibitors, such as anti-EGFR–selective agents, could be an effective novel anticancer strategy, which is less toxic and more tolerable than other clinical approaches for increasing the activity of cytotoxic drugs or radiotherapy *(55,56)*. Clinical trials are ongoing in a variety of tumor types, although the results of some of these trials have been controversial. However, the combined or the sequential use of EGFR-targeted agents and chemotherapy is currently under clinical investigation in human breast cancer. The effect of combining EGFR-targeted agents with radiotherapy has not been examined in detail in breast cancer, although it has been shown to be effective in other types of cancer *(57)*. A recent study, however, has reported that breast cancer cells expressing a dominant-negative EGFR were more sensitive to radiation, suggesting that EGFR disruption could increase the sensitivity to radiation therapy *(54)*. EGFR expression in breast cancer is generally associated with an increased likelihood of failure to respond to endocrine therapy *(58–61)*. A similar relationship between c-*erb*-B2 overexpression, a poor prognosis, and hormonotherapy resistance has also been observed, although these associations as yet remain controversial *(58,60–63)*. The concept that peptide growth factors can act as the growth mediating factors in the growth of hormone-sensitive breast cancer is not a new one. It had its origins in the late 1980s, when it was first recognized that estrogens were able to stimulate expression of a number of growth factors, including TGF-α, in hormone-sensitive human breast cancer cell lines *(64,65)*. Numerous studies have shown that key receptors in such pathways (e.g., ERs) are subject to activation by both estrogens and peptide growth factors *(66–68)*. The important significance of such convergence in hormone-sensitive breast cancer cells is that antihormonal drugs not only possess antiestrogenic activity through their ability to block ER signaling, but also have antigrowth factor actions by virtue of their ability to disrupt the intimate cross-talk between estrogen and growth factor signaling *(69,70)*. Expression of EGFR and c-*erb*-B2 is suppressed by long-term therapy with estrogens in vitro *(71–74)*. These data suggest that hormone-sensitive breast cancer cells possess control mechanisms to limit EGFR/*erb*-B2-mediated signaling. This concept may have significant clinical implications. It has been observed a time-dependent increases in the expression of EGFR and c-*erb*-B2 after antiestrogen treatment of MCF-7 human breast cancer cells in vitro. MCF-7 cells are estrogen responsive for their growth and are growth inhibited by many antiestrogenic drugs. However, their continuous culture in the presence of tamoxifen or faslodex eventually generates sublines that tolerate the presence of the antiestrogens, regrowing at rates equivalent to the original hormone-responsive parenteral cells *(75)*. McClelland et al. *(76)* have shown that antihormonal-resistant MCF-7 sublines express up to 10-fold increased amounts of EGFR mRNA and protein. A parallel increase in c-*erb*-B2 immunostaining in the antiestrogen-resistant MCF-7 cells was also observed. Furthermore, treatment with gefitinib of tamoxifen- or faslodex-resistant MCF-7 breast cancer cells determines inhibition of EGFR autophosphorylation and of cell growth, indicating that the autocrine EGFR loop is critical to the growth of these antihormonal-resistant cells. The increase in cellular expression of EGFR in hormone-resistant breast cancer cells thus appears to provide a promising molecular target for the effective treatment of endocrine-resistant human breast cancer. McClelland et al. have also shown that combination therapies with simultaneously target estrogen (tamoxifen) and EGFR signaling (gefitinib) may be more effective than the sequential use of such drugs. Moreover, these experimental studies suggest that anti-EGFR treatment of hormone-responsive breast cancer may contribute to prevention of the development of the hormone-resistant tumors.

There is experimental evidence that EGFR and c-*erb*-B2 coexpression confers a more aggressive clinical behavior *(77–79)*. The rationale for targeting simultaneously the two receptors stems from their frequent coexpression in breast cancer and their capacity to form heterodimers that activate signal transduction pathways. Four independent research groups have provided elegant experimental data showing that the EGFR-selective tyrosine kinase inhibitor gefitinib has potent in vitro and in vivo antitumor activity against human breast cancer cell lines that express the EGFR and that overexpress c-*erb*-B2 *(80–83)*. Gefitinib treatment efficiently blocks EGFR autophosphorylation and c-*erb*-B2 transphosphorylation *(80–83)*.

This effect is followed by inhibition of both MAPK and PI3K-akt signaling in breast cancer cells with subsequent growth inhibition and induction of apoptosis *(81,82)*. Furthermore, the combined treatment with gefitinib and trastuzumab is frankly synergistic both in inducing cell growth inhibition and apoptosis in vitro and in vivo *(81,82)*, suggesting that the simultaneous targeting of the EGFR and c-*erb*-B2 may result in an efficient tumor growth inhibition in breast cancer patients whose tumors coexpress both receptors. A possible biochemical and pharmacological explanation for the activity of gefitinib in EGFR and c-*erb*-B2 overexpressing breast cancer cells has been recently provided by Anido et al. *(83)*, who have demonstrated that gefitinib treatment blocks EGFR activation and also induces the formation of inactive EGFR/c-*erb*-B2 and EGFR/c-*erb*-B3 heterodimers and prevents HRG signaling. In this situation, gefitinib treatment significantly blocks signaling through the entire EGFR family of receptors because it also reduces the levels of c-*erb*-B2/c-*erb*-B3 that are potentially activable by HRG *(83,84)*. Collectively, these experimental evidence provide a strong rationale for studying the combination of gefitinib and trastuzumab in breast cancer patients who coexpress both the EGFR and c-*erb*-B2.

REFERENCES

1. Dickson RB, Lippman ME. Growth factors in breast cancer. *Endocr Rev* 1995;16:559–589.
2. Normanno N, Ciardiello F. EGF related peptides in the pathophysiology of the mammary gland. *J Mammary Gland Biol Neoplasia* 1997;2:143–151.
3. Osbore CK, Hamilton B, Titus G, Livingston RB. Epidermal growth factor stimulation of human breast cancer cells in culture. *Cancer Res* 1980;40:2361–2366.
4. Cohen S. Isolation of mouse submaxillary gland protein accelerating incisor eruptin and eyelid opening in the new-born animal. *J Biol Chem* 1962;237:1555–1562.
5. Gregory H. Isolation and structure of urogastrone and its relationship to epidermal growth factor. *Nature* 1975;257:325–327.
6. Mroczkowski B, Reich M, Chen K, Bell GI, Cohen S. Recombinant human EGF precursor is a glycosylated membrane protein with biological activity. *Mol Cell Biol* 1989;9:2771–2778.
7. Murphy LC, Murphy LJ, Dubik D, Bell GI, Shiu RPC. Epidermal growth factor gene expression in human breast cancer cells: regulation of expression by progestins. *Cancer Res* 1988;48:4555–4560.
8. Salomon DS, Brandt R, Ciardiello F, Normanno N. Epidermal growth factor-related peptides and their receptors in human malignancies. *Crit Rev Oncol/ Haematol* 1995;19:183–232.
9. Martinez-Lacaci I, Bianco C, De Santis M, Salomon DS. Epidermal growth factor related peptides and their cognate receptors in breast cancer. In: *Breast Cancer: Molecular Genetics, Pathogenesis, and Therapeutics.*
10. Klapper L, Glathe S, Vaisman N, et al. The ErbB-2/HER2 oncoprotein of human carcinomas may function solely as a shared coreceptor for multiple stroma-derived growth factor. *Proc Natl Acad Sci USA* 1999;96:4995–5000.

11. Riese DJ II, van Raaij TM, Plowman GD, Andrews GC, Stern DF. Cellular response to neuregulins is governed by complex interactions of the erbB receptor family. *Mol Cell Biol* 1995;15:5770–5776.
12. Salomon DS, Gullick W. The erbB family of receptors and their ligands: multiple targets for therapy. *Signal* 2001;2:4–11.
13. Kokai Y, Meyers JN, Wada T, et al. Synergistic interaction of p185 c-neu and the EGF receptor leads to transformation of rodent fibroblasts. *Cell* 1989;58:287–292.
14. Kuranagaran D, Tzahar E, Beerli R, et al. ErbB2 is a common auxiliary subunit of NDF and EGF receptors: implications for breast cancer. *EMBO J* 1996;15: 254–264.
15. Guy PM, Platko JV, Cantley LC, Cerione RA, Carraway KL III. Insect cell expressed p180erbB3 possesses an impaired tyrosine kinase activity. *Proc Natl Acad Sci USA* 1994;91:8132–8136.
16. Stem DF, Kamps MP. EGF-stimulated tyrosine phosphorylation of p185[neu]: a potential model for receptor interactions. *EMBO J* 1988;7:995–1001.
17. Yang Y, Spitzer E, Meyer D, et al. Sequential requirement of hepatocyte growth factor and neuregulin in the morphogenesis and differentiation of the mammary gland. *J Cell Biol* 1995;131:215–226.
18. Sebastian J, Richards RG, Walker MP, et al. Activation and function of the epidermal growth factor receptor and erbB2 during mammary gland morphogenesis. *Cell Growth Differ* 1998;9:777–785.
19. Schroeder JA, Lee DC. Dynamic expression and activation of ERBB receptors in the developing mouse mammary gland. *Cell Growth Differ* 1998;9:451–464.
20. Xie W, Paterson A, Chin E, Nabell L, Kudlow J. Targeted expression of a dominant negative epidermal growth factor receptor in mammary gland of transgenic mice inhibits pubertal mammary ductal development. *Mol Endocrinol* 1997;1:1766–1781.
21. Jones F, Sterm D. Expression of dominant negative ErbB2 in the mammary gland of transgenic mice reveals a rule in lobuloalveolar development and lactation. *Oncogene* 1999;18:3481–3490.
22. Jones FE, Welte T, Fu X-Y, Stern DF. ErbB4 signaling in the mammary gland is required for lobuloalveolar development and Stat5 activation during lactation. *J Cell Biol* 1999;147:77–88.
23. Nieman C, Brinkman V, Spitzer E, et al. Reconstitution of mammary gland development in vitro: requirement of c-met and c-erbB2 signaling for branching and alveolar morphogenesis. *J Cell Biol* 1998;143:533–545.
24. Walker RA, Dearing SJ. Expression of epidermal growth factor receptor mRNA and protein in primary breast carcinomas. *Breast Cancer Res Treat* 1999;53: 167–176.
25. Klijn JG, Berns PM, Schmitz PI, et al. The clinical significance of epidermal growth factor receptor (EGF-R) in human breast cancer: a review on 5232 patients. *Endocrinol Rev* 1992;13:3–17.
26. Chan KC, Gandhi A, Slamon DJ, et al. *Proc Am Assoc Cancer Res* 2000;41:482 (Abstr 3074).
27. Earp HS, Dawson TL, Li X, et al. Heterodimerization and functional interaction between EGF receptor family members: a new signaling paradigm with implications for breast cancer research. *Breast Cancer Res Treat* 1995;35:115–132.
28. Slamon DJ, Clark GM, Wong SG, et al. Human breast cancer: correlation of relapse and survival with amplification of the HER-2/neu oncogene. *Science* 1987;235:177–182.

29. Slamon DJ, Godolphin W, Jones LA, et al. Studies of the *HER-2/neu* proto-oncogene in human breast and ovarian cancer. *Science* 1989;244:707–712.
30. Seshadri R, Firgaira FA, Horsfall DJ, et al. Clinical significance of HER-2/neu oncogene amplification in primary breast cancer. The South Australian Breast Cancer Study Group. *J Clin Oncol* 1993;11:1936–1942.
31. Hynes NE, Sterm DF. The biology of *erbB2/neu/HER-2* and its role in cancer. *Biochem Biophys Acta Rev Cancer* 1994;1198:165–184.
32. Van de Vijver MJ, Peterse JL, et al. Neu-protein overexpression in breast cancer: association with comedo-type ductal carcinoma in situ and limited prognostic value in stage II breast cancer. *N Engl J Med* 1988;319:1239–1245.
33. Gullick WJ. The c-erbB3/HER3 receptor in human cancer. *Cancer Surv* 1996;27:339–349.
34. Srinivasan R, Poulsom R, Hurst H, Gullick W. Expression of the c-erbB-4/HER4 protein and mRNA in normal human fetal and adult tissues and in a survey of nine solid tumour types. *J Pathol* 1997;185:236–245.
35. Vogt U, Bielawski K, et al. Amplification of erbB-4 oncogene occurs less frequently than of erbB-2 in primary human breast cancer. *Gene* 1998;223:375–380.
36. Bacus SS, Chin D, Zelninick CR, et al. Type 1 receptor tyrosine kinases are differentially phosphorylated in mammary carcinoma and differentially associated with steroid receptors. *Am J Pathol* 1996;148:549–558.
37. Knowlden J, Gee J, Seery L, et al. c-erbB-3 and c-erbB-4 expression is a feature of the endocrine responsive phenotype in clinical breast cancer. *Oncogene* 1998;17:1949–1957.
38. Mendelsohn J. The epidermal growth factor receptor as target for cancer therapy. *Endocr Relat Cancer* 2001;8:3–9.
39. Baselga J, Tripathy D, Mendelsohn J, et al. Phase II study of weekly intravenous recombinant humanized anti-p185HER2 monoclonal antibody in patients with HER2/neu-overexpressing metastatic breast cancer. *J Clin Oncol* 1996; 14:737–744.
40. Cobleigh MA, Vogel CL, Tripathy D, et al. Multinational study of the efficacy and safety of humanized anti-HER2 monoclonal antibody in women who have HER2-overexpressing metastatic breast cancer that has progressed after chemotherapy for metastatic breast disease. *J Clin Oncol* 1999;17:2639–2648.
41. Slamon DJ, Leyland-Jones B, Shak S, et al. Use of chemotherapy plus a monoclonal antibody against HER2 for metastatic breast cancer that overexpresses HER2. *N Engl J Med* 2001;344:783–792.
42. Ernest VL, Barclay J, Kerlikowske K, et al. Incidence of and treatment for ductal carcinoma in situ of the breast. *JAMA* 1996;275:913–918.
43. Price P, Sinnett HD, Gusterson B, et al. Ductal carcinoma in situ: predictors of local recurrence and progression in patients treated by surgery alone. *Br J Cancer* 1990;61:869–872.
44. Silverstein MJ. Ductal carcinoma in situ of the breast. *Br Med J* 1998;317: 734–739.
45. Leal CB, Schmitt FC, Bento M. Ductal carcinoma in situ of the breast: histological categorisation and its relationship to ploidy and immunohistochemical expression of hormone receptors, p53, and c-erbB-2 protein. *Cancer* 1995;75:2123–2128.
46. Chan KC, Knox WF, Ghandhi A, Slamon DJ, et al. Blockade of growth factor receptors in ductal carcinoma in situ inhibits epithelial proliferation. *Br J Surg* 2001;88:412–418.

47. Dent P, Reardon DB, Park JS, et al. Radiation-induced release of transforming growth factor alpha activates the epidermal growth factor receptor and mitogen-activated protein kinase pathway in carcinoma cells, leading to increased proliferation and protection from radiation-induced cell death. *Mol Biol Cell* 1999; 10:2493–2506.

48. Schmidt-Ullrich RK, Mikkelsen RB, Dent P, et al. Radiation-induced proliferation of the human A431 squamous carcinoma cells is dependent on EGFR tyrosine phosphorylation. *Oncogene* 1997;15:1191–1197.

49. Dickstein BM, Wosikowski K, Bate SE. Increased resistance to cytotoxic agents in ZR75B human breast cancer cells transfected with epidermal growth factor receptor. *Mol Cell Endocrinol* 1995;110:205–211.

50. Newby JC, Johnston SR, Smith IE, et al. Expression of epidermal growth factor receptor and c-erbB2 during the development of tamoxifen resistance in human breast cancer. *Clin Cancer Res* 1997;3:1634–1651.

51. Wright C, Nicholson S, Angus B, et al. Relationship between c-erbB-2 protein product expression and response to endocrine therapy in advanced breast cancer. *Br J Cancer* 1992;65:118–121.

52. Fox SB, Harris AL. The epidermal growth factor receptor in breast cancer. *J Mammary Gland Biol Neoplasia* 1997;2:131–141.

53. Wosikowski K, Schuurhuis D, Kops GJ, et al. Altered gene expression in drug-resistant human breast cancer cells. *Clin Cancer Res* 1997;3:2405–2414.

54. Schmidt-Ullrich RK, Lammering J, Contessa K, et al. Presented at the 11th NCI-EORTC-AACR Symposium on New Drug in Cancer Therapy, Amsterdam, The Netherlands, 2000, Abstr 40.

55. Mendelsohn J, Fan, Z. Epidermal growth factor receptor family and chemo-sensitization. *J Natl Cancer Inst* 1997;89:341–343.

56. Ryan PD, Chabner BA. On receptor inhibitors and chemotherapy. *Clin Cancer Res* 2000;6:4607–4609.

57. Bonner J, Robert F, Raisch K, et al. Presented at the 11th NCI-EORTC-AACR Symposium on New Drug in Cancer Therapy, Amsterdam, The Netherlands, 2000, Abstr 38.

58. Nicholson RI, Manning DL, et al. New anti-hormonal approaches to breast cancer therapy. *Drugs Today* 1993;29:363–372.

59. Nicholson RI, McClelland RA, Gee JM, et al. Epidermal growth factor receptor expression in breast cancer: association with response to endocrine therapy. *Breast Cancer Res Treat* 1994;29:117–125.

60. Nicholson RI, Gee JMW, Harper ME, et al. ErbB signalling in clinical breast cancer: relationship to endocrine sensitivity. *Endocr Relat Cancer* 1997;4:1–9.

61. Nicholson RI, Gee JMW, Jones H, et al. ErbB signalling in clinical breast cancer. In: Ernst Schering Research Foundation Workshop 19: EGF Receptor in Tumour Growth and Progression, 1997, pp. 105–128.

62. Elledge RM, Green S, Ciocca D, et al. HER-2 expression and response to tamoxifen in estrogen receptor-positive breast cancer: a Southwest Oncology Group Study. *Clin Cancer Res* 1998;4:7–12.

63. Houston SJ, Plunkett TA, Barnes DM, et al. Over-expression of c-erbB2 is a independent marker of resistance to endocrine therapy in advanced breast cancer. *Br J Cancer* 1999;79:1220–1226.

64. Bates SE, Davidson NE, Valverius EM, et al. Expression of transforming growth factor alpha and its messenger ribonucleic acid in human breast cancer: its regulation by estrogen and ist possible functional significance. *Mol Endocrinol* 1988;2:543–555.

65. Lee AV, Darbre P, King RJ. Processing of insulin like growth factor-II (IGF-II) by human breast cancer cells. *Mol Cell Endocrinol* 1994;99:211–220.

66. Aronica SM, Katzenellenbogen BS. Stimulation of estrogen receptor-mediated transcription and alteration in the phosphorylation state of rat uterine estrogen receptor by estrogen, cyclic adenosinemonophosphate, and insulin-like growth factor-I. *Mol Endocrinol* 1993;7:743–752.

67. Bunone G, Briand PA, Miksicek RJ, Picard D. Activation of the unliganded estrogen receptor by EGF involves the MAP kinase pathway and direct phosphorylation. *EMBO J* 1996;15:2174–2183.

68. Richards RG, DiAugustine RP, Petrusz P, Clark GC, Sebastian J. Estradiol stimulates tyrosine phosphorylation of the insulin-like growth factor-1 receptor and insulin receptor substrate-1 in the uterus. *PNAS* 1996;93:12002–12007.

69. Freiss G, Rochefort H, Vignon F. Mechanisms of 4-hydroxytamoxifen anti-growth factor receptor binding sites and tyrosine kinase activity. *Biochem Biophy Res Commun* 1990;31:919–926.

70. Guvakova MA, Surmacz E. Tamoxifen interferes with the insulin-like growth factor I receptor (IGF-IR) signaling pathway in breast cancer cells. *Cancer Res* 1997;57:2606–2610.

71. Dati C, Antoniotti S, Taverna D, Perroteau I, De Bortoli M. Inhibition of c-erbB2 oncogene expression by oestrogens in human breast cancer cells. *Oncogene* 1990;5:1001–1006.

72. Chrysogelos SA, Yarden RI, Lauber AH, Murphy JM. Mechanisms of EGF receptor regulation in breast cancer cells. *Breast Cancer Res Treat* 1994;31:227–236.

73. Yarden RI, Lauber AH, EI-Ashry D, Chrysogelos SA. Bimodal regulation of epidermal growth factor receptor by estrogen in breast cancer cells. *Endocrinology* 1996;137:2739–2747.

74. De Fazio A, Chiew Ye, McEvoy M, Watts CK, Sutherland RL. Antisense estrogen receptor RNA expression increases epidermal growth factor receptor gene expression in breast cancer cells. *Cell Growth Differ* 1997;8:903–911.

75. Cheung KL, Willsher PC, Pinder SE, et al. Predictors of response to second-line endocrine therapy for breast cancer. *Breast Cancer Res Treat* 1997;45:219–224.

76. McClelland RA, Barrow D, Madden TA, et al. Enhanced epidermal growth factor receptor signalling in MCF-7 breast cancer cells after long-term culture in the presence of the pure antioestrogen ICI 182,780 (faslodex). *Endocrinology* 2001;142:2776–2788.

77. Salomon DS, Brandt R, Ciardiello F, Normanno N. Epidermal growth factor-related peptides and their receptors in human malignancies. *Crit Rev Oncol Hematol* 1995;19:183–232.

78. Slamon DJ, Clark GM, Wong SG, et al. Human breast cancer: correlation of relapse and survival with amplification of the HER-2/neu oncogene. *Science* 1987;235:177–182.

79. Harris AL, Nicholoson S, Sainsbury JR, et al. Epidermal growth factor receptor: a marker of early relapse in breast cancer and tumour stage progression in bladder cancer; interactions with neu. In: Furth M, Greaves M, eds. *The Molecular Diagnostics of Human Cancer*, Vol. 7: *Cancer Cells*. Cold Spring Harbor Laboratory Press, Cold Spring Harbor, NY, 1989;353–357.

80. Moasser MM, Basso A, Averbuch SD, Rosen N. The tyrosine kinase inhibitor ZD1839 (Iressa) inhibits HER2-driven signaling and suppresses the growth of HER2-overexpressing tumor cells. *Cancer Res* 2001;61:7184–7188.

81. Moulder SL, Yakes M, Muthuswamy SK, Bianco R, Simpson JF, Arteaga C. Epidermal growth factor receptor (HER1) tyrosine kinase inhibitor ZD1839 (Iressa) inhibits HER2/neu (erbB2)-overexpressing breast cancer cells in vitro and in vivo. *Cancer Res* 2001;61:8887–8895.

82. Normanno N, Campiglio M, De Luca A, et al. Cooperative inhibitory effect of ZD1839 (IRESSA) in combination with trastuzmab (Herceptin) on human breast cancer cell growth. *Ann Oncol* 2002;13:65–72.

83. Anido J, Albanell J, Rojo F, Guzman M, et al. ZD1839, a specific epidermal growth factor receptor (EGFR) tyrosine kinase inhibitor, induces the formation of inactive EGFR/HER2 and EGFR/HER3 heterodimers and prevents heregulin signaling in HER2-overexpressing breast cancer cells. *Clin Cancer Res* 2003;9:1274–1283.

84. Normanno N, Maiello MR, De Luca A. Epidermal growth factor receptor tyrosine kinase inhibitors (EGFR-TKIs): simple drugs with a complex mechanism of action? *J Cell Physiol* 2003;194:13–19.

11 *p53* as a Prognostic and Predictive Indicator

Daniela Kandioler, MD
and Raimund Jakesz, MD

CONTENTS

SUMMARY

Cancer is a disease of genes, and the *p53* gene appears to be the most frequently mutated gene associated with human cancer. *p53* is crucially involved in numerous central pathways determining the life and death of a cell. The information about the functional status of *p53* has been considered to be extremely important for estimation of prognosis and the need of further treatment as well as for prediction of response and the selection of the optimal therapy. The aim of this chapter is to evaluate why one of the most promising and most intensively studied markers is not recommended for routine clinical use to date. The pitfalls of the *p53* analysis and the challenges of well-designed *p53* studies are elucidated and the need of carefully planned studies using an optimal *p53* analysis method is pointed out.

Cancer Drug Discovery and Development: Biomarkers in Breast Cancer:
Molecular Diagnostics for Predicting and Monitoring Therapeutic Effect
Edited by: G. Gasparini and D. F. Hayes © Humana Press Inc., Totowa, NJ

Key Words: *p53*; biological marker; prognostic; predictive; *p53* sequencing; *p53* immunohistochemistry; *p53* study design.

1. INTRODUCTION: WHAT WENT WRONG WITH *p53*?

The treatment of breast cancer, a genetically heterogeneous malignant disease, has been greatly improved by providing individual treatment for the patient. While prognostic factors determine the need for further treatment, predictive factors are needed to select the appropriate therapy with the greatest likelihood of eliciting a response.

From a biological aspect, *p53* should a powerful predictive and prognostic marker. A *p53* has been shown to be responsible for the activation of the apoptotic machinery leading to cell death. The effect of most standard chemotherapies, tamoxifen, and also radiation treatment, is based on the induction of *p53*-dependent apoptosis. Thus, a defect in the *p53* pathway would cause resistance to treatment. Predicting either resistance or response to treatment is a key feature of a predictive marker. Furthermore, *p53* potently inhibits cell growth and provides protection from malignant progression. Taken together, these data suggest that *p53* should represent an independent prognostic marker.

However, in a review of *Molecular Markers in the Treatment of Breast Cancer* published in 2000, Hamilton and Piccart concluded that currently available data do not support the use of *p53* as a predictive factor in the therapy of breast cancer *(1)*. The prognostic impact of *p53* has been reported in numerous publications, which have been summarized in the 1999 consensus statement of the College of American Pathologists. Here, *p53* has been ranked as a category II factor, defined as "having been extensively studied but whose importance remains to be validated in statistically robust studies" *(2)*. So what went wrong with *p53*?

2. METHODOLOGICAL VARIABILITY

2.1. p53 *Immunohistochemistry (IHC)*

2.1.1. P53 IHC—BACKGROUND

The p53 protein is normally present at extremely low levels. One action of p53 is suppression of cellular proliferation; rapid degradation of the p53 protein after synthesis, regulated to a large extent by Mdm2, allows normal cells to grow *(3,4)*.

Stabilization of the p53 protein occurs as a common response to cellular stress including DNA damage, hypoxia, oncogene activation, pH, and temperature changes (heat shock). In response to these signals, p53 becomes active as a result of stabilization and mediates the inhibition of cell growth via cell cycle arrest, DNA repair, or cell death, to prevent the development and progression of malignant cells.

2.1.2. SIGNIFICANCE OF IHC RESULTS

Wild-type p53 protein has a very short cellular half-life. In contrast, mutated p53 appears relatively resistant to Mdm2-mediated degradation. Therefore, wild-type p53 protein is rarely detectable by routine IHC staining.

Mutation of the *p53* gene can result in the failure of normal degradation of p53 *(3)*. These proteins are dysfunctional, in contrast to proteins that are physiologically stabilized as a response to cellular stress. Because IHC detects stabilized p53 protein without further specification, this method is fraught with false-positive results, as it does not differentiate between pathological (due to gene mutation) and physiological (due to cellular stress) overexpression.

The majority of publications over the last 15 yr report IHC results founded on the assumption that the overexpression of p53 in tumors occurs due to gene mutation. The frequency of p53 overexpression in breast cancer ranges from 40% to 57% *(5)*, which is much higher than the frequency of *TP53* gene mutations in breast cancer (20–30%).

Comparative studies of IHC vs gene sequencing show that the concordance between the two methods is only 12–30% *(6–9)*.

IHC may also produce false-negative results. For instance, changes in the protein structure affecting the antibody-binding sites due to gene mutation; or the formation of a premature STOP codon most frequently occurring as a consequence of deletion or insertion mutations, causing a shift of the reading frame and preventing gene transcription and translation into protein at all.

Moreover mutations that do not result in greater expression of the p53 protein are termed "null mutations" and have been reported to occur at a frequency of 31% in breast cancer *(10)*. These may or may not alter p53 function.

2.1.3. STANDARDIZATION OF IHC

A number of antibodies to detect different epitopes of the p53 protein are available. Most groups use Mab 1801 (Oncogene Science) or DO-7 (DAKO), or both, for p53 IHC. The staining protocols, detection, and reporting procedure for positive staining are not standardized. A number of parameters are variously reported: the staining intensity, the percentage of tumor cell nuclei, the staining index (=product of staining intensity and area), or the staining score (=sum of staining intensity and positive tumor cell nuclei). Different cutoff points ranging from 0% to 75% further complicate the issue *(11,12)*. The role of interobserver variability, which is linked to microscopic detection methods, can be estimated only after the method itself has been standardized.

Although p53 IHC promises to be a simple and inexpensive method, it currently bears all the major disadvantages of a marker analysis method with respect to significance and standardization. This is a major hindrance to correct estimation of the clinical importance and the independence of p53 IHC as a marker. In the absence of comparative studies, it is currently not even clear whether the standardization of IHC can improve the situation.

2.2. Direct Detection of p53 Genetic Abnormalities

2.2.1. SCREENING METHODS

Various screening methods have been applied in different studies, promising high-throughput screening for mutations. These are based on the analysis of sequence-dependent changes in the conformation of single- and double-stranded DNA using capillary electrophoresis *(13,14)*. The specificity, sensitivity, and reproducibility of these methods are controversial. In some studies, when compared to direct sequencing, these methods will not detect up to 50% of mutations. Moreover, these methods are unable to distinguish between polymorphisms and relevant mutations *(15,16)*. In most articles, screening results are compared with the clinical outcome. Consecutive sequencing is performed only for tumors which proved to be positive at initial screening. Tumors with negative screening are disclosed from sequencing and often incorrectly adjudged to have a normal genotype. In this regard, the rate of detected *p53* abnormality using the most common of these methods, SSCP, is 20%, but the concordance of SSCP with sequencing is only 50%. Thus the mutation frequencies derived from studies using screening methods prior to sequencing may not reflect true frequencies, as a significant fraction of mutations may have been missed.

Commercially available array-based technologies are gaining popularity as a screening method for mutations *(17,18)*. However, comparative studies concerning sensitivity, specificity, and reproducibility have not yet been published. To promote this technology, one has to carefully design studies that permit comparisons with the most sensitive technique at the present time, namely *p53* sequencing.

2.3. p53 Sequencing

The *p53* tumor suppressor gene encodes a nuclear phosphoprotein that directly binds to DNA. Directly interacting with DNA as a transcription factor, p53 controls numerous genes involved in DNA repair, cell division, and apoptosis. To allow abnormal proliferation and progression, cells dedicated to become malignant have to be deprived of their tumor suppressor ability. The most commonly used pathway to inactivate *p53* in human cancer is mutation of the gene itself. In breast cancer 20% of tumors appear to be mutated.

2.3.1. STANDARDIZATION OF SEQUENCING

Although IHC or SSCP are more appealing methods to evaluate *p53* abnormalities, the preceding paragraphs illustrate the inaccuracies of these approaches. Currently, the gold standard to detect *p53* abnormalities is sequencing of the gene.

Sequencing has the reputation of being time consuming and cost ineffective. Today, however automated capillary sequencing provides a high throughput, a computerized standardized interpretation, and characterization of mutations *(6–8)*.

Sequencing results can either be positive (mutated) or negative (normal, wild-type). Thus, problems related to different scoring systems, cutoff points, and interobserver variability do not exist. For *p53* analysis it is now generally accepted that, to achieve highest sensitivity, direct sequencing has to be applied to the entire *p53* gene including splice sites. In older studies, sequencing was limited to hot spot regions spanning exons 5–8. These studies might not reflect true frequencies, in consideration of the fact that up to 20% of mutations are missed in breast cancer *(24)*.

Reproducibility and correct interpretation are ensured by a standardized number of reanalyses and by sequencing the opposite DNA strand in order to confirm mutations. Routine coamplification of positive and negative controls has disclosed problems related to the contamination or fidelity of the DNA polymerase (enzyme) used for polymerase chain reaction. Characterization of mutation ensures standardized reporting of mutations and identification of polymorphisms.

In contrast to IHC, sequencing is highly sensitive and specific and can be applied to various materials including fine-needle aspirates and paraffin-embedded and frozen tissue *(25)*.

Sequencing will not detect inactivation of *p53* by mechanisms other than mutation, for example, cytoplasmatic sequestration: p53 protein imprisoned in the cytoplasm fails to activate transcription of target genes and cannot mediate cell cycle arrest or apoptosis. To date there are no studies demonstrating the frequency and cancer-specific relevance of such finding. It is unclear whether the sequestration is stable and what happens when *p53* is up-regulated in response to DNA damage. So far mutation of the *p53* gene, and not cytoplasmatic sequestration of the protein, is the most commonly known path to inactivate the *p53* tumor suppressor function in human cancer.

3. ARE ALL GENE MUTATIONS OF CLINICAL RELEVANCE?

3.1. Significance of p53 *Gene Mutation*

In multivariate analysis, the presence of *TP53* mutations is consistently associated with an increased risk of relapse and death from breast cancer

(19). In addition, a mutant *p53* genotype appeared to be clearly associated with a lack of response to DNA-damaging treatment in different cancer types, including breast cancer *(6–8,10)* (Tables 1; *[8,10,16,20–23]* and 2 *[6–8]*).

However, it has become increasingly clear that not all *p53* mutations are of equal significance, almost certainly owing to the pleiotrophic features of this gene and its protein. Certain data indicate functional differences between the central and peripheral coding regions. The highly conserved region located in the middle of the protein is responsible for DNA binding and is affected most frequently by mutations (80%).

There are some reports of mutations that show that the L2 and L3 loops of the *p53* gene may have a distinct tumorigenic potential *(26)*. In contrast, only 4% of mutations occur in the tetramerization domain. However, for this region, germline mutations in Li–Fraumeni cancer syndrome families have been published, proving the clinical relevance of such rare mutations *(27)*.

A specific sensitivity to chemotherapeutic agents has been reported for certain mutations *(28)*. Even if the different types of mutations as well as the different location of mutations confer a specific grade of treatment sensitivity, clinically this does not seem to impair the prognostic and predictive implications of *p53*. While the response to (*p53*-dependent) treatment was shown to be related to the *p53* genotype in more than 168 patients from neoadjuvant studies, we were unable to identify a single tumor that responded to treatment in the presence of a *p53* mutation (Table 2; *[6–8]*). This was found to be true for more than 70 different mutations in the *p53* gene. The results were reproducible in three different tumor types (breast, colorectal, lung cancer).

4. *p53* AND RESPONSE PREDICTION

4.1. Biologic Rationale

The effect of the majority of currently used chemotherapeutic drugs is based on the induction of DNA damage, which favors rapidly growing cells. These drugs share a final common pathway: apoptosis. *p53* plays a central role in this pathway: DNA damage is the strongest promoter of *p53* activation. The latter is responsible for the induction of apoptosis in response to DNA damage *(29)*.

Therefore, in several preclinical studies, *TP53* gene mutation represents a crucial defect in the apoptosis pathway and results in drug resistance *(30,31)*.

These studies suggest that *p53*-mediated drug resistance is important for several agents, including anthracylines (doxorubicin, epirubicin), antimetabolites (5-fluorouracil, methotrexate, gemcitabine), topoisomerase blockers (CPT-11), alkylating substances (cyclophosphamide, ifosfamide, cisplatin), hormonal therapies such as tamoxifen and aromatase inhibitors, and radiation therapy *(32)* (Fig. 1).

Table 1
Studies Providing Adequate Designs for Evaluating the Predictive Power of *p53*

Authors (ref.)	Journal	No. of patients	Technique	Technical specificities	Therapy	Design	Prospective	Relation of p53 and response	p-value
Anelli (20)	Ann Oncol 2003	73	Sequencing		Paclitaxel + docorubincin	Neoadjuvant	Yes	Predictive	0.004
Berns (10)	Cancer Res 2000	202	Sequencing	Exons 2–11	TAM	Metastatic	No	Predictive	0.0001
Kandioler (8)	Clin Cancer Res 2000	25	Sequencing	Exons 2–11 + splice sites	FEC	Neoadjuvant	No	Predictive	0.0029
Elledge (16)	Breast Cancer Res Treat 1998	360	IHC	Pab 1801	TAM	Metastatic	No	No	
Makris (21)	Clin Cancer Res 1997	80	IHC	PAb240, PAb1801	Various therapies	Neoadjuvant	No	No	
Formenti (22)	I J Radiat Oncol Biol Phys 1997	35	IHC		5-FU + RT	Neoadjuvant	Yes	Predictive	0.01

The table includes studies with neoadjuvant or metastatic design only. This design allows direct assessment of response to treatment and therefore estimation of the predictive power of *p53*. Results of studies using immunohistochemistry (IHC) are compared to those using sequencing for *p53* analysis.

Table 2
Relationship of *p53* Sequencing and Response to Neoadjuvant Treatment in Cancer Patients

Author (ref.)	Journal	No. of patients	Cancer type neoadjuvant therapy	Response	Sequencing result			Immunohistochemistry	
					Mutant	Normal	p-value	Positive	Negative
Kandioler et al. (8)	Clin Cancer Res 2000	25	Breast cancer 5-FU/epirubicine/ cyclophosphamide	CR PR SD PD	0 7	18 10	0.0029	1 14	17 3
Kandioler et al. (7)	JTCVS 1999	58	Lung cancer Cisplatin/ifosfamide	CR PR SD PD	0 18	32 8	0.001	9[a] 5[a]	7[a] 3[a]
Kandioler et al. (6)	Ann Surg 2002	68	Rectal cancer Short-term radiation	CR PR SD PD	0 29	14 21	0.000	na na	na na

[a]Immunohistochemistry was available for a limited number of patients in this study.

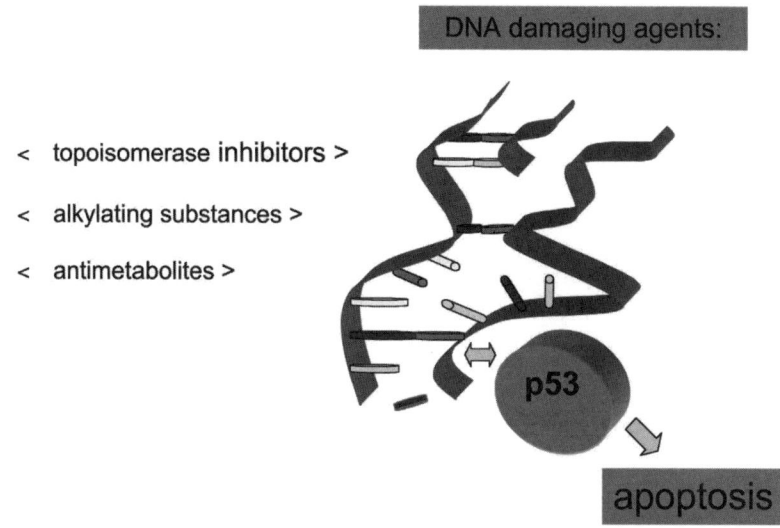

Doxorubicin, Cyclophosphamid, 5-FU, Methotrexate, Gemcytabine
Radiation...

Fig. 1. Functional *p53* is required to respond to DNA-damaging substances.
DNA damage is the most important trigger for *p53* transcription. The p53 protein binds directly to DNA and initiates apoptosis. Loss of *p53* function will
therefore result in treatment resistance.

4.1.1. P53-INDEPENDENT SUBSTANCES

Paclitaxel exhibits significant antitumor activity in breast cancer patients
in prospective randomized studies *(33)*. In vitro experiments show cells
lacking functional *p53* to be particularly sensitive to paclitaxel *(34)*. Because
paclitaxel blocks cells in the G_2/M phase of the cell cycle, this agent has been
proposed as a radiosensitizer.

In a small analysis of a breast cancer patient cohort treated neoadjuvantly with paclitaxel monotherapy, we were able to show in the
clinical setting that the response to paclitaxel was positively related to the
presence of *TP53* gene mutations (detected with sequencing), and was not
related to apoptosis (detected with the TUNEL assay), suggesting that cell
death caused by paclitaxel occurs in a *p53*-independent manner *(8)*. As the
response to paclitaxel occurred preferentially in *p53* mutants, we hypothesized that it might be the defect in the G1 cell cycle checkpoint which
increases sensitivity to taxanes in *p53* mutants, probably due to accumulation of cells in the phase of mitosis (Fig. 2).

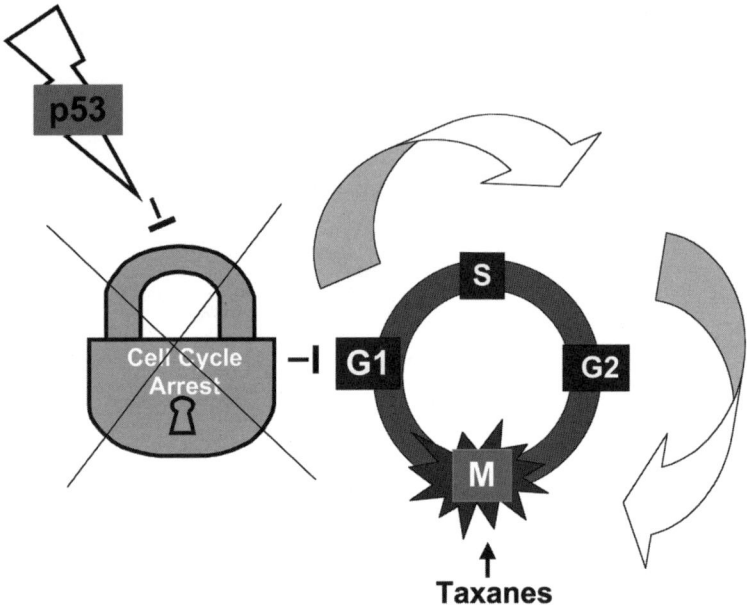

Taxanes

Fig. 2. Mutant, dysfunctional *p53* may improve response to taxanes. During mitosis, taxanes are effective against tumor cells, inducing a *p53*-independent cell death. Tumor cells harboring a mutant *p53* gene will not be arrested in the G_1 phase. These cells remain unobstructed and can reach the phase of mitosis in a more synchronized way. Therefore mutant tumor cells may respond even better to taxanes.

4.2. Study Design

As predictive markers are used to estimate the likelihood of sensitivity or resistance to a distinct therapy, the end point of studies evaluating predictive markers should be the response to treatment *(35)*. The neoadjuvant setting is ideal to measure tumor response directly. Adjuvant trials offer only indirect parameters of response, namely disease-free and overall survival. In the adjuvant setting, a survival advantage can be attributed only indirectly to treatment response, on the condition that an untreated control group is coevaluated. An untreated control arm is not needed in neoadjuvant trials, as there is unlikely to be a response to no treatment. In this regard, several studies have shown that complete pathologic response after several cycles of therapy is highly associated with disease-free and overall survival *(39,40)*. Therefore retrospective *p53* analyses from patients who are prospectively entered into neoadjuvant trials might achieve a high level of evidence (see clinical utility score of tumor markers) *(35–37)*. Such studies are cost effective and time saving, provided all patients of the initial study can be included.

Berns reviewed 26 reports from 1995 to 2000 that correlated *p53* status and response to treatment, including nearly 6000 breast cancer patients. This review included five studies using *p53* sequencing analysis, but unfortunately these were all adjuvant trials and, in addition, patients were treated with multiple agents. All five sequencing studies were reported as being predictive of response to tamoxifen or *p53*-dependent chemotherapy. The results from the 21 reviewed IHC studies were conflicting (6 predictive, 15 not predictive). The reviewed studies included four neoadjuvant trials, all of which unfortunately used IHC for *p53* analysis and were all negative for the prediction of response *(10,21,43)*.

Furthermore, the review included five trials with second-line treatment in the metastatic setting, which also allows direct response assessment, although most frequently clinical and not pathohistological response is evaluated in such studies. However, in the two studies which used sequencing, the *p53* genotype was reported to be predictive. In the three IHC studies *p53* results did not provide predictive information *(10)*.

Currently, no reported studies of *p53* as a predictive factor takes into account all of these issues; monotherapy, evaluation of a reliable end point, and issues regarding the technical aspects of the assay for *p53* abnormalities *(35–37)*.

In Table 1 we reviewed recent studies that meet the minimum requirements to assess the predictive value of *p53* in breast cancer. These studies provide a neoadjuvant or metastatic setting, allowing a direct response assessment.

All studies using *p53* sequencing technique proved to be predictive of response to *p53*-dependent therapies. Results from the listed IHC studies were found to be inconsistent; the majority were not predictive for response. However, most of the studies were retrospective and did not include the complete cohort from the initial prospective trial.

In three retrospective studies on three different cancers we evaluated the predictive power of *p53*. Using *p53* sequence analysis in neoadjuvantly treated patients only, we found that the *p53* genotype consistently and completely demarcated a group of patients who did not respond to treatment (Table 2; *[6–8]*). Sequencing analysis of these 168 patients who had received *p53*-dependent neoadjuvant treatment revealed no single patient harboring a *p53* mutation among those who responded to treatment. The probability that a mutant *p53* genotype indicates treatment failure (=specificity) was 100% in breast, lung, and rectal cancer, respectively. In these studies the *p53* genotype proved to be a powerful predictor of treatment failure. The complete identification of a group of patients (i.e., responders or nonresponders) is a prerequisite for the clinical utility of a predictive marker, as it allows the clinician to make treatment decisions *(44)*.

5. *p53* AND PROGNOSIS

The *p53* gene appears to be involved in a vast number of essential cellular functions. As a transcription factor it binds to a number of genes, either turning them on or off. Cells with inactivated *p53* generally exhibit an increased proliferation rate owing to loss of cell cycle control and a higher genomic instability secondary to loss of DNA repair.

p53 also appears to be involved in the inhibition of angiogenesis, affecting tumor spread and invasion. Therefore *p53* would also be expected to be indicative of the tumor-inherent biological aggressiveness determining the outcome and the prognosis, independent of therapy (or in the absence of systemic therapy). Because *p53* may interact positively or negatively with different systemic therapies, the pure prognostic value of *p53* can be assessed only by analysis of untreated patient cohorts. The majority of prognostic results derive from retrospective studies, and most of them contained patients who received one or more systemic therapies.

Nonetheless, several studies have tried to address *p53* as a prognostic factor (Table 3; *[5,11,16,46,48–53]*)1996 mutations in the *p53* gene were reported to constitute the single most important indicator for recurrence and death in breast cancer *(45)*. Blaszyk reviewed 14 studies published between 1993 and 1998, correlating *p53* gene mutation and prognosis in breast cancer. Eleven of theses studies used screening methods for *p53* analysis. Overall the relative risks reported by the authors were between 2.2 and 3.3 *(46)*.

Elledge reviewed a large number of studies relating the *p53* status to prognosis in breast cancer *(16)*. In these 57 studies published from 1992 to 1997, different methods for *p53* analysis were used: IHC in 43, screening methods (SSCP, CDGE) in 12, and sequencing in 2 studies only. The authors state that a positive *p53* IHC appeared to be consistently associated with other poor prognostic factors such as estrogen and progesterone receptor negativity, a poor grade, and a high proliferative fraction, and was not associated with size or nodal status. The authors concluded that positive *p53* IHC appeared to be independently associated with a worse prognosis and increases the relative risk of relapse by 1.5. Overall, the authors considered the risk difference to be too small to decide on adjuvant therapy based on the *p53* IHC alone.

6. CONCLUSIONS

The *p53* gene is one of the most intensively studied molecules in the human genome. From a biologic aspect, *p53* is an extraordinary molecule. It has led many researchers to believe that probably every cancer cell has to inherit a defect in the *p53* pathway. Thousands of changes may contribute to the malignant phenotype *(54)*. In any case, *p53* appears to be involved in a plethora of cell-inherent systems determining cellular proliferation and

Table 3
Studies Meeting Some Important Requirements (Bold) to Assess the Prognostic Value of p53 in Breast Cancer

Author (ref.)	Journal	No. of patients	Technique	Technical specifics	Untreated control	Adjuvant therapy	Prospective for marker question	Multivariate analysis	DFS	OS	Authors' conclusions
Elledge (16)	*Breast Cancer Res Treat* 1998	694	IHC	PAb 1801+ PAb240	Yes	TAM	No	Independent	0.008	0.056	Prognostic but weak
Beenken (48)	*Ann Surg* 2001	90	IHC	DACO	Yes	CMF	No	Independent		0.011	Coexpression of *p53* and *c-erb*-B2 has even more prognostic significance than T or N stage
Balszyk (46)	*Int J Cancer* 2000	90	Screening / IHC	ddf+exons 4-10 + splice sites / Pab1801+ Pab240+ Pab421		CMF or CAF +/- TAM	Yes	Independent	0.0032 0.02	0.0001 0.003	Gene mutations associated with adverse outcome
Elkhuizen (49)	*JCO* 2000	361	IHC	Mab DO7	Yes	FU, Doxo, Cyclophosph	No	Independent	0.05		Associated with higher local relapse rate
Degeorges (50)	*BCRT* 1998	282	IHC	Mab DO7	Yes	CMF	No	ns	ns	ns	
Geisler (11)	*Cancer Res* 2001	91	Screening	TTGE + sequencing+ Mab DO7	No	doxorubicin	Yes	ns	0.0002	0.0034	
Thor (52)	*JNCI* 1998	595	IHC		No	CAF	No	Independent	0.035	0.023	
Takahashi (53)	*IJC* 2000	76	Screening	Yeast functional assay	No	5 FU + TAM	No	Independent	ns	0.032	*p53* mutation + loss of estrogen receptor affect prognosis
Dublin (5)	*IJC* 1997	277	IHC	Mab DO1	Yes	CMF	No	ns	ns	ns	

Only studies providing multivariate analysis were selected. Other important challenges for prognostic marker studies as untreated control group and prospective design are only incompletely met. Methods for *p53* analysis do not include sequencing and antibodies used for IHC and screening methods are different as well as the treatment regimens.

DFS, Disease-free survival; OS, overall survival. ns, not significant.

death. During cancer development, tumor cells select against the tumor-suppressor functions of *p53*. Disruption of *p53*-dependent apoptosis confers a selective advantage during carcinogenesis. Considering the biologic rationale, *p53* appears to be an ideal prognostic and predictive factor. However, more than 10 yr of *p53* research have not resulted in a reliable demonstration of the true prognostic and predictive value of *p53* and its clinical usefulness in breast cancer or other malignancies. Reviewing the plethora of clinical studies, which are not comparable in many respects, preventing meta-analysis, it would appear that future studies should be planned more carefully to promote the *p53* story.

- To assess the true predictive value of *p53* (or any other predictive marker) an *optimal study design* is essential: ideally, *p53* should be analyzed on the basis of monotherapeutic neoadjuvant studies, as the parameter of interest is *response* to treatment with the agent of interest.
- Careful attention is required to *the optimal analysis method.* Any new method to be introduced has to be compared in carefully planned studies to sequencing, which remains the gold standard method.
- As the marker information is needed prior to therapy, it has to be considered that *p53* has to be assessable on biopsy.

Nonetheless, clinical application of *p53* status as a criterion for treatment decisions and selection of appropriate therapy could potentially help the clinician to increase response rates to chemo- and radiation therapy, and subsequently increase the rate of radical resection. In addition, patients will be spared the discomfort of ineffective treatment as well as unpleasant side effects.

After all these years of clinical *p53* research the final statement has not yet changed: To implement *p53* in clinical cancer treatment, well-designed prospective randomized neoadjuvant studies using carefully selected methods of *p53* analysis are urgently needed.

REFERENCES

1. Hamilton A, Piccart M. The contribution of molecular markers to the prediction of response in the treatment of breast cancer: a review of the literature on HER-2, p53 and BCL-2. *Ann Oncol* 2000;11:647–663.
2. Fitzgibbons PL, Page DL, Weaver D, et al. Prognostic factors in breast cancer. College of American Pathologists Consensus Statement 1999. *Arch Pathol Lab Med* 2000;124:966–978.
3. Ashcroft M, Vousden KH. Regulation of p53 stability. *Oncogene* 1999;18:7637–7643.
4. Harris CC. 1995 Deichmann Lecture—p53 tumor suppressor gene: at the crossroads of molecular carcinogenesis, molecular epidemiology and cancer risk assessment. *Toxicol Lett* 1995;82–83:1–7.

5. Dublin EA, Miles DW, Rubens RD, Smith P, Barnes DM. p53 immunohistochemical staining and survival after adjuvant chemotherapy for breast cancer. *Int J Cancer* 1997;74:605–608.

6. Kandioler D, Zwrtek R, Ludwig C, et al. TP53 genotype but not p53 immunohistochemical result predicts response to preoperative short-term radiotherapy in rectal cancer. *Ann Surg* 2002;235:493–498.

7. Kandioler-Eckersberger D, Kappel S, Mittlbock M, et al. The TP53 genotype but not immunohistochemical result is predictive of response to cisplatin-based neoadjuvant therapy in stage III non-small cell lung cancer. *J Thorac Cardiovasc Surg* 1999;117:744–750.

8. Kandioler-Eckersberger D, Ludwig C, Rudas M, et al. TP53 mutation and p53 overexpression for prediction of response to neoadjuvant treatment in breast cancer patients. *Clin Cancer Res* 2000;6:50–56.

9. Bergh J. Clinical studies of p53 in treatment and benefit of breast cancer patients. *Endocr Relat Cancer* 1999;6:51–59.

10. Berns EM, Foekens JA, Vossen R, et al. Complete sequencing of TP53 predicts poor response to systemic therapy of advanced breast cancer. *Cancer Res* 2000;60:2155–2162.

11. Geisler S, Lonning PE, Aas T, et al. Influence of TP53 gene alterations and c-erbB-2 expression on the response to treatment with doxorubicin in locally advanced breast cancer. *Cancer Res* 2001;61:2505–2512.

12. Clahsen PC, van de Velde CJ, Duval C, et al. p53 protein accumulation and response to adjuvant chemotherapy in premenopausal women with node-negative early breast cancer. *J Clin Oncol* 1998;16:470–479.

13. Andersen PS, Jespersgaard C, Vuust J, Christiansen M, Larsen LA. Capillary electrophoresis-based single strand DNA conformation analysis in high-throughput mutation screening. *Hum Mutat* 2003;21:455–465.

14. Iacopetta B, Elsaleh H, Grieu F, Joseph D, Sterrett G, Robbins P. Routine analysis of p53 mutation in clinical breast tumor specimens using fluorescence-based polymerase chain reaction and single strand conformation polymorphism. *Diagn Mol Pathol* 2000;9:20–25.

15. Bosserhoff AK, Buettner R, Hellerbrand C. Use of capillary electrophoresis for high throughput screening in biomedical applications. A minireview. *Comb Chem High Throughput Screen* 2000;3:455–466.

16. Elledge RM, Allred DC. Prognostic and predictive value of p53 and p21 in breast cancer. *Breast Cancer Res Treat* 1998;52:79–98.

17. Lu ML, Wikman F, Orntoft TF, et al. Impact of alterations affecting the p53 pathway in bladder cancer on clinical outcome, assessed by conventional and array-based methods. *Clin Cancer Res* 2002;8:171–179.

18. Torhorst J, Bucher C, Kononen J, et al. Tissue microarrays for rapid linking of molecular changes to clinical endpoints. *Am J Pathol* 2001;159:2249–2256.

19. Sjogren S, Inganas M, Norberg T, et al. The p53 gene in breast cancer: prognostic value of complementary DNA sequencing versus immunohistochemistry. *J Natl Cancer Inst* 1996;88:173–182.

20. Anelli A, Brentani RR, Gadelha AP, Amorim De Albuquerque A, Soares F. Correlation of p53 status with outcome of neoadjuvant chemotherapy using paclitaxel and doxorubicin in stage IIIB breast cancer. *Ann Oncol* 2003;14:428–432.

21. Makris A, Powles TJ, Dowsett M, et al. Prediction of response to neoadjuvant chemoendocrine therapy in primary breast carcinomas. *Clin Cancer Res* 1997;3:593–600.

22. Formenti SC, Dunnington G, Uzieli B, et al. Original p53 status predicts for patho-logical response in locally advanced breast cancer patients treated preoperatively with continuous infusion 5-fluorouracil and radiation therapy. *Int J Radiat Oncol Biol Phys* 1997;39:1059–1068.

23. Bergh J, Norberg T, Sjogren S, Lindgren A, Holmberg L. Complete sequencing of the p53 gene provides prognostic information in breast cancer patients, particu-larly in relation to adjuvant systemic therapy and radiotherapy. *Nat Med* 1995;1:1029–1034.

24. Hartmann A, Blaszyk H, Kovach JS, Sommer SS. The molecular epidemiology of p53 gene mutations in human breast cancer. *Trends Genet* 1997;13:27–33.

25. Masood S. Assessment of prognostic factors in breast fine-needle aspirates. *Am J Clin Pathol* 2000;113:S84–S96.

26. Powell B, Soong R, Iacopetta B, Seshadri R, Smith DR. Prognostic significance of mutations to different structural and functional regions of the p53 gene in breast cancer. *Clin Cancer Res* 2000;6:443–451.

27. Chene P. The role of tetramerization in p53 function. *Oncogene* 2001;20:2611–2617.

28. Aas T, Borresen AL, Geisler S, et al. Specific P53 mutations are associated with de novo resistance to doxorubicin in breast cancer patients. *Nat Med* 1996;2:811–814.

29. Bates S, Vousden KH. Mechanisms of p53-mediated apoptosis. *Cell Mol Life Sci* 1999;55:28–37.

30. Lowe SW, Bodis S, McClatchey A, et al. p53 status and the efficacy of cancer therapy in vivo. *Science* 1994;266:807–810.

31. Fisher DE. Apoptosis in cancer therapy: crossing the threshold. *Cell* 1994;78:539–542.

32. Cleator S, Parton M, Dowsett M. The biology of neoadjuvant chemotherapy for breast cancer. *Endocr Relat Cancer* 2002;9:183–195.

33. Buzdar AU, Singletary SE, Theriault RL, et al. Prospective evaluation of paclitaxel versus combination chemotherapy with fluorouracil, doxorubicin, and cyclophos-phamide as neoadjuvant therapy in patients with operable breast cancer. *J Clin Oncol* 1999;17:3412–3417.

34. Rakovitch E, Mellado W, Hall EJ, Pandita TK, Sawant S, Geard CR. Paclitaxel sensitivity correlates with p53 status and DNA fragmentation, but not G2/M accu-mulation. *Int J Radiat Oncol Biol Phys* 1999;44:1119–1124.

35. Yamauchi H, Stearns V, Hayes DF. When is a tumor marker ready for prime time? A case study of c-erbB-2 as a predictive factor in breast cancer. *J Clin Oncol* 2001;19:2334–2356.

36. Hayes DF. Designing tumor marker studies: will the results provide clinically useful information. *Arch Pathol Lab Med* 2000;124:952–954.

37. Concato J, Shah N, Horwitz RI. Randomized, controlled trials, observational studies, and the hierarchy of research designs. *N Engl J Med* 2000;342:1887–1892.

38. Faneyte IF, Schrama JG, Peterse JL, Remijnse PL, Rodenhuis S, van de Vijver MJ. Breast cancer response to neoadjuvant chemotherapy: predictive markers and relation with outcome. *Br J Cancer* 2003;88:406–412.

39. Fisher B, Brown A, Mamounas E, et al. Effect of preoperative chemotherapy on local-regional disease in women with operable breast cancer: findings from National Surgical Adjuvant Breast and Bowel Project B-18. *J Clin Oncol* 1997;15:2483–2493.

40. Fisher B, Bryant J, Wolmark N, et al. Effect of preoperative chemotherapy on the outcome of women with operable breast cancer. *J Clin Oncol* 1998;16:2672–2685.
41. van der Hage JA, van de Velde CJ, Julien JP, Tubiana-Hulin M, Vandervelden C, Duchateau L. Preoperative chemotherapy in primary operable breast cancer: results from the European Organization for Research and Treatment of Cancer trial 10902. *J Clin Oncol* 2001;19:4224–4237.
42. Stearns V, Singh B, Tsangaris T, et al. A prospective randomized pilot study to evaluate predictors of response in serial core biopsies to single agent neoadjuvant doxorubicin or paclitaxel for patients with locally advanced breast cancer. *Clin Cancer Res* 2003;9:124–133.
43. Chang J, Powles TJ, Allred DC, et al. Biologic markers as predictors of clinical outcome from systemic therapy for primary operable breast cancer. *J Clin Oncol* 1999;17:3058–3063.
44. Hayes DF, Thor AD. c-erbB-2 in breast cancer: development of a clinically useful marker. *Semin Oncol* 2002;29:231–245.
45. Kovach JS, Hartmann A, Blaszyk H, Cunningham J, Schaid D, Sommer SS. Mutation detection by highly sensitive methods indicates that p53 gene mutations in breast cancer can have important prognostic value. *Proc Natl Acad Sci USA* 1996;93:1093–1096.
46. Blaszyk H, Hartmann A, Cunningham JM, et al. A prospective trial of midwest breast cancer patients: a p53 gene mutation is the most important predictor of adverse outcome. *Int J Cancer* 2000;89:32–38.
47. Hilsenbeck SG, Ravdin PM, de Moor CA, Chamness GC, Osborne CK, Clark GM. Time-dependence of hazard ratios for prognostic factors in primary breast cancer. *Breast Cancer Res Treat* 1998;52:227–237.
48. Beenken SW, Grizzle WE, Crowe DR, et al. Molecular biomarkers for breast cancer prognosis: coexpression of c-erbB-2 and p53. *Ann Surg* 2001;233: 630–638.
49. Elkhuizen PH, van Slooten HJ, Clahsen PC, et al. High local recurrence risk after breast-conserving therapy in node-negative premenopausal breast cancer patients is greatly reduced by one course of perioperative chemotherapy: A European Organization for Research and Treatment of Cancer Breast Cancer Cooperative Group Study. *J Clin Oncol* 2000;18:1075–1083.
50. Degeorges A, de Roquancourt A, Extra JM, et al. Is p53 a protein that predicts the response to chemotherapy in node negative breast cancer? *Breast Cancer Res Treat* 1998;47:47–55.
51. Rahko E, Blanco G, Soini Y, Bloigu R, Jukkola A. A mutant TP53 gene status is associated with a poor prognosis and anthracycline-resistance in breast cancer patients. *Eur J Cancer* 2002;39:447–453.
52. Thor AD, Berry DA, Budman DR, et al. erbB-2, p53, and efficacy of adjuvant therapy in lymph node-positive breast cancer. *J Natl Cancer Inst* 1998;90:1346–1360.
53. Takahashi M, Tonoki H, Tada M, et al. Distinct prognostic values of p53 mutations and loss of estrogen receptor and their cumulative effect in primary breast cancers. *Int J Cancer* 2000;89:92–99.
54. Schmitt CA, Fridman JS, Yang M, Baranov E, Hoffman RM, Lowe SW. Dissecting p53 tumor suppressor functions in vivo. *Cancer Cell* 2002;1:289–298.

V PREDICTIVE BIOMARKERS IN BODY FLUIDS

12 Occult Metastatic Cells in Breast Cancer Patients

State of the Art, Pitfalls, and Promises

Stephan Braun, MD, Julia Seeber, MD, and Christian Marth, MD

SUMMARY

Blood-borne distant metastasis is the leading cause of cancer-related death in patients with breast cancer. The onset of this fundamental process can now be assessed in cancer patients using immunocytochemical and molecular assays able to detect even single metastatic cells. However, careful validation of technically confounding variables, including choice of detection antibody, preparation of cellular samples, and size of analyzed sample volumes, is mandatory for reproducible and comparable results. In studies with validated assays, analyses of bone marrow samples show that disseminated cells are present in 20–40% of primary breast cancer patients without any

Cancer Drug Discovery and Development: Biomarkers in Breast Cancer:
Molecular Diagnostics for Predicting and Monitoring Therapeutic Effect
Edited by: G. Gasparini and D. F. Hayes © Humana Press Inc., Totowa, NJ

clinical or histopathological signs of metastasis. The common homing of circulating breast cancer cells in bone marrow is indicative of systemic tumor cell spread and growth of overt metastases in relevant organ sites such as bone, lung, or liver. Recent clinical studies involving more than 3000 breast cancer patients demonstrated that presence of tumor cells in bone marrow at primary diagnosis is an independent prognostic factor for unfavorable clinical outcome. To date, sampling of bone marrow, however, is not a routine procedure in clinical management of breast cancer patients. In this chapter, we review the existing tumor cell assays and discuss their current clinical relevance and perspectives for the clinical management of breast cancer patients.

Key Words: Breast cancer; disseminated tumor cells; circulating tumor cells; prevalence; prognosis.

INTRODUCTION

In breast cancer, recent guidelines for adjuvant systemic therapy result in treatment recommendations for more than 90% of patients even in case of a negative lymph-node status (1,2). The risk of tumor relapse in these patients is considered high enough to recommend adjuvant therapy, even though up to 70% of early stage breast cancer patients are cured by locoregional surgery alone. Therefore, the availability of additional factors enabling individual risk assessment would be desirable to improve identification of patients at risk for relapse.

Although the presence of lymph-node metastasis is a negative prognostic factor for breast cancer and other cancers, it is still not possible to reliably identify those patients who will eventually relapse with metastatic disease only by their lymph node status at primary therapy, indicating that other ways of metastatic tumor cell spread also play an important role. Gene expression profiling (3) and clinical studies (4,5) further indicate that during early stages of breast cancer tumors are more likely to disseminate either via the lymphatic or the hematogenous route rather than simultaneously via both routes.

Advances in the development of immunocytochemical and molecular assays now enable specific detection of metastatic tumor cells even at the single cell stage and thus allow to address the important question of systemic tumor cell dissemination as one of the first crucial steps in the metastatic cascade. Using these technologies, it has become evident that 20–40% of patients with breast cancer harbor occult metastatic cells in their bone marrow even in the absence of any lymph node metastases (stage N0) and clinical signs of overt distant metastases (stage M0). However, these techniques for detection of metastatic cells are not yet established in clinical routine practice, and no international consensus has been reached to recommend a single standardized protocol as benchmark technology.

Several studies on breast cancer patients suggested that presence of disseminated tumor cells (DTCs) in bone marrow represents an additional clinical marker that may be capable to identify those patients who are cured by surgery alone (in the absence of such cells) or may require more specific therapy (in the presence of such cells). One of the intriguing opportunities of this marker might therefore be its use for clinical decision making in risk adapted adjuvant treatment strategies. Another important and (in comparison to other markers) unique application might be the monitoring of therapeutic efficacy in the adjuvant setting with no measurable disease. In this overview, we discuss usefulness and clinical relevance of immunologic and molecular analyses applied for diagnosis of DTCs in bone marrow of breast cancer patients.

2. STATE OF THE ART AND PITFALLS IN TUMOR CELL DETECTION

2.1. Histopathology

Using conventional histopathologic techniques at time of primary diagnosis without clinical signs of metastatic bone disease, the likelihood of identifying DTCs in bone marrow is as low as 4% *(6,7)*. These findings suggest that histopathologic evaluation might not be sensitive enough for the indicated purpose.

2.2. Immunocytochemistry

2.2.1. TUMOR CELLS IN BONE MARROW

To date, most experience with bone marrow screening for DTCs exists for immunocytochemical analyses (Table 1). Numerous studies reported a strong prognostic impact of the presence of DTCs *(4,5,8–14)*, while other investigations failed to do so (Table 2) *(15–22)*. One reason for the discrepant results of clinical follow-up studies is a substantial methodological variation (e.g., sensitivity and specificity of detection antibody, lower detection rate of bone marrow biopsy as compared to bone marrow aspiration, considerable variation in the number of cells analyzed) resulting in a wide range of detection rates between study populations (Tables 1 and 2). Nevertheless, the six most recent studies *(5,8–10,12,23)* comprising more than 3000 patients consistently reported that the presence of DTCs in bone marrow has a strong prognostic impact on patient survival (Table 2). However, even in these studies, at least three confounding technical factors varied considerably: (1) consistent and blinded analysis of noncarcinoma control patients, (2) diversity of antibodies used for identification of epithelial cells in bone marrow, and (3) number of cells analyzed per patient sample.

Table 1
Technical and Clinical Variability in Bone Marrow Micrometastasis Studies[a]

Variables		No. of studies (%)
Technical type		
Tissue collection	Bone marrow biopsy	5 (24)
	Bone marrow aspiration	16 (76)
Assay	Immunocytochemistry	17 (81)
	RT-PCR	4 (19)
Antigens	Mucin-like antigens	5 (24)
	Cytokeratin	11 (52)
	Mixed	5 (24)
Quantitation of tumor cells	Yes (cytospin)	6 (29)
	No (biopsy)	5 (24)
	No (cell smears)	6 (29)
	No (RT-PCR)	4 (19)
Detection rates	<10%	2 (9)
	10–19%	4 (19)
	20–29%	4 (19)
	30–40%	6 (29)
	>40%	5 (24)
Clinical type		
Investigated subgroups	All subgroups	20 (95)
	Node-negative, only	1 (5)
	Node-positive, only	—
Study type	Mono-center	20 (95)
	Oligo-/multicenter	1 (5)
	Controlled clinical trial	—
	Prospective prevalence study	21 (100)
Size of study population	≤100	8 (38)
	101–500	9 (43)
	>500	4 (19)

[a]Data from refs. *4,5,8–15,17–23,78,80–82.*

Pantel et al. *(24)* designed a study to evaluate some of the variables affecting the immunocytochemical detection of individual epithelial tumor cells in bone marrow. Bone marrow aspirates were taken from 368 patients with primary carcinomas of the breast, lung, prostate, or colon–rectum using an alkaline phosphatase antialkaline phosphatase staining technique. DTCs were detected with specificity proven monoclonal antibodies CK2 and

A45-B/B3. In the first line, detection rate was affected by blood contamination of the aspirates, the number of aspirates analyzed, and the number of marrow cells screened per aspiration site. The significantly lower detection rate by monospecific anti-CK-18 antibody CK2 as compared to antibody A45-B/B3, which detects heterodimers CK-8/18 and CK8/19, indicated that assay sensitivity may, however, be further affected by factors of the microenvironment or altered gene expression during metastasis. Several recent studies analyzing gene expression *(3)* and protein expression *(25,26)* indicated that down-regulation of single CK peptides (e.g., CK-18) may be necessary to alter cell plasticity in order to increase invasiveness and metastasis. Thus, beyond mere basic technical aspects (e.g., sensitivity and specificity), tumor-related processes significantly influence assay validity.

Sufficient methodological validation of the detection antibodies has only been reported for anticytokeratin antibodies *(7,24,27–29)*. The rare occurrence of single CK-positive cells in aspirates of noncarcinoma control patients *(9)* points to minimal—yet acceptable—technical variations within a biological system. The resulting risk of false-positive findings in cancer patients can be minimized by using morphological criteria in addition to immunostaining for diagnosis of DTCs *(27,28)*. Additional justification for using cytokeratin-specific antibodies in screening assays for occult breast carcinoma cells can be derived from several recent studies, describing phenotypic characteristics of CK-positive DTCs as similar to those usually found in malignant solid tumors *(30–33)*. Furthermore, in single CK-positive DTCs, numerical chromosome aberrations were detected by interphase fluorescent *in situ* hybridization analysis *(34)*; multiple mutations by whole-genome amplification *(35)*; and multiple chromosomal aberrations by combined transcriptome and genome analysis of single micrometastatic cells *(36–38)*.

Both the International Society of Cell Therapy (ISCT) and the National Cancer Institute (NCI) have recognized the need for standardization of the immunocytochemical assay and for its evaluation in prospective studies *(27,39)*. On the basis of data available from published methodological analyses *(9,24,27,29)* such a standardized assay may consist of a specificity-proven, anti-CK monoclonal antibody (i.e., A45–B/B3) and a sufficient sample size (i.e., 2×10^6 mononucleated cells per patient) obtained from two aspiration sites. The use of new automated devices for the microscopic screening of immunostained slides may help to read slides more rapidly and to increase reproducibility of the read-out process *(40–42)*.

2.2.2. Tumor Cells in Peripheral Blood

Peripheral blood would be an ideal source for the detection of disseminated tumor cells because of an easy sampling procedure. The presence of malignant cells in peripheral blood was described several decades ago

Table 2
Occult Metastatic Cancer Cells in Bone Marrow and Peripheral Blood of Breast Cancer Patients in Selected Studies

Authors (ref.)	Antigens	Preparation	Technique	No. of patients	Detection rate (%)	Prognostic value
Bone marrow						
Porro et al. (22)	Mucin	Biopsy	ICC	159	16	None
Salvadori et al. (21)	Mucin	Biopsy	ICC	121	17	None
Mathieu et al. (20)	Mucin/CK	Biopsy	ICC	93	1	None
Courtemanche et al. (18)	Mucin	Biopsy	ICC	50	8	None
Singletary et al. (19)	Mucin/CK	Cell smears	ICC	71	38	None
Cote et al. (14)	Mucin/CK	Cell smears	ICC	49	37	DFS, OS
Harbeck et al. (13)	Mucin/CK	Cell smears	ICC	100	38	DFS[a], OS[a]
Diel et al. (12)	Mucin	Cell smears	ICC	727	43	DFS[a], OS[a]
Funke et al. (17)	CK	Cytospins	ICC	234	38	n.d.
Landys et al. (11)	CK	Biopsy	ICC	128	19	DFS[a], OS[a]
Mansi et al. (10)	Mucin	Cell smears	ICC	350	25	DFS, OS
Untch et al. (15)	CK	Cytospins	ICC	581	28	None
Braun et al. (9)	CK	Cytospins	ICC	552	36	DDFS[a], OS[a]
Braun et al. (4)	CK	Cytospins	ICC	150	29	DDFS, OS[a]
Gerber et al. (5)	CK	Cytospins	ICC	484	31	DFS[a], OS[a]
Gebauer et al. (8)	Mucin/CK	Cell smears	ICC	393	42	DFS[a], OS
Wiedswang et al. (23)	CK	Cytospins	ICC	817	13	DDFS[a], BCSS[a]
Datta et al. (82)	CK19	Cell suspension	RT-PCR	34	26	DFS
Fields et al. (81)	CK19	Cell suspension	RT-PCR	83	71	DFS

Vannucchi et al. (80)	CK19	Cell suspension	RT-PCR	33	DFS
Slade et al. (78)	CK19	Cell suspension	RT-PCR	23	None
Peripheral blood					
Mapara et al. (86)	CK19, EGF-R	Cell suspension	RT-PCR	21	None
Smith et al. (59)	CK 8./18/19	Cytospins	ICC	22 (133)[b]	na
Smith et al. (59)	CK19	Cell suspension	RT-PCR	22 (145)[b]	na
Stathopoulou et al. (57)	CK 19	Cell suspension	RT-PCR	148	DFS[a], OS[a]
Zach et al. (79)	hMAM	Cell suspension	RT-PCR	114	None
Racila et al. (71)	CK	Cell suspension	FC	30	na
Witzig et al. (106)	CK	Cytospins	ICC	75	na

BCSS, Breast cancer specific survival; CK, cytokeratin; DFS, disease-free survival; DDFS, distant disease-free survival; FC, flow cytometry; H&E, hematoxylin and eosin staining; hMAM, human mammaglobin; ICC, immunocytochemistry; IHC, immunohistochemistry; OS, overall survival; RT-PCR, reverse-transcriptase polymerase chain reaction; na, not analyzed.

[a]Prognostic value supported by multivariate analysis.
[b]Number of samples analyzed.

(43,44), and concerns toward intraoperative manipulation of the tumor causing uncontrolled tumor shedding were supported by studies on gastrointestinal and prostate cancer patients *(45–50)*. More recent reports have confirmed the malignant nature of the detected cells using cytogenetic or molecular analysis *(51,52)*. From model systems, it was estimated that about 10^6 tumor cells/g of tumor tissue are shed daily into the blood, although such model calculations might overestimate the number actually shed in vivo *(53–55)*. Yet, for circulating tumor cells (CTCs), blood is only a temporary compartment in which no decision on the subsequent fate of CTCs per se is made, except for trapping of tumor emboli in the first capillary bed these cells encounter. Yet despite the fact that most cells that once entered the blood circulation survive the blood passage, metastasis remains an inefficient process with successful onset of micrometastasis by only a limited number of cells *(56)*. In consequence, from currently available studies it remains unknown, which fraction of CTCs survive and inherit the potential for metastatic growth in the new secondary microenvironment. This ignorance, which in part is due to the nature of the analysis of CTCs, hence probably less clonally selected, and in part to an enormous discrepancy between the actual circulating tumor load and the fraction available for analysis, explains the undetermined clinical value of presence of CTCs (Table 2). In breast cancer, few relatively small studies with different technical approaches suggested that presence of CTCs correlated with stage and course of the disease *(57–59)*. For other solid tumors, several reports have also shown a prognostic impact of CTCs in blood *(60–64)*. However, it remains debatable if these studies are empowered enough to answer the question of prognostic impact with a reasonably low β-type error, in view of relatively small study populations and sole focus on p-values for α-type error.

2.3. Specific Tumor Cell Enrichment and Depletion

Some of the discordant results from studies examining the role of DTCs and CTCs might be also due to the low frequency of these cells, and hence the technique-related variable degree of the sampling error. New enrichment techniques based on improved density gradient methods *(65)* and immunomagnetic procedures *(66,67)* may increase assay sensitivity in parallel reducing the degree of sampling error, which in consequence might help to increase data consistency of the clinical significance of DTCs and CTCs. Immunomagnetic enrichment utilizes differential expression of either tumor- or tissue-specific antigens by tumor cells as compared to mesenchymal cells in bone marrow and peripheral blood. For positive separation of tumor cells, beads coated with tumor- or tissue-specific antigens select DTCs and CTCs, while for negative separation, antibodies directed against hematopoietic or mesenchymal markers are coated to ferromagnetic beads *(67–72)*. These selection strategies have the additional advantage that the tumor cells are still viable and can be used for additional studies including the propagation of malignant cells in vitro *(73)*. At present, these new techniques are costly, time consuming, and their benefit over "standard" Ficoll gradients remains to be substantiated in further studies.

2.4. Genetic and Epigenetic-Based Assays

The lack of a unique genetic marker for solid cancers such as breast cancer requires sufficient sensitivity and specificity of tumor-cell associated genetic markers used for detection of DTCs and CTCs within a body compartment. The major limiting factor in detection of DTCs and CTCs by reverse transcriptase polymerase chain reaction (RT-PCR) is illegitimate transcription of tumor-associated or epithelial-specific genes reported for mesenchymal cells *(74,75)*. Moreover, owing to the extreme genetic instability of breast carcinoma cells, deficient expression of the marker gene in DTCs and CTCs may lower the actual sensitivity in vivo as compared to experimental model systems that use tumor cell lines to estimate assay sensitivity. Quantitative real-time PCR provides interesting prospects for better quantification of the tumor cell load, provided specific markers are available. The studies conducted so far in bone marrow and peripheral blood (Table 1) applied CK-19, mucin, and human mammaglobin (hMAM) mRNA markers *(57,59,76–82)* yet with uncertain specificity *(57,75,83–87)*. To date, the marker most extensively investigated for the detection of tumor cell (i.e., DTC/CTC) derived transcripts is CK-19. Using nested RT-PCR or competitive quantitative RT-PCR, with the number of CK-19 transcripts being normalized to the number of (breast cancer unrelated) *ABL* transcripts, several investigators found CK-19 transcripts in bone marrow and peripheral blood of early or metastatic breast cancer patients in 63–74% and 30–52%, respectively *(57,59,78)*. In establishing a quantitative real-time RT-PCR assay, however, we encountered serious difficulties being unable to obtain discernible crossing-points for samples from 129 cancer and 16 control patients *(83)*, strongly suggesting that CK-19 transcripts in BM—to some extent—are not of epithelial/tumor origin. Our assay used CK-19 primers with known absence of reactivity with CK-19a/CK-19b pseudogenes in lymphoid tissues *(88)*. These real-time RT-PCR data essentially confirm our previous results using nested RT-PCR. While in all breast cancer tissues hMAM, EGF-R, and CK-19 transcripts were detectable, blood samples from 31 healthy controls and 20 patients with hematological malignancies revealed absence of hMAM transcripts but presence of CK-19 transcripts in 27% and EGF-R transcripts in 10% of these cases *(84)*. These data are in contrast to the above cited studies on prevalence and assumed clinical relevance of CK-19 transcript detection in peripheral blood and bone marrow. The data on the limited value of currently propagated RT-PCR assays for the detection of DTC and CTC-derived transcripts point to the urgent need of improved approaches and studies demonstrating the actual value.

Beyond genetic characteristics, with the prevailing uncertainty about their specificity in solid tumors, changes in the status of DNA methylation, known as epigenetic alterations, are among the most common molecular alterations in human neoplasia *(89)*, including breast cancer *(90)*. Cytosine methylation occurs after DNA synthesis by enzymatic transfer of a methyl group from the methyl donor *S*-adenosylmethionine to the carbon-5 position of cytosine. Cytosines (C) are methylated in the human genome mostly when located 5' to a guanosine (G). Regions with a high G:C content are so-called CpG islands. It has been increasingly recognized over the past 4–5 yr that the CpG islands of many genes, which are mostly unmethylated in normal tissue, are methylated to various degrees in human cancers, thus representing tumor-specific alterations *(89,91)*. In a recent study on the prognostic value of DNA methylation in serum of breast cancer patients, methylated serum DNA for RASSF1A and/or APC was found to discriminate significantly and independently of established clinical factors between patients with more favorable (unmethylated serum DNA) and those with poor prognosis (methylated serum DNA) *(92)*. The tumor specificity and the possibility to use blood tests, together with the option for specific therapy using demethylating agents *(93)*, suggest the potential of this approach for diagnosis and monitoring patients' course of the disease. Yet, it still remains to be shown whether the assessment of epigenetic alterations and their specific treatment play the assumed functional role that determines metastatic growth, and hence the fate of the patient.

3. CLINICAL RELEVANCE
OF TUMOR CELL DETECTION

So far, studies on the prognostic value of DTCs in bone marrow are almost exclusively based on immunocytochemical data (Table 1). An important initial question was whether the presence of epithelial antigen-positive cells is correlated with established risk factors in breast cancer, such as tumor size or lymph node involvement. Diel et al. *(12)* found a significant correlation between bone marrow positivity, as assessed by antitumor-associated glycoprotein-12 (TAG-12) immunocytochemistry, and tumor size, nodal status, histopathologic tumor grading, as well as postmenopausal status. The London Ludwig Cancer Institute Group described that presence of EMA-positive cells in bone marrow was significantly related to lymph node involvement, peritumoral vascular invasion, and primary tumor size *(94)*. Studies using different anticytokeratin monoclonal antibodies demonstrated merely a tendency toward correlation between detection of cytokeratin-positive cells in bone marrow and locoregional lymph node involvement *(7,95)*. Applying the broad-spectrum anticytokeratin monoclonal antibody A45-B/B3 for DTC detection *(9)*, a significant association of such cells in bone marrow with the diagnosis of inflammatory breast cancer, tumor size, extensive lymph node metastasis of >10 nodes, and tumor grade was reported.

To assess the clinical significance of DTCs in bone marrow, follow-up studies were initiated. Using a polyclonal EMA antibody, Mansi et al. *(10)* detected metastatic cells in 25% of bone marrow samples. In their 6-yr follow-up analysis, univariate statistics revealed that the immunocytochemical finding predicts for an increased rate of relapse in bone and other distant sites, as well as decreased overall survival. Multivariate analysis both after 6 *(96)* and more than 12 yr of clinical follow-up *(10)* indicated that the prognostic impact of EMA-positive cells was not independent of established risk factors, such as tumor size, grade, and lymph node status. Using another mucin marker TAG-12, Diel et al. *(12)* reported a detection rate of 43% in a collective of 727 primary breast cancer patients. After a median follow-up time of 36 mo (3–108 mo), the presence of TAG-12-positive cells was described as being superior to axillary lymph node status, tumor stage, and tumor grade as an independent prognostic indicator for both metastasis-free and overall survival. But in contrast Gebauer et al. *(8)* detected metastatic cells in 42% of 393 breast cancer patients. Follow-up data were available for up to 10 yr after surgery. The multivariate analysis revealed independent prognostic relevance for bone marrow status, although tumor size and axillary lymph node status were superior prognostic factors.

Using different cocktails of monoclonal antibodies to cell-surface antigens and cytokeratins, Cote et al. *(14)*, Harbeck et al. *(13)*, and Gebauer et al. *(8)* were able to derive prognostic information from the presence of occult metastatic cells in bone marrow. A potential disadvantage of some of the earlier studies is substantial methodological variation. Therefore, a prospective two-center study in 552 primary breast cancer patients was initiated, using a validated immunoassay *(24,29)*. The test results could be reproduced independently at both study centers *(9)*. In this study, multivariate regression analysis verified that the presence of DTCs in bone marrow predicts poor prognosis overall (Fig. 1) and independent of the lymph node status (Fig. 2). These findings demonstrate for the first time that by using an identical assay for detection of DTC, reproducible results can be generated. In parallel to our study, a Norwegian study was launched and recently published, as the currently largest available single center study (817 patients), with a median follow-up of 49 mo *(23)*. The independent prognostic value of DTC in bone marrow was clearly confirmed for distant metastasis-free and breast cancer-specific survival. In combination of independent prognostic factors, such as tumor size, grading, and lymph node status, they were able to classify subgroups of both node-negative and node-positive patients

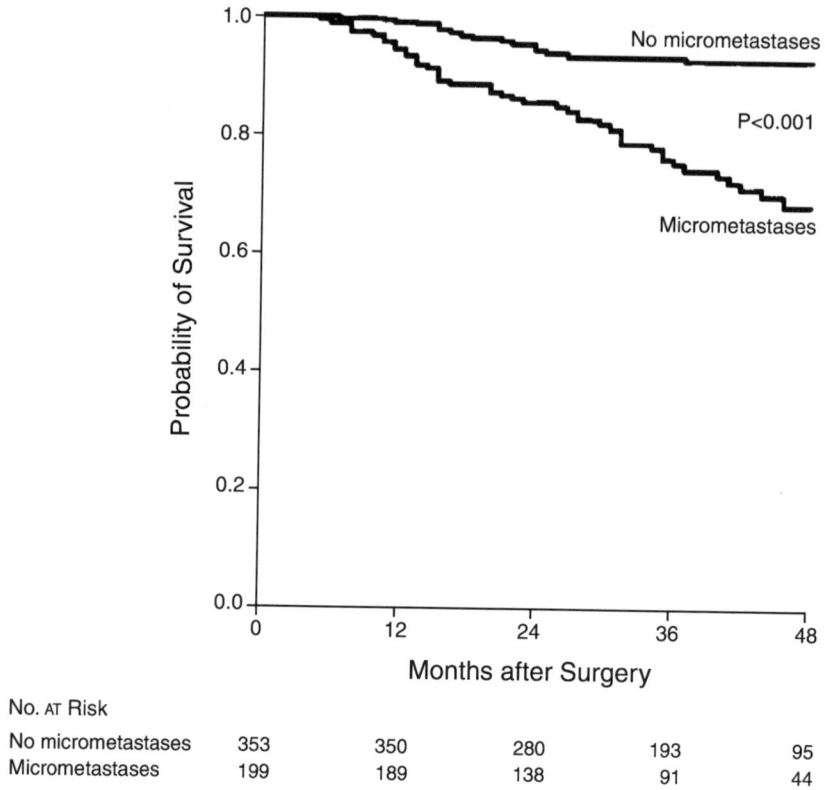

No. AT Risk				
No micrometastases	353	350	280	193	95
Micrometastases	199	189	138	91	44

Fig. 1. Overall survival of 552 breast cancer patients according to presence or absence of DTC in bone marrow, after a median observation time of 38 mo (log-rank test). (Adapted from ref. 9.)

into excellent and high-risk prognosis groups (Fig. 2), supporting the usefulness of DTC screening for patient stratification.

4. CONCLUSIONS AND PERSPECTIVES

Various immunocytochemical and molecular methods have been applied to detect occult hematogenous tumor cell spread in breast cancer patients. Numerous studies have marked the prognostic implications associated with the presence of occult metastatic cells (OMCs) at the time of diagnosis. Yet, screening of bone marrow micrometastasis is currently not accepted as a routine diagnostic tool. Reasons for this are the lack of international consensus and consequently the lack of studies demonstrating both improved risk stratification and patient outcome in the setting of clinical trials. International consensus is now urgently needed regarding quality control issues

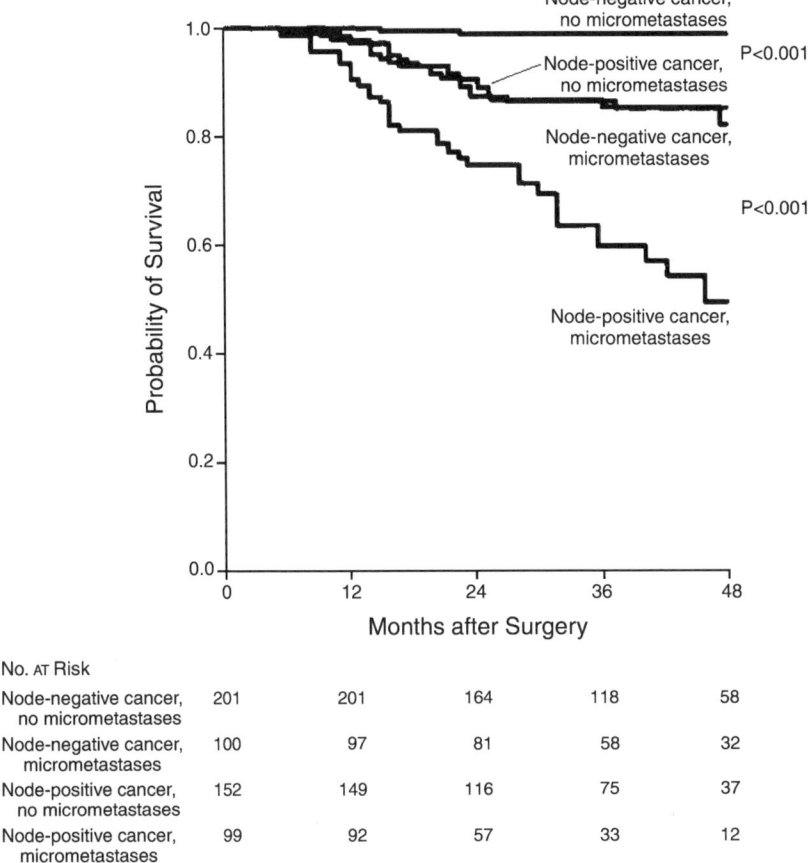

Fig. 2. Overall survival of 552 breast cancer patients according to presence or absence of DTC in bone marrow and lymph-node status, after a median observation time of 38 mo (log-rank test). (Adapted from ref. *9*.)

and criteria for acceptable technical assay performance, such as false-negative and false-positive rates, for clinically applicable assays to permit comparisons between different assay platforms. Finally, to support efforts on clinical trial design, marker implementation into current risk classification systems, such as the Tumor–Node–Metastasis (TNM) classification system is needed. A useful proposal has recently been made by the International Union Against Cancer (UICC) *(97)*. The most recent TNM classification for breast cancer *(98)* does not qualify the presence of single cancer cells in peripheral blood or bone marrow as metastasis (stage M0), but it optionally reports the presence of such cells together with their detection method (e.g., M0[i+] or [mol+]).

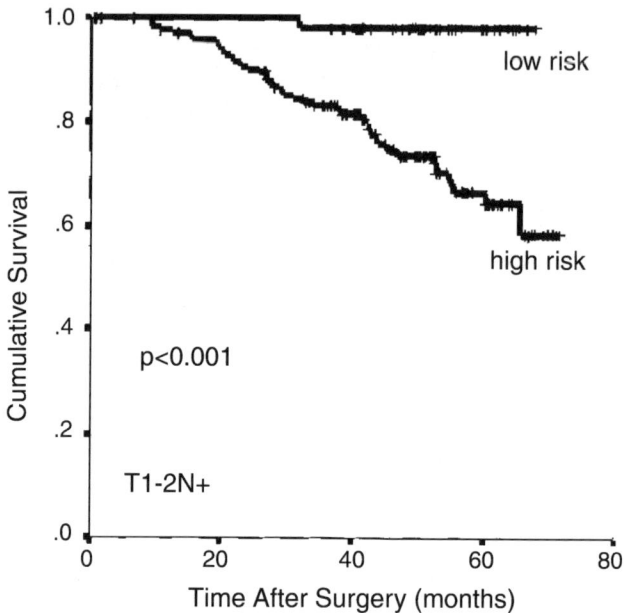

Fig. 3. Overall survival of breast cancer patients according to presence or absence of independent prognostic factors, after a median observation time of 49 mo (log-rank test). Low-risk profile (tumor size <2 cm, estrogen/progesterone receptor-positive and bone marrow-negative) vs high-risk profile (tumor size >2 cm and/or estrogen/progesterone receptor-negative and/or bone marrow-positive). (Adapted from ref. *23*.)

Beyond merely adding another prognostic factor to the plethora of such markers in breast cancer, it needs to be emphasized that assessment of occult hematogenous tumor cell spread inherits the potential for a tool for prediction and monitoring of efficacy of systemic therapy *(99–103)*. In contrast to lymph nodes, which are generally accepted as "indirect" marker of hematogenous tumor cell spread and, hence, risk of systemic spread but which are also generally removed at primary surgery and unavailable for follow-up evaluations, bone marrow and blood can be obtained repeatedly in the postoperative course of the patient. In Fig. 3, for example, the only prognostic factor available for follow-up risk assessment is the presence of bone marrow micrometastasis. The clinical value of such examinations has been strongly suggested by clinical studies on a total of almost 500 patients, which identified the prognostic relevance of OMC present in bone marrow several months after diagnosis or treatment when no relapse has occurred until that date *(100,104,105)*. The potential of a surrogate marker assay that permits immediate assessment of therapy-induced cytotoxic effects on occult metastatic cells is therefore evident, as indicated previously *(100)*. Since repeated bone marrow sampling might not be easily implemented into clinical study protocols for breast cancer, serial examinations of blood for CTCs or tumor cell-associated nucleic acids might be more acceptable for most patients and clinical investigators than repeated bone marrow aspirations. The detection and characterization of CTCs in peripheral blood of cancer patients has therefore received much attention in recent years and could lead to strategies for evaluation of therapeutic efficacy. The availability of a standardized, reliable blood test could enable implementation of CTCs as a surrogate marker for clinical development of new anticancer agents and optimization of existing treatment protocols. For the time being and with validated assays being available for the evaluation of bone marrow only, prospective clinical studies are now required to evaluate whether eradication of DTCs in bone marrow after systemic therapy translates into a longer disease-free period and overall survival.

ACKNOWLEDGMENT

This work was supported by Jubilaeumsfonds der Österreichischen Nationalbank.

REFERENCES

1. Goldhirsch A, Glick JH, Gelber RD, Coates AS, Senn HJ. Meeting highlights: international consensus panel on the treatment of primary breast cancer. *J Clin Oncol* 2001;19:3817–3827.
2. Goldhirsch A, Wood WC, Gelber RD, Coates AS, Thurlimann B, Senn H-J. Meeting highlights: Updated International Expert Consensus on the Primary Therapy of Early Breast Cancer. *J Clin Oncol* 2003;21:3357–3365.
3. Woelfle U, Cloos J, Sauter G, et al. Molecular signature associated with bone marrow micrometastasis in human breast cancer. *Cancer Res* 2003;63:5679–5684.
4. Braun S, Cevatli BS, Assemi C, et al. Comparative analysis of micrometastasis to the bone marrow and lymph nodes of node-negative breast cancer patients receiving no adjuvant therapy. *J Clin Oncol* 2001;19:1468–1475.
5. Gerber B, Krause A, Muller H, et al. Simultaneous immunohistochemical detection of tumor cells in lymph nodes and bone marrow aspirates in breast cancer and its correlation with other prognostic factors. *J Clin Oncol* 2001;19:960–971.
6. Ridell B, Landys K. Incidence and histopathology of metastases of mammary carcinoma in biopsies from the posterior iliac crest. *Cancer* 1979;44:1782–1788.
7. Schlimok G, Funke I, Holzmann B, et al. Micrometastatic cancer cells in bone marrow: in vitro detection with anti-cytokeratin and in vivo labeling with anti-17-1A monoclonal antibodies. *Proc Natl Acad Sci USA* 1987;84:8672–8676.
8. Gebauer G, Fehm T, Merkle E, Beck EP, Lang N, Jager W. Epithelial cells in bone marrow of breast cancer patients at time of primary surgery: clinical outcome during long-term follow-up. *J Clin Oncol* 2001;19:3669–3674.

9. Braun S, Pantel K, Müller P, et al. Cytokeratin-positive cells in the bone marrow and survival of patients with stage I, II or III breast cancer. *N Engl J Med* 2000;342:525–533.

10. Mansi JL, Gogas H, Bliss JM, Gazet JC, Berger U, Coombes RC. Outcome of primary-breast-cancer patients with micrometastases: a long-term follow-up. *Lancet* 1999;354:197–202.

11. Landys K, Persson S, Kovarik J, Hultborn R, Holmberg E. Prognostic value of bone marrow biopsy in operable breast cancer patients at the time of initial diagnosis: results of a 20-year median follow-up. *Breast Cancer Res Treat* 1998; 49:27–33.

12. Diel IJ, Kaufmann M, Costa SD, et al. Micrometastatic breast cancer cells in bone marrow at primary surgery: prognostic value in comparison with nodal status. *J Natl Cancer Inst* 1996;88:1652–1664.

13. Harbeck N, Untch M, Pache L, Eiermann W. Tumour cell detection in the bone marrow of breast cancer patients at primary therapy: results of a 3-year median follow-up. *Br J Cancer* 1994;69:566–571.

14. Cote RJ, Rosen PP, Lesser ML, Old LJ, Osborne MP. Prediction of early relapse in patients with operable breast cancer by detection of occult bone marrow micrometastases. *J Clin Oncol* 1991;9:1749–1756.

15. Untch M, Kahlert S, Funke I, et al. Detection of cytokeratin 18-positive cells in bone marrow of breast cancer patients: no prediction of bad outcome. *Proc ASCO* 1999;18:639a (Abstr 2472).

16. Molino A, pelosi G, Turazza M, et al. Bone marrow micrometastases in 109 breast cancer patients: correlations with clinical and pathological features. *Breast Cancer Res Treat* 1997;42:23–30.

17. Funke I, Fries S, Rolle M, et al. Comparative analyses of bone marrow micrometastases in breast and gastric cancer. *Int J Cancer* 1996;65:755–761.

18. Courtemanche DJ, Worth AJ, Coupland RW, Rowell JL, MacFarlane JK. Monoclonal antibody LICR-LON-M8 does not predict the outcome of operable breast cancer. *Can J Surg* 1991;34:21–26.

19. Singletary SE, Larry L, Trucker SL, Spitzer G. Detection of micrometastatic tumor cells in bone marrow of breast carcinoma patients. *J Surg Oncol* 1991;47:32–36.

20. Mathieu MC, Friedman S, Bosq J, et al. Immunohistochemical staining of bone marrow biopsies for detection of occult metastasis in breast cancer. *Breast Cancer Res Treat* 1990;15:21–26.

21. Salvadori B, Squicciarini P, Rovini D, et al. Use of monoclonal antibody MBr1 to detect micrometastases in bone marrow specimens of breast cancer patients. *Eur J Cancer* 1990;26:865–867.

22. Porro G, Menard S, Tagliabue E, et al. Monoclonal antibody detection of carcinoma cells in bone marrow biopsy specimens from breast cancer patients. *Cancer* 1988;61:2407–2411.

23. Wiedswang G, Borgen E, Karesen R, et al. Detection of isolated tumor cells in bone marrow is an independent prognostic factor in breast cancer. *J Clin Oncol* 2003;21:3469–3478.

24. Pantel K, Schlimok G, Angstwurm M, et al. Methodological analysis of immunocytochemical screening for disseminated epithelial tumor cells in bone marrow. *J Hematother* 1994;3:165–173.

25. Schaller G, Fuchs I, Pritze W, et al. Elevated keratin 18 protein expression indicates a favorable prognosis in patients with breast cancer. *Clin Cancer Res* 1996;2:1879–1885.

26. Zajchowski DA, Bartholdi MF, Gong Y, et al. Identification of gene expression profiles that predict the aggressive behavior of breast cancer cells. *Cancer Res* 2001;61:5168–5178.
27. Borgen E, Naume B, Nesland JM, et al. Standardisation of the immunocytochemical detection of cancer cells in bone marrow and blood: I. Establishment of objective criteria for the evaluation of immunostained cells. *Cytotherapy* 1999;1: 377–388.
28. Borgen E, Beiske K, Trachsel S, et al. Immunocytochemical detection of isolated epithelial cells in bone marrow: non-specific staining and contribution by plasma cells directly reactive to alkaline phosphatase. *J Pathol* 1998;185:427–434.
29. Braun S, Müller M, Hepp F, Schlimok G, Riethmüller G, Pantel K. Re: Micrometastatic breast cancer cells in bone marrow at primary surgery: prognostic value in comparison with nodal status. *J Natl Cancer Inst* 1998;90:1099–1100.
30. Putz E, Witter K, Offner S, et al. Phenotypic characteristics of cell lines derived from disseminated cancer cells in bone marrow of patients with solid epithelial tumors: establishment of working models for human micrometastases. *Cancer Res* 1999;59:241–248.
31. Pantel K, Dickmanns A, Zippelius A, et al. Establishment of micrometastatic carcinoma cell lines: a novel source of tumor cell vaccines. *J Natl Cancer Inst* 1995;87:1162–1168.
32. Pantel K, Schlimok G, Braun S, et al. Differential expression of proliferation-associated molecules in individual micrometastatic carcinoma cells. *J Natl Cancer Inst* 1993;85:1419–1424.
33. Pantel K, Izbicki JR, Angstwurm M, et al. Immunocytochemical detection of bone marrow micrometastasis in operable non-small cell lung cancer. *Cancer Res* 1993;53:1027–1031.
34. Müller P, Carroll P, Bowers E, et al. Low frequency epithelial cells in bone marrow from prostate carcinoma patients are cytogenetically aberrant. *Cancer* 1998;83: 538–546.
35. Dietmaier W, Hartmann A, Wallinger S, et al. Multiple mutation analyses in single tumor cells with improved whole genome amplification. *Am J Pathol* 1999;154:83–95.
36. Schmidt-Kittler O, Ragg T, Daskalakis A, et al. From latent disseminated cells to overt metastasis: Genetic analysis of systemic breast cancer progression. *Proc Natl Acad Sci USA* 2003;100:7737–7742.
37. Klein CA, Seidl S, Petat-Dutter K, et al. Combined transcriptome and genome analysis of single micrometastatic cells. *Nat Biotech* 2002;20:387–392.
38. Klein CA, Schmidt-Kittler O, Schardt JA, Pantel K, Speicher MR, Riethmüller G. Comparative genomic hybridization, loss of heterozygosity, and DNA sequence analysis of single cells. *Proc Natl Acad Sci USA* 1999;96:4494–4499.
39. Lugo TG, Braun S, Cote RJ, Pantel K, Rusch V. Detection and measurement of occult disease for the prognosis of solid tumors. *J Clin Oncol* 2003;21:2609–2615.
40. Borgen E, Naume B, Nesland JM, et al. Use of automated microscopy for the detection of disseminated tumor cells in bone marrow samples. *Cytometry* 2001;46:215–221.
41. Kraeft S-K, Sutherland R, Gravelin L, et al. Detection and analysis of cancer cells in blood and bone marrow using a rare event imaging system. *Clin Cancer Res* 2000;6:434–442.
42. Bauer KD, de la Torre-Bueno J, Diel IJ, et al. Reliable and sensitive analysis of occult bone marrow metastases using automated cellular imaging. *Clin Cancer Res* 2000;6:3552–3559.

43. Zeidman I. The fate of circulating tumors cells. I. Passage of cells through capillaries. *Cancer Res* 1961;21:38–39.
44. Fidler IJ. Quantitative analysis of distribution and fate of tumor emboli labeled with ^{125}I-5-iodo-2'-desoxyuridine. *J Natl Cancer Inst* 1970;145:773–782.
45. Hansen E, Wolff N, Knuechel R, Ruschoff J, Hofstaedter F, Taeger K. Tumor cells in blood shed from the surgical field. *Arch Surg* 1995;130:387–393.
46. Denis MG, Lipart C, Leborgne J, et al. Detection of disseminated tumor cells in peripheral blood of colorectal cancer patients. *Int J Cancer* 1997;74:540–544.
47. Eschwege P, Dumas F, Blanchet P, et al. Haematogenous dissemination of prostatic epithelial cells during radical prostatectomy. *Lancet* 1995;346:1528–1530.
48. Weitz J, Kienle P, Magener A, et al. Detection of disseminated colorectal cancer cells in lymph nodes, blood and bone marrow. *Clin Cancer Res* 1999;5:1830–1836.
49. Weitz J, Kienle P, Lacroix J, et al. Dissemination of tumour cells in patients undergoing surgery for colorectal cancer. *Clin Cancer Res* 1998;4:343–348.
50. Uchikura K, Takao S, Nakajo A, et al. Intraoperative molecular detection of circulating tumor cells by reverse transcription-polymerase chain reaction in patients with biliary-pancreatic cancer is associated with hematogenous metastasis. *Ann Surg Oncol* 2002;9:364–370.
51. Engel H, Kleespies C, Friedrich J, et al. Detection of circulating tumour cells in patients with breast or ovarian cancer by molecular cytogenetics. *Br J Cancer* 1999;81:1165–1173.
52. Fehm T, Sagalowsky A, Clifford E, et al. Cytogenetic evidence that circulating epithelial cells in patients with carcinoma are malignant. *Clin Cancer Res* 2002;8:2073–2084.
53. Liotta LA, Kleinerman J, Saidel GM. Quantitative relationships of intravascular tumor cells, tumor vessels, and pulmonary metastases following tumor implantation. *Cancer Res* 1974;34:997–1004.
54. Butler TP, Gullino PM. Quantitation of cell shedding into efferent blood of mammary adenocarcinoma. *Cancer Res* 1975;35:512–516.
55. Chang YS, di Tomaso E, McDonald DM, Jones R, Jain RK, Munn LLM. osaic blood vessels in tumors: frequency of cancer cells in contact with flowing blood. *Proc Natl Acad Sci USA* 2000;97:14608–14613.
56. Chambers AF, Groom AC, MacDonald IC. Dissemination and growth of cancer cells in metastatic sites. *Nat Rev Cancer* 2002;2:563–572.
57. Stathopoulou A, Vlachonikolis I, Mavroudis D, et al. Molecular detection of cytokeratin-19-positive cells in the peripheral blood of patients with operable breast cancer: evaluation of their prognostic significance. *J Clin Oncol* 2002;20:3404–3412.
58. Terstappen LW, Rao C, Gross S, Weiss AJ. Peripheral blood tumor cell load reflects the clinical activity of the disease in patients with carcinoma of the breast. *Int J Oncol* 2000;17:573–578.
59. Smith BM, Slade MJ, English J, et al. Response of circulating tumor cells to systemic therapy in patients with metastatic breast cancer: comparison of quantitative polymerase chain reaction and immunocytochemical techniques. *J Clin Oncol* 2000;18:1432–1439.
60. Ghossein RA, Rosai J, Scher HI, et al. Prognostic significance of detection of prostate-specific antigen transcripts in the peripheral blood of patients with metastatic androgen-independent prostatic carcinoma. *Urology* 1997;50:100–105.

61. Thorban S, Rosenberg R, Busch R, Roder RJ. Epithelial cells in bone marrow of oesophageal cancer patients: a significant prognostic factor in multivariate analysis. *Br J Cancer* 2000;83:35–39.

62. Hoon DSB, Wang Y, Dale PS, et al. Detection of occult melanoma cells in blood with a multiple-marker polymerase chain reaction assay. *J Clin Oncol* 1995;13: 2109–2116.

63. Hoon DSB, Bostick P, Kuo C, et al. Molecular markers in blood as surrogate prognostic indicators of melanoma recurrence. *Cancer Res* 2000;60:2253–2257.

64. de la Taille A, Olsson CA, Buttyan R, et al. Blood-based reverse transcriptase polymerase chain reaction assays for prostatic specific antigen: long term follow-up confirms the potential utility of this assay in identifying patients more likely to have biochemical recurrence (rising PSA) following radical prostatectomy. *Int J Cancer* 1999;84:360–364.

65. Ellis WJ, Pfitzenmaier J, Colli J, Arfman E, Lange PH, Vessella RLU-hwscsaB-X-a. Detection and isolation of prostate cancer cells from peripheral blood and bone marrow. *Urology* 2003;61:277–281.

66. Bilkenroth U, Taubert H, Riemann D, Rebmann U, Heynemann H, Meye A. Detection and enrichment of disseminated renal carcinoma cells from peripheral blood by immunomagnetic cell separation. *Int J Cancer* 2001;92:577–582.

67. Flatmark K, Bjornland K, Johannessen HO, et al. Immunomagnetic detection of micrometastatic cells in bone marrow of colorectal cancer patients. *Clin Cancer Res* 2002;8:444–449.

68. Naume B, Borgen E, Beiske K, et al. Immunomagnetic techniques for the enrichment and detection of isolated breast carcinoma cells in bone marrow and peripheral blood. *J Hematother* 1997;6:103–114.

69. Martin VM, Siewert C, Scharl A, et al. Immunomagnetic enrichment of disseminated epithelial tumor cells from peripheral blood by MACS. *Exp Hematol* 1998;26:252–264.

70. Naume B, Borgen E, Nesland JM, et al. Increased sensitivity for detection of micrometastases in bone marrow/peripheral-blood stem-cell products from breast cancer patients by negative immunomagnetic separation. *Int J Cancer* 1998;78: 556–560.

71. Racila E, Euhus D, Weiss AJ, et al. Detection and characterization of carcinoma cells in the blood. *PNAS* 1998;95:4589–4594.

72. Kruger WH, Kroger N, Togel F, et al. Disseminated breast cancer cells prior to and after high-dose therapy. *J Hematother Stem Cell Res* 2001;10:681–689.

73. Rye PD, Hoifodt HK, Overli GE, Fodstad O. Immunobead filtration: a novel approach for the isolation and propagation of tumor cells. *Am J Pathol* 1997;150: 99–106.

74. Zippelius A, Lutterbuse R, Riethmuller G, Pantel K. Analytical variables of reverse transcription-polymerase chain reaction-based detection of disseminated prostate cancer cells. *Clin Cancer Res* 2000;6:2741–2750.

75. Zippelius A, Kufer P, Honold G, et al. Limitations of reverse transcriptase-polymerase chain reaction for detection of micrometastatic epithelial cancer cells in bone marrow. *J Clin Oncol* 1997;15:2701–2708.

76. Bosma AJ, Weigelt B, Lambrechts AC, et al. Detection of circulating breast tumor cells by differential expression of marker genes. *Clin Cancer Res* 2002;8:1871–1877.

77. Taback B, Chan AD, Kuo CT, et al. Detection of occult metastatic breast cancer cells in blood by a multimolecular marker assay: correlation with clinical stage of disease. *Cancer Res* 2001;61:8845–8850.

78. Slade MJ, Smith BM, Sinnett HD, Cross NCP, Coombes RC. Quantitative polymerase chain reaction for the detection of micrometastases in patients with breast cancer. *J Clin Oncol* 1999;17:870–879.

79. Zach O, Kasparu H, Krieger O, Hehenwarter W, Girschikofsky M, Lutz D. Detection of circulating mammary carcinoma cells in the peripheral blood of breast cancer patients via a nested reverse transcriptase polymerase chain reaction assay for mammaglobin mRNA. *J Clin Oncol* 1999;17:2015–2019.

80. Vannucchi AM, Bosi A, Glinz S, et al. Evaluation of breast tumour cell contamination in the bone marrow and leukapheresis collections by RT-PCR for cytokeratin-19 mRNA. *Br J Haematol* 1998;103:610–617.

81. Fields KK, Elfenbein GJ, Trudeau WL, Perlinss JB, Jansen WE, Moscinski LC. Clinical significance of bone marrow metastases as detected using polymerase chain reaction in patients with breast cancer undergoing high-dose chemotherapy and autologous bone marrow transplantation. *J Clin Oncol* 1996;14:1868–1876.

82. Datta YH, Adams PT, Drobyski WR. Sensitive detection of occult breast cancer by the reverse-transcriptase polymerase chain reaction. *J Clin Oncol* 1994;12:475–482.

83. Auer M, Fiegl H, Riha K, Daxenbichler G, Braun S, Marth C. Parallel immunomagnetic enrichment and cytokeratin-19 reverse transcriptase PCR for occult metastatic tumor cell detection in bone marrow of breast and ovarian cancer patients. *Proc AACR* 2003;44:782–783 (Abstr 3424).

84. Grunewald K, Haun M, Urbanek M, et al. Mammaglobin gene expression: a superior marker of breast cancer cells in peripheral blood in comparison to epidermal-growth-factor receptor and cytokeratin-19. *Lab Invest* 2000;80:1071–1077.

85. Lambrechts AC, Bosma AJ, Klaver SG, et al. Comparison of immunocytochemistry, reverse transcriptase polymerase chain reaction, and nucleic acid sequence-based amplification for the detection of circulating breast cancer cells. *Breast Cancer Res Treat* 1999;56:219–231.

86. Mapara MY, Körner IJ, Hildebrandt M, et al. Monitoring of tumor cell purging after highly efficient immunomagnetic selection of CD34 cells from leukapheresis products in breast cancer patients: comparison of immunocytochemical tumor cell staining and reverse transcriptase-polymerase chain reaction. *Blood* 1997;89:337–344.

87. Krismann M, Todt B, Schröder J, et al. Low specificity of cytokeratin 19 reverse transcriptase-polymerase chain reaction analyses for detection of hematogenous lung cancer dissemination. *J Clin Oncol* 1995;13:2769–2775.

88. van Trappen PO, Gyselman VG, Lowe DG, et al. Molecular quantification and mapping of lymph-node micrometastases in cervical cancer. *Lancet* 2001;357:15–20.

89. Jones PA, Baylin SB. The fundamental role of epigenetic events in cancer. *Nat Rev Genet* 2002;3:415–428.

90. Widschwendter M, Jones PA. DNA methylation and breast carcinogenesis. *Oncogene* 2002;21:5462–5482.

91. Laird PW. Early detection: the power and the promise of DNA methylation markers. *Nat Rev Cancer* 2003;3:253–266.

92. Muller HM, Widschwendter A, Fiegl H, et al. DNA Methylation in serum of breast cancer patients: an independent prognostic marker. *Cancer Res* 2003;63:7641–7645.

93. Daskalakis M, Nguyen TT, Nguyen C, et al. Demethylation of a hypermethylated P15/INK4B gene in patients with myelodysplastic syndrome by 5-aza-2'-deoxycytidine (decitabine) treatment. *Blood* 2002;100:2957–2964.

94. Berger U, Bettelheim R, Mansi JL, Easton D, Coombes RC, Neville AM. The relationship between micrometastases in the bone marrow, histopathologic features of the primary tumor in breast cancer and prognosis. *Am J Clin Pathol* 1988;90:1–6.

95. Cote RJ, Rosen PP, Hakes TB, et al. Monoclonal antibodies detect occult breast carcinoma metastases in the bone marrow of patients with early stage disease. *Am J Surg Pathol* 1988;12:333–340.

96. Mansi JL, Easton D, Berger U, et al. Bone marrow micrometastases in primary breast cancer: prognostic significance after 6 years' follow-up. *Eur J Cancer* 1991;27:1552–1555.

97. Hermanek P, Hutter RV, Sobin LH, Wittekind C. Classification of isolated tumor cells and micrometastases. *Cancer* 1999;86:2668–2673.

98. Singletary SE, Allred C, Ashley P, et al. Revision of the American Joint Committee on Cancer Staging System for Breast Cancer. *J Clin Oncol* 2002;20:3628–3636.

99. Thurm H, Ebel S, Kentenich C, et al. Rare expression of epithelial cell adhesion molecule on residual micrometastatic breast cancer cells after adjuvant chemotherapy. *Clin Cancer Res* 2003;9:2598–2604.

100. Braun S, Kentenich CRM, Janni W, et al. Lack of effect of adjuvant chemotherapy on the elimination of single dormant tumor cells in bone marrow of high-risk breast cancer patients. *J Clin Oncol* 2000;18:80–86.

101. Braun S, Hepp F, Kentenich CRM, et al. Monoclonal antibody therapy with edrecolomab in breast cancer patients: monitoring of elimination of disseminated cytokeratin-positive tumor cells in bone marrow. *Clin Cancer Res* 1999;5:3999–4004.

102. Pantel K, Enzmann T, Köllermann J, Caprano J, Riethmüller G, Köllermann MW. Immunocytochemical monitoring of micrometastatic disease: reduction of prostate cancer cells in bone marrow by androgen deprivation. *Int J Cancer* 1997;71:521–525.

103. Schlimok G, Pantel K, Loibner H, Fackler-Schwalbe I, Riethmüller G. Reduction of metastatic carcinoma cells in bone marrow by intravenously administered monoclonal antibody: towards a novel surrogate test to monitor adjuvant therapies of solid tumours. *Eur J Cancer* 1995;31A:1799–1803.

104. Janni W, Hepp F, Rjosk D, et al. The fate and prognostic value of occult metastatic cells in the bone marrow of patients with breast carcinoma between primary treatment and recurrence. *Cancer* 2001;92:46–53.

105. Wiedswang G, Borgen E, Kåresen R, et al. Isolated tumor cells in bone marrow three years after diagnosis in disease free breast cancer patients predict unfavourable clinical outcome. *Breast Cancer Res Treat* 2003;82:S8 (Abstr 8).

106. Witzig TE, Bossy B, Kimlinger T, et al. Detection of circulating cytokeratin-positive cells in blood of breast cancer patients using immunomagnetic enrichment and digital microscopy. *Clin Cancer Res* 2001;8:1085–1091.

13 Circulating HER2/neu

Clinical Utility

Allan Lipton, MD,
Laurence Demers, PHD,
Kim Leitzel, MS,
Suhail M. Ali, MD,
Rainer Neumann, PHD,
Christopher P. Price, PHD,
and Walter P. Carney, PHD

Cancer Drug Discovery and Development: Biomarkers in Breast Cancer:
Molecular Diagnostics for Predicting and Monitoring Therapeutic Effect
Edited by: G. Gasparini and D. F. Hayes © Humana Press Inc., Totowa, NJ

SUMMARY

The *HER2/neu* oncogene and its p185 receptor protein is an indicator of a more aggressive form of breast cancer. The HER2/neu status guides Herceptin® therapy, specifically directed to the extracellular domain (ECD) of the HER2/neu oncoprotein. The HER2/neu ECD is shed from cancer cells into the circulation and is measurable by immunoassay. We performed an in-depth review of the peer-reviewed literature on circulating ECD levels with respect to prevalence, prognosis, prediction of response to therapy, and monitoring of breast cancer. Studies showed that the prevalence of an elevated ECD in patients with primary breast cancer varied between 0% and 38% (mean 18.5%) while in metastatic breast cancer the range was from 23% to 80% (mean 43%). Some women who have HER2/neu–negative tumors by tissue testing develop elevated ECD levels in metastatic disease. Elevated ECD levels have been correlated with indicators of poor prognosis, for example, overall survival and disease-free survival. Elevated ECD levels predict a poor response to hormone therapy and some chemotherapy regimens but can predict improved response to combinations of Herceptin and chemotherapy. Many studies support the value of monitoring ECD levels during breast cancer progression, as serial increases precede the appearance of metastases using imaging techniques, and longitudinal ECD changes paralleled the clinical course of disease. The monitoring of circulating HER2/neu ECD levels provides a tool for assessing prognosis, predicting the response to therapy and for earlier detection of disease progression and intervention with appropriate therapy. Additional prospective studies are required to validate these potential applications.

Key Words: HER2/neu; extracellular domain; oncoprotein; breast cancer.

1. INTRODUCTION

The activation and overexpression of cellular oncogenes has been considered to play an important role in the development of human cancer *(1)*. An important member of the oncogene family is the growth factor receptor known as the Human Epidermal Growth Factor Receptor-2 (HER2) *(2)*, which is also referred to as *HER2/neu* or c-*erb*-B2. *HER2/neu* is structurally and functionally related to the v-*erb*-B retroviral oncogene *(3)* and is part of the *HER* family which also includes HER1 or EGFR (epidermal growth factor receptor) and *HER3* and *HER4 (4)*.

The *HER2/neu* oncogene has been localized to chromosome 17q and encodes a transmembrane tyrosine kinase growth factor receptor that is expressed on cells of epithelial origin. The full-length glycoprotein has a

HER-2 Activation

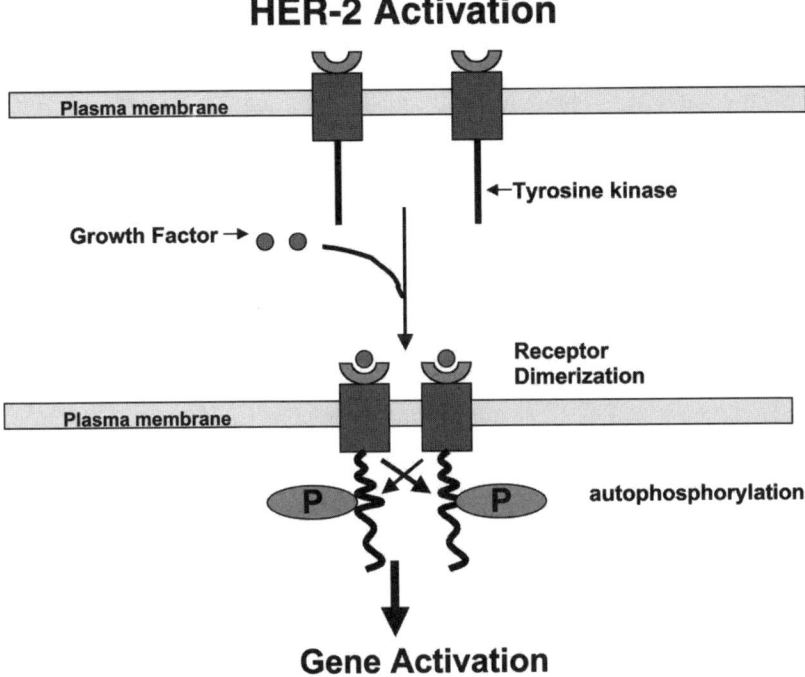

Fig. 1. HER2/neu signaling pathways are activated by homo- and hetero-dimerizations with extracellular domains of the other HER family members.

molecular weight of 185,000 daltons (p185) and is composed of the internal tyrosine kinase domain, a short transmembrane portion, and has an extracellular domain (ECD) similar to the three other members of the *HER* family *(2,5)*. The ECD portion of the receptor protein is heavily glycosylated, has a molecular weight in the 97–115-Kda range and has been shown to be shed into cultured fluids of SKBR-3 cells *(6)*, as well as plasma *(7)* and serum *(8,9)* from normal individuals and patients with breast cancer *(7–9)*.

The mechanism of activation of the HER2/neu pathway is not completely understood but studies have shown that the ECDs of the *HER* family of receptor tyrosine kinases form homodimers and heterodimers and that receptor dimerization activates a cascade of events in the HER-2/neu signaling pathway *(4)*. A ligand that binds to the HER2/neu receptor has not been identified but a family of peptide ligands named *neu* differentiation factors or heregulins have been identified that bind to the HER3 and HER4 receptors, inducing heterodimerization with the HER2/neu receptor and therefore inducing transphosphorylation and thus activation of the HER2/neu receptor (Fig. 1). Heterodimers between the EGFR and HER2/neu can also form upon binding of a ligand such as epidermal growth factor or transforming growth factor-α to the EGF receptor *(10)*. Dimerization of the receptor results in tyrosine phosphorylation of the HER2/neu kinase with subsequent activation of downstream transduction pathways and signaling through ras, c-Src, phosphatidylinosital 3 kinase (PI3K), and phospholipase C (PLC)-γ pathways. Formation of heterodimers increases the affinity of the partnering receptor for its ligand and results in potentiation of the mitogenic signal *(11)*.

In a report by Codony-Servat et al. *(12)*, it was demonstrated that cleavage of the HER2/neu ECD involves metalloproteinase (MMP) activity and that the process of cleavage was inhibited by the MMP inhibitor TIMP-1 but not by TIMP-2. They also showed that HER-2/neu ECD shedding was inhibited by broad spectrum MMP inhibitors such as EDTA (ethylenediamine tetracetic acid), TAPI-2 and Batimastat. The report also confirmed data from Christianson et al., showing that HER2/neu ECD cleavage results in the release of a truncated membrane-bound phosphorylated p95 fragment *(13)*.

Molina et al., showed in a 2001 report *(14)* that HER2/neu shedding was activated by 4-aminophenylmercuric acetate (APMA, a well known MMP activator) in HER2/neu overexpressing breast cancer cells and it could be blocked by the MMP inhibitor Batimastat. The increase in ECD shedding also enhanced the production of the p95 fragment. In the same report, Molina et al. *(14)*, demonstrated that Herceptin®, an anti-HER2/neu therapy, had a direct inhibitory effect on the basal and activated processes involved in HER2/neu cleavage from HER2/neu-overexpressing breast cancer cells. The HER2/neu ECD shedding that was activated by APMA could be blocked with Herceptin, leading to a reduction in the release of the p95 fragment. The analysis of 24 human breast tumors by this group showed that the p95 fragment could be detected in only 14 out of 24 of the specimens, and the p95 band was highly variable. Studies continue to determine the potential clinical value of the phosphorylated membrane fragment *(14)*.

Trastuzumab (commonly referred to as Herceptin, manufactured by Genentech, San Francisco, California, USA) is a humanized monoclonal antibody (MAb) developed to target the HER2/neu receptor that is overexpressed on some cancer cells, including 25–30% of breast cancers as well as a variety of other epithelial cancers. Herceptin binds with high affinity to the ECD of HER2/neu and inhibits proliferation of tumor cells that overexpress HER2/neu protein. The results of a large multicenter phase III clinical trial demonstrated that Herceptin, when added to conventional chemotherapy, can provide benefit to patients with metastatic breast cancer that overexpresses HER2/neu. As compared with the best available standard chemotherapy, concurrent treatment with Herceptin and first line chemotherapy was associated with significantly longer time to disease progression, a higher rate of response, longer duration of response, and improved overall survival *(15)*.

In this chapter, we will review HER2/neu circulating ECD levels in relation to prevalence, prognosis, prediction of response to therapy, monitoring in metastatic breast cancer, and monitoring for early detection of recurrence.

2. METHODS OF DETERMINING HER2/neu STATUS

The most widely accepted method for measuring HER2/neu protein (p185) overexpression is immunohistochemistry (IHC) *(16,17)* whereas the number of *HER2/neu* gene copies or gene amplification is determined by using a fluorescence *in situ* hybridization (FISH) assay *(16,17)*. Enzyme-linked immunoabsorbent assays (ELISAs) have been used since 1991 to quantitate either the full length p185 in tumor tissue *(7)* or the soluble circulating HER2/neu ECD in serum *(8)* or plasma *(7)*.

However, there are limitations to tissue testing, the most important being that they are one-time tests used to determine the HER2/neu status of the primary breast cancer which in turn determines eligibility for Herceptin. Herceptin is given primarily in the metastatic setting, yet the HER2/neu status is determined from the original breast tumor, which may have been removed many years earlier. It is clear from this review of the literature (and will be discussed later) that the HER2/neu status of a breast cancer patient can change from the primary to the metastatic phase.

Tissue testing for HER2/neu protein overexpression by IHC and FISH testing for DNA amplification are subject to technical problems. These include, but are not limited to, differences in the methodology between laboratories and the operator, variability in operator interpretation, and variation in reagents. Although the FISH technology is reproducible, the major drawback is that the FISH equipment is expensive and not widely available in diagnostic pathology laboratories.

The third method used to quantitate full length p185 in tumor tissue or the circulating ECD in serum or plasma is the immunoassay. Zabrecky et al. *(6)*, using MAb directed to the ECD *(20)*, demonstrated that the ECD was shed into the culture supernatant of SK-BR-3 breast cancer cells. Studies employing specific MAbs against the HER2/neu protein and using immunoprecipitation and Western blot techniques showed that the ECD was a glycoprotein with molecular weight between 97 and 115kDa *(6)*. Subsequent studies illustrated that the ECD could be detected in the plasma of healthy subjects and is elevated in women with primary and metastatic breast cancer *(7)*. These observations were later confirmed by Leitzel et al. *(8)* and Pupa et al. *(9)*.

In the last several years, many reports have described a variety of ELISA formats that have been used to quantitate the ECD in serum or plasma of breast cancer patients and control groups. However, it has been difficult to compare results between publications owing to a lack of standardization between the ELISAs. For example, three publications reporting ECD results with one particular commercial assay (Triton-Ciba Corning-Chiron) used at least three different cutoff levels (3 U/mL, 12 U/mL and 30 U/mL) to separate normal and diseased populations *(8,21,22)*. In some reports, antibody specificity or assay validation for HER2/neu has not been demonstrated *(23)*, nor have adequate references been provided to demonstrate that the antibodies in the ELISAs specifically detect the HER2/neu ECD.

In summary, IHC and FISH testing can be used to determine the HER2/neu status in primary tumor tissue but are not adequate for assessing HER2/neu status of a woman after the tumor is removed by surgery. In contrast, the immunoassay method for measuring the circulating HER2/neu ECD is the only way to obtain a real-time status of HER2/neu and the only practical way to monitor changes in the HER2/neu ECD levels.

3. PREVALENCE OF CIRCULATING HER2/neu LEVELS IN BREAST CANCER

We reviewed a total of 55 publications from which data on the prevalence *(7,8,22–73)* of elevated levels of circulating HER2/neu could be extracted. The data are summarized in Fig. 2 and represent circulating HER2/neu ECD measurements in more than 6500 patients with breast cancer. A review of 24 references used to evaluate ECD levels in primary breast cancer showed that approx 18.5% of the 1923 patients had circulating HER2/neu ECD levels that were above the control cutoff described in each publication.

In contrast, a review of 45 references and 4622 patients with metastatic breast cancer (MBC) showed that 43% of the patients had circulating HER2/neu ECD values above the normal cutoff for the control group. In 15 of the 45 publications ECD levels were elevated above the control group in over 50% of the patients studied.

It is interesting to note that the data in Fig. 2 came from essentially six different assays. The automated Immuno-1 HER2/neu test (manufactured by Bayer Health Care, Tarrytown, NY) and the Oncogene Science manual microtiter plate HER2/neu test (manufactured by Oncogene Science, Cambridge, MA) are essentially the same assays since both use anti-HER2/neu MAbs NB-3 and TA-1 *(20)*, a soluble p97–115-kDa standard, and a 15 ng/mL cutoff *(35,65,74)*. It should also be noted that there was a strong correlation between the automated and manual HER2/neu assays *(35,65,74)*. Both the automated and manual HER2/neu assays have been cleared by the US Food and Drug Administration (FDA) for use in the management and monitoring of women with metastatic breast cancer. These are the only two assays currently cleared for the measurement of the circulating p97–115-kDa HER2/neu ECD. There were 20 publications in Fig. 2 that used the two methods described above. There were 21 references to the Triton/Ciba/Chiron

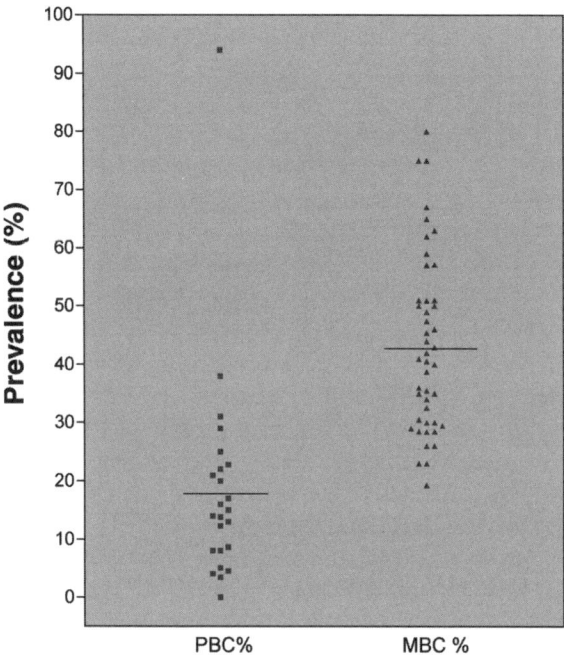

Fig. 2. Circulating HER2/neu ECD measurements in more than 6500 patients with breast cancer. PBC % = % of primary breast cancer patients who had HER2/neu ECD levels above the control cutoff described in each publication (each square = 1 publication; 24 references, n = 1923 patients total, mean = 18.5% above cutoff). MBC % = % of metastatic breast cancer patients who had HER2/neu ECD levels above the control cutoff described in each publication (each triangle = 1 publication; 45 references, n = 4622 patients total, mean = 43% above cutoff).

assays with 11 different cutoffs ranging from 5 to 30 U/mL as well as a 120 fmol/mL or 450 fmol/mL cutoff. These assays are essentially the same and are no longer commercially available. There were five references to the Nicherei assay, three references to the Calbiochem or ORP assay, three references to the Dianova assay, and two references to the Bender assay. We could not find any references that described the antibody specificities or standard material used in the Calbiochem, Dianova or the Bender assays nor could we find any references that validated biochemically that the assays clearly measured the circulating HER2/neu ECD. The Calbiochem, Dianova, and Bender assays are available as research use only assays, which means that their performance characteristics have not been determined. In fact, the Bender assay claims to measure the circulating soluble p185; however, there has never been a scientific report of a circulating full-length p185 nor does the manufacturer present data to support their claim. Several other reports, however, have reproducibly demonstrated that the only HER2/neu fragment found circulating is the truncated p97–115-kDa *(6–9)* ECD, so it is unclear what the Bender assay actually measures.

In a report by Andersen et al. *(25)*, it was shown that elevated HER2/neu ECD levels were detected in the serum of 8% of preoperative breast cancer patients and in only 3% of postoperative sera from patients without recurrent breast cancer. In contrast, 59% (55 out of 93) of patients with recurrent breast cancer developed elevated HER2/neu ECD levels. It was also reported that elevated ECD levels were detected significantly more often in patients with distant metastases than in patients with recurrent disease restricted to local metastasis (68% vs 19%). This observation was supported by Watanabe et al. *(21)*, who concluded that the circulating HER2/neu ECD level was closely related to tumor mass, since the HER2/neu ECD level in recurrent disease was found to be significantly higher than in nonrecurrent disease.

In the report by Andersen *(25)* it was shown that 14 of 24 patients who had immunohistochemistry (IHC)-positive breast tumors also had elevated HER2/neu serum levels during the metastatic phase of the disease. In contrast, 28 of 82 (34%) patients, who had IHC-negative primary breast tumors, developed elevated serum levels during the metastatic phase. Kandl et al. *(48)* also reported that some patients with negative HER2/neu tumor staining developed extremely high serum levels of HER2/neu during the evolution of metastatic disease which also correlated with extensive MBC. Molina also reported that 23% of patients with recurrent breast cancer with no tissue overexpression had elevated ECD levels, once again supporting the concept that there is a subpopulation of women with HER2/neu–positive tumors that are not identified by tissue testing of the primary breast cancer.

4. SERUM HER2/neu AS A PROGNOSTIC INDICATOR

We analyzed 20 publications and outcomes data from 4430 breast cancer patients (3338 metastatic patients and 1092 primary breast cancer patients) to see if elevated serum HER2/neu ECD levels correlated with poor prognosis. This analysis took into account several indicators of prognosis including time to progression (TTP), overall survival (OS), and disease-free survival (DFS). The data is summarized in Table 1 and in some cases, where available, the hazard ratios had also been calculated and these have been summarized in Fig. 3.

Bewick et al. examined the clinical significance of shed ECD plasma levels in metastatic breast cancer (MBC) patients *(27)* and showed that 46% of the patients receiving high-dose chemotherapy (HDCT) had elevated ECD levels compared to controls. The results showed that patients with high levels of ECD had a significantly poorer overall survival and progression-

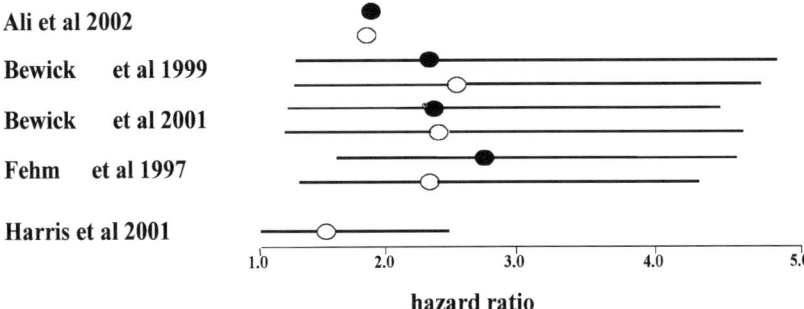

Fig. 3. Summary of the hazard ratios and 95% confidence intervals calculated in the respective publications quoted for serum HER2/neu as a prognostic marker in patients with breast cancer. Overall survival (closed circle) and disease-free survival (open circle).

free interval following high-dose therapy with paclitaxel and autologous stem cell transplantation compared to individuals without elevated ECD levels. For instance, the median overall survival of patients with a low ECD level was 29.8 mo, significantly longer than the 15.9 mo seen in patients with high ECD levels. In addition, the progression-free survival period was significantly longer at 13 mo for patients with low ECD levels than the 8.6 mo observed for patients with high ECD levels *(27)*. In a similar study by Harris et al., patients treated with HDCT and bone marrow transplant who had high ECD levels did worse than patients receiving the same treatment but with low ECD levels *(43)*.

When the prognostic value of this oncoprotein was evaluated by Molina et al., the patients with abnormally high presurgical serum HER2/neu levels had a worse prognosis than those patients with normal levels, in both node-negative and node-positive patients *(57)*. In addition, serum ECD levels in patients with advanced breast cancer were related to the site of recurrence with significantly higher values in patients with metastases (45.4%) than in those with locoregional recurrence (9.2%). In 2002, a report by Ali et al. demonstrated that the median overall survival for MBC patients with elevated serum HER2/neu was 17.1 mo. In contrast, women with normal levels of serum HER2/neu ECD had a median overall survival of 29.0 mo, indicating that elevated HER2/neu levels correlated with poor clinical outcome *(24)*.

In summary, the collective evidence presented in Table 1 from more than 4000 breast cancer patients shows a strong correlation between elevated HER2/neu ECD levels and worse prognosis as demonstrated by a decrease in time to progression, decreased overall survival and decreased disease-free progression.

Table 1
Summary of Data Showing HER2/neu Relationship to Indicators of Prognosis in Patients With Breast Cancer

Authors (ref.)	Patients	Therapy	Prognostic indices (elevated vs nonelevated)	Significance
Ali et al. 2002 (24)	566 MBC	Megestrol or fadrozole; 2nd line	TTP median 89 vs 176 d	$p < 0.0001$
			OS 515 vs 869 d	$p < 0.00001$
Bewick et al. 1999 (26)	57 MBC	High dose chemotherapy	TTP median 7.3 vs 14.3 mo	$p = 0.004$
			OS median 17.2 vs 28.9 mo	$p = 0.002$
Bewick et al. 2001 (27)	46 MBC	High dose chemotherapy	TTP median 8.6 vs 13.0 mo	$p = 0.009$
			OS median 15.9 vs 29.8 mo	$p = 0.009$
Classen et al. 2002 (33)		2nd line chemo or hormonal	TTP median 23.4 vs 56.7 mo	$p = 0.002$
Fehm et al. 1997 (38)	211 MBC	Anthracyclines and CMF	DFS median 11.0 vs 49.0 mo	$p = 0.01$
			5 year OS 41% vs 61%	$p = 0.01$
Fehm et al. 1998 (39)	80 MBC	CMF, NC or FNC	DFS less when elevated	$p = 0.01$
Fehm et al. 2002 (40)	52 PBC and 52 MBC	Chemo or hormonal therapy	DFS 22 vs 27 mo	$p = 0.04$
Harris et al. 2001 (43)	425 MBC	High dose chemotherapy	DFS less when elevated	$p = 0.13$
			OS less when elevated	$p = 0.0096$
		AFM	DFS less when elevated	$p = 0.061$
			OS less when elevated	$p = 0.045$
Hayes et al. 2001 (44)	103 MBC	Chemo and hormonal therapy	OS median 16.4 vs 22.7 mo	$p = 0.002$
			TTP median 6.0 vs 7.03 mo	$p = 0.096$
Kandl et al. 1994 (48)	79 MBC	Chemo and hormonal therapy	OS median 21 vs 64 mo	$p = 0.03$
Leitzel et al. 1995 (76)	300 MBC	Megestrol or fadrozole; 2nd line	OS median 15.0 vs 28.0 mo	$p < 0.0001$

Study	Sample	Treatment	Outcome	p value
Lipton et al. 2002 (54)	719 MBC	Megestrol or fadrozole; 2nd line	TTP 90 vs 180 d	$p < 0.0001$
			TTF median 93 vs 175 d	$p < 0.0001$
			OS median 17.2 vs 29.6 mo	$p < 0.0001$
Lipton et al. 2003 (55)	562 MBC	Letrozole or tamoxifen	TTP median 5.7 vs 9.4 mo	$p = 0.0001$
Mehta et al. 1998 (78)	79 PBC	CMF or CMFVP	DFS less when elevated	$p = 0.045$
Molina et al. 1996 (57)	412 PBC	dna	OS less when elevated	$p < 0.0001$
			DFS less when elevated	$p < 0.0001$
Narita et al. 1994 (61)	81 PBC	dna	OS less when elevated	$p < 0.05$
			DFS less when elevated	$p < 0.01$
Nugent et al. 1992 (62)	161 PBC and 6 MBC	dna	OS less when elevated	$p < 0.001$
			DFS less when elevated	$p < 0.001$
Willsher et al. 1996 (23)	81 PBC and 38 MBC	Tamoxifen	Stage I, II: OS median 27 vs >84 mo	$p = 0.002$
			DFS median 11 vs >84 mo	$p = 0.002$
			Stage III: OS 24 vs 64 mo	$p = 0.04$
			Stage IV: OS 18 vs 31 mo	$p = 0.27$
Wu et al. 1999 (72)	226 PBC	Chemo and tamoxifen	OS less when elevated	$p = 0.0004$
Yamauchi et al. 1997 (73)	94 MBC	Droloxifene 1st line	TTP shorter when elevated	$p = 0.001$
			OS less when elevated	$p = 0.058$

DNA, Data not available; MBC, metastatic breast cancer; PBC, primary breast cancer.

5. SERUM HER2/neu AS A PREDICTIVE INDICATOR

5.1. Hormone Therapy

In the early 1990's Wright et al. *(75)*, using IHC, reported that patients with metastatic breast cancer who demonstrated HER2/neu overexpression and estrogen receptor (ER) positivity, had a response rate of only 20% to first-line hormone therapy whereas 48% of the metastatic breast cancer patients who were ER positive but had a normal IHC expression of HER2/neu responded to the first-line hormone therapy.

Since that report there have been several publications concerning HER2/neu ECD levels and the response rate of metastatic breast cancer patients to first- and second-line hormone therapies. Table 2 lists several published studies representing 1778 metastatic breast cancer patients and 119 patients with primary breast cancer, and their response rates to hormone therapy with respect to serum HER2/neu ECD levels.

In the 2002 report by Lipton et al. *(54)*, it was shown that MBC patients ($n = 711$) who were treated with second-line hormonal therapy (either the progestin megestrol acetate, or the aromatase inhibitor fadrozole) and who had a pretreatment serum HER2/neu level above the normal cutoff of 15 ng/mL were less likely to respond to the therapy (20.7%) compared to the 40.9% response of metastatic breast cancer patients who had serum HER2/neu levels below the normal cutoff of 15 ng/mL. The response rates reported here were nearly identical to those reported by the Wright et al. IHC studies mentioned earlier. The Lipton et al. studies also showed that patients with elevated pretreatment HER2/neu ECD levels had a shorter duration of response, a shorter TTP (illustrated in Fig. 4), and a shorter overall survival than ER-positive patients who had pretreatment serum ECD levels below the 15 ng/mL cutoff. In a recent report of first-line hormonal therapy, Lipton et al. *(55)* also demonstrated that metastatic breast cancer patients ($n = 562$) treated with either an aromatase inhibitor (letrozole) or an antiestrogen (tamoxifen) and who had elevated pretreatment serum HER2/neu levels, had a shorter time to progression, a shorter time to treatment failure, a decreased objective response rate (complete response plus partial response) and a decreased clinical benefit rate (complete response plus partial response plus stable disease greater than 24 wk) than similar patients who had serum HER2/neu levels below the normal cutoff of 15 ng/mL. Thus both forms of hormonal therapy were less effective if the pretreatment ECD levels were above the 15 ng/mL cutoff value. This study also showed that patients with normal serum HER2/neu ECD levels responded better to letrozole than to tamoxifen. However, there was no significant difference in response rate to letrozole or tamoxifen if the serum HER2/neu level was elevated. Therefore the superiority of letrozole was the greatest in those patients with normal serum HER2/neu levels.

Table 2
Summary of Data on HER2/neu as a Predictor of Response to Hormonal Therapy in Patients With Breast Cancer

Authors (ref.)	Patients	Therapy	Predictive indices (elevated vs nonelevated)	Significance
Hayes et al. 2001 (44)	103 MBC	Megestrol or fadrozole	RR 28% vs 37%	$p = 0.041$
Leitzel et al. 1995 (76)	300 MBC	Megestrol or fadrozole	RR 20.7% vs 40.9%	$p = 0.004$
			DR 11.6 vs 15.5 mo	$p < 0.0001$
Lipton et al. 2002 (54)	719 MBC	Megestrol, letrozole or fadrozole	RR 23% vs 45%	$p < 0.0001$
Lipton et al. 2003 (55)	562 MBC	Letrozole or tamoxifen	RR 15% vs 32%	$p < 0.0001$
			DR 18.5 vs 25.3 mo	$p = 0.014$
Willsher et al. 1999 (23)	119 PBC	Tamoxifen	RR 70% vs 70%	$p = 0.71$
Yamauchi et al. 1997 (73)	94 MBC	Droloxifene	RR 9% vs 56%	$p = 0.00001$

DR, Duration of response; RR, response rate.

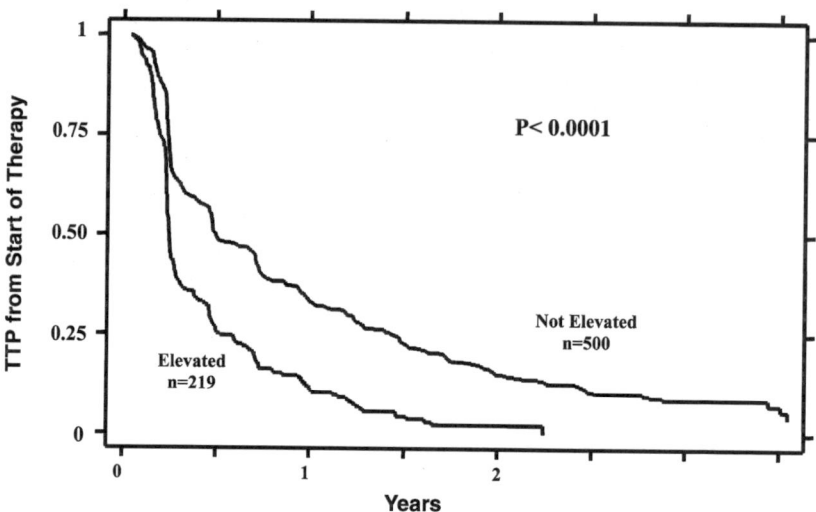

Fig. 4. Kaplan–Meier plot of TTP as a function of pretreatment serum HER2/neu level. These data are derived from three studies of patients with metastatic disease treated with second-line hormone therapy (two separate studies of fadrozole vs megestrol acetate; one study of letrozole vs megestrol acetate). HER2/neu not elevated, <15 ng/mL (n = 500) HER2/neu elevated, >15 ng/mL (n = 219).

5.2. Chemotherapy

Early studies by Gusterson et al. *(79)* and Muss et al. *(80)* reported that overexpression of HER2/neu correlated with a decreased responsiveness to combination therapy of cyclophosphamide/methotrexate 5-fluorouracil (CMF).

In 1995, Tsai et al. *(81)* demonstrated that an increased expression of p185neu resulted in enhanced chemoresistance following transfection of HER2/neu into non-small–cell lung cancer (NSCLC) cell lines established from untreated patients. In a follow-up 1996 report, the same investigators examined a panel of 20 NSCLC cell lines for HER2/neu ECD levels in the cell culture supernatant and then correlated the ECD levels with chemoresistance or chemosensitivity *(82)*. Various cytotoxic drugs were used such as doxorubicin, cisplatin, etoposide, and malphalan. The results showed that high HER2/neu ECD levels correlated with chemoresistance and cell lines expressing low ECD levels were relatively chemosensitive. In this report, multivariate analysis revealed that the level of p185 neu was the only predictor for chemoresistance to doxorubicin and etoposide. In a 1997 report by Fehm et al., they showed that in node-positive breast cancer patients, those with elevated HER2/neu ECD levels had a worse outcome than patients with nonelevated HER2/neu levels when treated with adjuvant CMF or cyclophosphamide–Novantrone–5-fluorouracil *(38)*.

In 1997 Pegram et al. also reported that HER2/neu overexpression altered chemotherapeutic drug sensitivity in a variety of human breast and ovarian cancer cells *(78)*. The next step in the analysis of the predictive role of HER2/neu expression and response to various regimens of chemotherapy was to examine published data concerning chemotherapy responses and HER2/neu ECD levels. These data are summarized in Table 3. We reviewed 12 publications, which contained data on 131 primary breast cancer patients and 1228 patients with metastatic disease.

In the report by Colomer et al. *(34)*, 58 MBC patients were studied and it was shown that the probability of obtaining a complete response to a paclitaxel–doxorubicin chemotherapy regimen was significantly lower in patients with elevated HER2/neu ECD levels compared to patients with nonelevated levels. In addition, the duration of clinical response was significantly shorter in patients with elevated HER2/neu ECD levels compared with the cases with nonelevated levels. For instance the duration of response was only 7.5 mo for patients with ECD elevations compared to 11 mo for patients with normal ECD levels. Overall, elevated levels of the ECD correlated with reduced efficacy of a paclitaxel–doxorubicin chemotherapy combination.

In a report by Mehta et al. *(83)*, it was concluded that breast cancer patients with more than three positive lymph nodes would benefit from determining the prechemotherapy levels of HER2/neu ECD and this could serve as an important marker to predict the response of breast cancer patients to chemotherapy. Postchemotherapy c-*erb*-B2 levels were also a prognostic indicator for disease-free survival in patients who received chemotherapy. Both the Mehta et al. *(83)* and Fehm et al. reports *(40)* concluded that patients with elevated HER2/neu ECD levels had a lower response to first-line therapy than breast cancer patients with normal serum HER2/neu ECD levels.

Nunes and Harris *(11)* as well as Kaptain et al. *(10)* reviewed the role of HER2/neu ECD in relation to alkylating-containing regimens, anthracycline-containing regimens, and taxanes. Overall they concluded that HER2/neu–positive tumors are relatively resistant to CMF-containing regimens but had an increased sensitivity to anthracycline-containing regimens. The clinical value of HER2/neu ECD testing and response to various chemotherapeutic regimens continues to be an area of research investigation. Therefore, the availability of an FDA-cleared serum HER2/neu ECD test will allow standardized studies to be conducted for the comparison of data between laboratories.

Yu et al. *(84)* showed that HER2/neu-transfected cells are more resistant to paclitaxel. However, the effect of taxanes in xenograft models in conjunc-

Table 3
Summary of Data on HER2/neu as a Predictor of Response to Chemotherapy in Patients With Breast Cancer

Authors (ref.)	Patients	Therapy	Predictive indices (elevated vs nonelevated)	Significance
Bewick et al. 1999 (26)	57 MBC	HDCT and ABSC	DFS 7.5 vs 14.3 mo	$p = 0.004$
Classen et al. 2002 (33)	64 MBC	Tamoxifen, adriamycin+ cyclophospan or CMF	RR 11.5% vs 84.2%	$p < 0.001$
Colomer et al. 2000 (34)	58 MBC	Paclitaxel and doxorubicin	CR 0% vs 26%	$p = 0.021$
			No response 37% vs 23%	
Fehm et al. 1997 (38)	211 MBC	NC or FNC, CMF	DFS 11.0 vs 49.0 mo	$p = 0.01$
Fehm et al. 1998 (39)	80 MBC	CMF, NC or FNC	RR 29% vs 59%	
Fehm et al. 2002 (40)	52 PBC and 52 MBC	Chemo and hormonal therapy	80% levels corresponded with response	
Harris et al. 2001 (43)	425 MBC	Doxorubicin, 5FU, methotrexate	Lower response when elevated	$p = 0.061$
Hayes et al. 2001 (44)	139 MBC	Anthracyclines	RR 29% vs 38%	$p = 0.26$
Kandl et al. 1994 (48)	74 MBC	No details	RR 50% vs 50%	NS
Luftner et al. 1999 (56)	35 MBC	Dose intensified paclitaxel monotherapy	Higher response (69%) when elevated	
Mehta et al. 1998 (78)	79 PBC	CMF, CMFVP	Lower response when elevated	$p = 0.04$
Revillon et al. 1996 (63)	33 MBC	Vinorelbine	RR 90% vs 61%	$0.5 < p < 0.9$

CR, Complete response; DFS, disease-free survival; RR, response rate.

tion with Herceptin appeared to reverse the resistance to both paclitaxel and docetaxel *(86)*, which is especially interesting because some of the best current response rates are seen when Herceptin is combined with docetaxel or paclitaxel *(86,87)*.

5.3. Herceptin-Based Therapy

In a report in 2002, Esteva et al. analyzed the response rate of 30 MBC patients (all shown to be HER2/neu–positive by tissue testing) treated with docetaxel and Herceptin who were separated into responders with high or low ECD levels *(86)*. The circulating HER2/neu ECD levels were measured at baseline and at the time of response evaluation for all 30 patients. The median level at baseline was 41.9 ng/mL (range, 7.1 ng/mL to 666.5 ng/mL). Twenty-one patients (70%) had elevated HER2/neu levels at baseline. The patients with high ECD baseline levels had the highest response rate to Herceptin-based therapy (76%) whereas only 33% of those with low ECD levels responded. In comparison, 67% of the FISH-positive patients responded. The overall response rate achieved was 63%; however, when patients with minor responses and stable disease were considered, 83% of the patients obtained some clinical benefit from the combination of weekly docetaxel and Herceptin. Esteva et al. also reported that serial changes in serum HER2/neu ECD levels correlated very well with clinical response to weekly docetaxel and Herceptin therapy. The authors concluded that additional research is warranted to determine the value of serum HER2/neu ECD testing in selecting and monitoring patients undergoing Herceptin-based therapy.

In a retrospective study designed to determine whether HER2/neu levels could predict outcomes of Herceptin-based therapy, Hoopman et al. *(87)* examined plasma samples from 20 MBC patients. HER2/neu ECD levels were measured in samples collected at the beginning of Herceptin-based therapy and at the time of first diagnostic imaging. HER2/neu levels were evaluated in relation to the clinical course of each patient and using imaging results, and then the data were analyzed with respect to prediction of the patient response to therapy defined as the time to progression. The data presented showed that the change in plasma HER2/neu levels were predictive of clinical course in 16 of 20 patients (80%) and that all therapy responders had normal ECD levels at the time of first diagnostic imaging. The patients with permanently elevated or increasing serum HER2/neu levels displayed a poor clinical outcome in 6 of the 10 cases. Based on these results the authors concluded that plasma HER2/neu levels might be an early predictor of response to Herceptin-based therapies.

Finally, in a report by Dnistrian et al. *(37)* metastatic breast cancer patients were stratified according to pretreatment serum HER2/neu levels to determine whether ECD levels could predict the response to Herceptin-based therapies. Of 18 patients treated with Herceptin and Taxol who had pretreatment ECD levels less than the cutoff (15 ng/mL), 6 responded favorably to Herceptin-based therapy. In contrast, 30 of the 36 patients (83%) who had elevated pretreatment serum HER-2/neu levels (mean 344 ng/mL), had a favorable response. Furthermore, in all patients with abnormally high pretreatment serum HER2/neu levels, the ECD level decreased significantly with disease regression and in most cases it returned to normal.

The observation that elevated serum HER2/neu levels may be predictive of response to Herceptin-based therapy (summarized in Table 4) is interesting in light of the publications demonstrating that elevated pretreatment HER2/neu ECD levels predict poor response to hormone therapy and some regimens of chemotherapy. It is not entirely unexpected, however, that high levels can predict response to Herceptin because the HER2/neu receptor provides the binding site for Herceptin which is necessary for its action. The shed ECD may therefore provide an indication of the amount of receptor that is available for binding, as well as the activity of the malignancy. Additional studies will need to be done to clarify this possibility.

6. MONITORING HER2/neu ECD LEVELS IN MBC PATIENTS TREATED WITH HORMONE OR CHEMOTHERAPY

In this section (summarized in Table 5), we reviewed 16 references (14 related to MBC and 4 related to PBC) representing 1148 breast cancer patients. The 1148 patients were divided into 499 MBC patients and 649 primary breast cancer patients. In these studies serial or longitudinal changes in serum HER2/neu ECD values were compared to the clinical course of disease in women with MBC. The clinical course of a patient's disease (defined as progression, response or stable disease) was determined by monitoring results of clinical tests such as X-ray films or CT scans. Patients were then classified as to whether changes in serum HER2/neu levels did or did not correspond to the clinical course of disease. For example, it was determined whether the serum value increased with progression or decreased with response to therapy to determine correspondence.

In a report by Cook et al. *(35)*, longitudinal monitoring was performed on 103 stage IV breast cancer patients who were being treated with various regimens of hormonal or chemotherapy, to determine whether serum HER2/neu changes correlated with changes in the clinical course of disease. Thirty-eight (36.9%) of the 103 stage IV patients had an elevated ECD, 33 of whom showed longitudinal HER2/neu values which paralleled the clinical course of disease, thus giving an overall sensitivity of 86.8%.

Schwartz et al. *(65)* reported serum HER2/neu levels in patients with MBC who were receiving a variety of conventional therapeutic regimens.

Table 4
Summary of Data on Serum HER2/neu as a Predictor of Response to Herceptin-Based Therapies in Patients With Metastatic Breast Cancer

Authors (ref.)	Patients	Therapy	Prognostic indices	Significance
Dnistrian et al. 2003 (37)	54 MBC	Herceptin ± paclitaxel	RR 86% in elevated, 61% in nonelevated	p < 0.001
Esteva et al. 2002 (86)	30 MBC	Doxetaxel and herceptin	RR 76% in elevated, 33% in nonelevated	p = 0.04
Hoopmann et al. 2003 (87)	20 MBC	Various chemotherapies and herceptin	Predicted clinical course in 80% of patients	
Schoendorf et al. 2002 (64)	23 MBC	Various chemotherapies and herceptin	Corresponded with clinical course in 74% of clinical events	

RR, Response rate.

Table 5
Summary of Data on HER2/neu for Monitoring Therapy and Early Detection of Metastases

Authors (ref.)	Patients	Therapy	Monitoring observation	Significance
Cook et al. 2001 (35)	38 MBC	No details given	86.8% concordance between changes and clinical course	
Cheung et al. 2000 (32)	30 MBC	Docetaxel/Doxorubicin based	100% concordance with course in all with elevated levels Earlier detection of progression; median 4 mo	
Dnistrian et al. 2003 (37)	54 MBC	Herceptin ± paclitaxel	87.5% concordance between changes and clinical course	
Isola et al. 1994 (47)	8 MBC	No details given	100% concordance between changes and clinical course	
Fehm et al. 2002 (40)	52 PBC and 52 MBC	Chemo or hormonal therapy	27% and 50% of patients had elevated HER2/neu 6 and 3 mo before metastases	
Hoopmann et al. 2003 (87)	20 MBC	Various chemotherapies and herceptin	Predicted clinical course in 80% of patients Level increased in 35% of patients at time of detection of metastases by imaging	
Kath et al. 1993 (50)	8 MBC	Various chemo and hormonal therapies	100% concordance with clinical course	
Luftner et al. 1999 (56)	35 MBC	Dose intensified Paclitaxel	Levels follow clinical course	

Study	Patients	Therapy	Results	
Mansour et al. 1997 (88)	18 MBC	No details given	Elevated levels associated with relapse, lead time 6–9 mo	$p = 0.007$
Molina et al. 1996 (57)	200 PBC	No details given	Lead time to detection of relapse 2–9 mo	
Molina et al. 1999 (60)	250 PBC	No details given	Lead time to relapse 4.5 ± 2.5 mo	
Narita et al. 1992 (61)	4 MBC	No details given	Lead time to relapse 4.8 ± 2.4 mo	
Schoendorf et al. 2002 (64)	23 MBC	Various chemo and hormonal therapies and herceptin	Levels followed clinical course Levels paralleled course in 74% of events	
Schwartz et al. 2000 (65)	147 PBC and 138 MBC	Various chemo and hormonal therapies and herceptin	Levels reflect clinical course	
Sugano et al. 2000 (68)	3 MBC	Tamoxifen, CAF	Indicator of relapse sens 58.3% spec 85.2%	
Volas et al. 1996 (22)	48 MBC	Fadrozole, megestrol acetate	58% of patients showed concordance with clinical course	

All patients had a pretherapy serum specimen and four posttherapy specimens. Longitudinal testing of the serum HER2/neu levels showed clearly that women who expressed HER2/neu in their tissue had elevated serum levels and that changes in the ECD levels reflected the clinical course of the patients' disease. This report also investigated whether there were serial changes in normal individuals over a several month period. In the study, six specimens were drawn monthly from seven premenopausal and eight postmenopausal women and tested for serum HER2/neu levels. These studies demonstrated that the serial HER2/neu values were consistent for a given person over a several month period. In one representative example, the serum HER2/neu values over several months were found to be very consistent and with very little variation. The serum values were 8.2 ng/mL, 8.3 ng/mL, 7.7 ng/mL, 8.3 ng/mL, 8.1 ng/mL, and 8.1 ng/mL. Similar data was demonstrated with the remaining normal individuals, and was therefore a good basis for comparative monitoring studies in MBC patients.

Cheung et al. (32) examined serial changes in serum HER2/neu levels in 30 MBC patients from 2 multicentered trials in which patients received either docetaxel-based therapy or doxorubicin-based therapy. The authors concluded that among the patients with positive tissue staining, sequential changes in serum completely paralleled the initial response to therapy.

In a report by Lueftner et al. (56), serum samples were taken weekly from 35 patients to monitor changes in the serum HER2/neu ECD levels and to correlate those changes to the clinical course of disease. The MBC patients received dose-intense paclitaxel treatment. In this study the overall response rate was 36% but the response rate among the HER2/neu-positive patients was 62%, showing a high sensitivity of the HER2/neu-positive patients to dose-intense paclitaxel treatment. In all responders, the HER2/neu level decreased below the detection limit either before the clinical diagnosis of response or by the end of the next cycle. However, in this cohort of patients normalization of the HER2/neu levels also occurred in patients that were stable or had progressive disease. The authors speculate that this could be explained by the fact that the chemotherapy is effective against the HER2/neu-positive tumor cells but not against the HER2/neu-negative tumor cells that could be responsible for the progressive disease. It was also pointed out by the authors that chemotherapy may alter the mechanisms by which the ECD is shed, but no data was presented to support this hypothesis.

In summary, numerous reports of patients receiving hormone or chemotherapy showed that longitudinal changes in serum HER2/neu levels paralleled the clinical course of a patient's disease. Overall, several studies showed that increases in serum HER2/neu levels were reflective of progressive breast cancer while decreasing serum HER2/neu levels were reflective of response to therapy or a prolonged lack of disease progression.

7. MONITORING METASTATIC BREAST CANCER PATIENTS TREATED WITH HERCEPTIN-BASED THERAPIES

In studies presented in Table 5, women with MBC being treated with Herceptin and various chemotherapies ($n = 110$) were monitored for changes in HER2/neu ECD levels. HER2/neu ECD levels were determined prior to treatment and then serially thereafter. Previous studies reported by Payne et al. have shown that Herceptin does not interfere with measuring ECD levels in the HER2/neu assay used in all three of these studies described below (74). In an initial report by Schwartz et al., in 2000, it was suggested that changes in serum HER2/neu during Herceptin-based therapy might parallel the clinical course of disease; however, there were too few patients in the report to make a valid conclusion (65).

In a 2002 report by Esteva et al. (86), 30 MBC patients treated with docetaxel (Taxotere) and Herceptin were monitored for changes in serum HER2/neu to see if serial changes would reflect the clinical course of disease. Studies showed that ECD levels decreased in 14 of 16 (87%) of responding patients. As seen in studies of patients receiving conventional therapies, serial changes in serum HER2/neu levels did parallel the clinical course of disease after Herceptin treatment.

In a report by Schoendorf et al. (64), 23 MBC patients treated with Herceptin and chemotherapy (for a median time of 13 mo, with a range of 4–22) were monitored serially for the change in serum HER2/neu ECD. The changes in HER2/neu ECD level were then evaluated in conjunction with response or lack of response to therapy. In the group of patients with elevated levels (12 of 19), 35 events of either response or progression were documented. The serial changes in serum HER2/neu correlated with remission or disease progression in 74% of the patients. The correlation between serial ECD changes and clinical changes was increased when the analysis was focused on MBC patients with visceral metastasis. This group of clinical investigators concluded that serial changes in plasma HER2/neu ECD levels did parallel changes in the clinical course of disease.

In a 2003 report (89) a group of 57 MBC patients treated over a 2-year period with Herceptin and Taxol were monitored for changes in serum HER2/neu and the data was correlated with clinical changes. The studies clearly showed that serum HER2/neu ECD changes paralleled the clinical course of disease. The women with serially decreasing ECD levels responded to Herceptin-based therapy while women with progressing breast cancer that did not respond to the combined therapy had serially increasing ECD levels. These data were consistent with the observations made in MBC patients who were treated with conventional hormone and chemotherapies.

In summary, these four publications collectively studied a small number of women with MBC who received Herceptin-based therapies and who had their serum HER2/neu levels monitored for up to 2 yr. All four publications showed that serial changes in the ECD levels reflected the clinical course of disease. Women who had serially decreasing ECD levels responded to Herceptin-based therapy whereas women with progressive breast cancer had serially increasing ECD levels.

8. SERUM HER2/neu LEVELS AND DETECTION OF EARLY RECURRENCE

In the 1996 report by Molina et al. *(58)*, they evaluated the utility of measuring HER2/neu, carcinoembryonic antigen (CEA), and CA 15-3 in the early diagnosis of recurrence. Serial serum measurements were performed in 200 primary breast cancer patients (no evidence of residual disease) followed for 1– 4 yr with a median of 2.2 yr. Of the 89 patients who developed metastasis, 28% had a serum HER2/neu above the cutoff, 30% had a CEA that was above the normal cutoff and 47% demonstrated elevated levels of CA 15-3. The lead time prior to diagnosis was 4.5 ± 2.4 mo for HER2/neu, CEA was 4.9 ± 2.4 mo and CA 15-3 was 4.8 ± 2.4 mo. However, sensitivity was clearly related to the site of recurrence, with the lowest sensitivity found in locoregional relapse and the highest in patients with visceral metastasis. When patients with locoregional relapse were excluded, the sensitivity for HER2/neu improved to 31% and the overall sensitivity of early detection with all three markers combined was 76%. This data and others are summarized in Table 5. The increased sensitivity observation was also supported by Watanabe *(21)* and Schwartz *(65)*, however, Eskilinen only reported limited value in measuring serum CEA, CA 15-3, and HER2/neu in conjunction with other cancer tests *(90)*.

In the study by Dnistrian et al. *(37)* HER2/neu, CA 15-3 and CEA were all measured serially from baseline to investigate the changes in 54 metastatic breast cancer patients undergoing Herceptin and Taxol therapy. When the individual data was combined the concordance with monitoring for response was 76%, similar to Molina et al. *(58)*, but individually the concordance was 67% (only 31% in the Molina report) for HER2/neu, 54% for CA 15-3 and 43% for CEA.

In a report by Ali et al. *(24)*, a study was done to measure CA 15-3 (a surrogate marker for disease burden) with serum HER2/neu in 566 ER/PR-positive metastatic breast cancer patients. These patients were treated with second-line hormone therapy, megestrol acetate, or an aromatase inhibitor, Fadrozole. Overall, 30% of the patients had an elevated HER2/neu ECD level ($n = 168$) and 60% had an increased CA 15-3; however, there was only a weak correlation between the two. Similar to a previous report, the clinical benefit (complete response plus partial response plus stable disease greater than 24 wk) of endocrine therapy was significantly lower in patients with elevated HER2/neu ECD levels. The investigators concluded that HER2/neu was a significant independent predictive and prognostic factor in hormone receptor-positive MBC patients even when adjusted for tumor burden as measured by CA 15-3. The combination of an elevated HER2/neu and CA15-3 predicted a worse prognosis for MBC patients than did an elevated CA 15-3 alone.

The Colomer report *(34)* suggests that a panel of tumor tests such as CEA, CA 15-3 and HER2/neu could be used to monitor patients postoperatively to increase the sensitivity of detecting early recurrence. The value of early detection will increase with the introduction of a variety of targeted therapy used as either monotherapy or in conjunction with hormonal or chemotherapies.

9. CONCLUSIONS

This chapter has shown that the prevalence of an elevated serum HER2/neu ECD is highly variable in breast cancer, which probably reflects the differing time of sampling in relation to the evolution and aggressiveness of the disease. As might be expected, there is a higher prevalence of elevated levels in the metastatic phase of the disease, conforming with the view that increased HER2/neu amplification is associated with a more aggressive form of the disease. There is strong data to show that an elevated serum HER2/neu ECD is an indicator of poor prognosis and furthermore is a predictor of poor response to therapy using chemotherapeutic and hormonal treatment regimens. Conversely an elevated serum HER2/neu ECD level is a predictor of improved response to Herceptin-based therapy, as it reflects the presence of an increased population of target molecules for the drug to bind to the malignant cell.

This chapter has also demonstrated an interesting observation regarding the potential use of serum HER2/neu ECD measurement as a tool for detecting the development of metastatic disease, ahead of conventional indicators, as well as monitoring of response to a variety of therapies administered in the metastatic phase of breast cancer. The review has also clearly established the need for more studies to clarify the clinical value of HER2/neu ECD testing in breast cancer patients. The review has also established the relationship between serum HER2/neu ECD levels and the presentation of breast cancer. It has identified several potential roles for the HER2/neu oncoprotein in clinical decision-making with respect to the diagnosis and management of breast cancer. In turn this could lead to improvement in clinical outcome. Prospective studies are also required in which the use of the HER2/neu oncoprotein test is used as a decision-making tool to demonstrate improved clinical outcomes.

REFERENCES

1. Aaronson SA. Growth factors and cancer. *Science* 1991;254:1146–1153.
2. Coussens L, Yang-Feng TL, Liao Y-C, et al. Tyrosine kinase receptor with extensive homology to EGF receptor shares chromosomal location with *neu* oncogene. *Science* 1985;230:1132–1139.
3. Bargmann CI, Hung MC, Weinberg RA. The *neu* oncogene encodes an epidermal growth factor receptor related protein. *Nature* 1986;319:226–230.
4. Kurebayshi J. Biological and clinical significance of HER2 overexpression in breast cancer. *Breast Cancer* 2001;8:45–51.
5. Brandt-Rauf PW, Pincus MR, Carney WP. The c-erbB-2 protein in oncogenesis: molecular structure to molecular epidemiology. *Crit Rev Oncogenesis* 1994;5:313–329.
6. Zabrecky JR, Lam T, McKenzie SJ, Carney W. The extracellular domain of p185 is released from the surface of human breast carcinoma cells, SK-BR-3. *J Biol Chem* 1991;266:1716–1720.
7. Carney WP, Hamer PJ, Petit D, et al. Detection and quantitation of the human *neu* oncoprotein. *J Tumor Marker Oncol* 1991;6:53–72.
8. Leitzel K, Teramoto Y, Sampson E, et al. Elevated soluble c-erbB-2 antigen levels in the serum and effusions of a proportion of breast cancer patients. *J Clin Oncol* 1992;10: 436–443.
9. Pupa SM, Menard S, Morelli D, Pozzi B, De Palo G, Colnaghi MI. The extracellular domain of the c-erbB-2 oncoprotein is released from tumor cells by proteolytic cleavage. *Oncogene* 1993;8:2917–2923.
10. Kaptain S, Tan LK, Chen B. HER-2/*neu* and breast cancer. *Diag Mol Pathol* 2001;10:139–152.
11. Nunes RA, Harris LN. The HER2 extracellular domain as a prognostic and predictive factor in breast cancer. *Clin Breast Cancer* 2002;3:125–135.
12. Codony-Servat J, Albanell J, Lopez-Talavera JC, Arribas J, Baselga J. Cleavage of the HER2 ectodomain is a pervanadate-activable process that is inhibited by the tissue inhibitor of metalloproteases-1 in breast cancer cells. *Cancer Res* 1999;59:1196–1201.
13. Christianson TA, Doherty JK, Lin YJ, et al. NH2-terminally truncated HER-2/*neu* protein: relationship with shedding of the extracellular domain and with prognostic factors in breast cancer. *Cancer Res* 1998;58:5123–5129.
14. Molina MA, Codony-Servat J, Albanell J, Rojo F, Arribas J, Baselga J. Trastuzumb (Herceptin), a humanized anti-HER-2/*neu* receptor monoclonal antibody inhibits basal and activated HER2 ectodomain cleavage in breast cancer cells. *Cancer Res* 2001;61:4744–4749.
15. Slamon DJ, Leyland-Jones B, Shak S, et al. Use of chemotherapy plus a monoclonal antibody against HER2 for metastatic breast cancer that overexpresses HER2. *N Engl J Med* 2001;344:783–792.
16. Ross JS, Fletcher JA. HER-2/*neu* (c-erbB2) gene and protein in breast cancer. *Am J Clin Pathol* 1999;112:S53–67.
17. Schaller G, Evers K, Papadopoulos S, Ebert A, Buhler H. Current use of HER2 tests. *Ann Oncol* 2001;12:S97–100.
18. Slamon DJ, Clark GM, Wong SG, Levin WJ, Ullrich A, McGuire Wl. Human breast cancer: correlation of relapse and survival with amplification of the HER-2/*neu* oncogene. *Science* 1987;235:177–182.
19. Slamon DJ, Godolphin W, Jones LA, et al. Studies of the HER-2/*neu* proto-oncogene in human breast and ovarian cancer. *Science* 1989;244:707–712.

20. McKenzie SJ, Marks PJ, Lam T, et al. Generation and characterization of mono-clonal antibodies specific for the human *neu* oncogene product, p185. *Oncogene* 1989;4:43–48.
21. Watanabe N, Mityamoto M, Tokuda Y, et al. Serum c-erbB-2 in breast cancer patients. *Acta Oncol* 1994;33:901–904.
22. Volas GH, Leitzel K, Teramoto Y, Grossberg H, Demers L, Lipton A. Serial serum c-erbB-2 levels in patients with breast carcinoma. *Cancer* 1996;78:267–272.
23. Willsher PC, Beaver J, Pinder S, et al. Prognostic significance of serum c-erbB-2 protein in breast cancer patients. *Breast Cancer Res Treat* 1996;40:251–255.
24. Ali SA, Leitzel K, Chinchilli VM, et al. Relationship of serum HER-2/*neu* and serum CA 15-3 in patients with metastatic breast cancer. *Clin Chem* 2002;48:1314–1320.
25. Andersen TI, Paus E, Nesland JM, McKenzie SJ, Borresen AL. Detection of c-erbB-2 related protein in sera from breast cancer patients. *Acta Oncol* 1995; 34:499–504.
26. Bewick M, Chadderton T, Conlon M, et al. Expression of c-erbB-2/HER-2 in patients with metastatic breast cancer undergoing high-dose chemotherapy and autologous blood stem cell support. *Bone Marrow Transpl* 1999;24:377–384.
27. Bewick M, Conlon M, Gerard S, et al. HER-2 expression is a prognostic factor in patients with metastatic breast cancer treated with a combination of high dose cyclophosphamide, mitoxantrone, paclitaxel and autologous blood stem cell support. *Bone Marrow Transplantation* 2001;27:847–853.
28. Breuer B, Luo JC, DeVivo I, et al. Detection of elevated c-erbB-2 oncoprotein in the serum and tissue in breast cancer. *Med Sci* 1993;21:383–384.
29. Breuer B, DeVivo I, Luo JC, et al. ErbB-2 and myc oncoproteins in sera and tumors of breast cancer patients. *Cancer Epidemiol Biomarkers Prevention* 1994;3:63–66.
30. Breuer B, Smith S, Thor A, et al. ErbB-2 protein in sera and tumors of breast cancer patients. *Breast Cancer Res Treat* 1998;49:261–270.
31. Chearskul S, Bhothisuwan K, Ornrhebroi S, et al. Serum c-erbB-2 protein in breast cancer patients. *J Med Assoc Thai* 2000;83:886–893.
32. Cheung KL, Pinder SE, Paish C, et al. The role of blood tumor marker measure-ment (using a biochemical index score and c-erB2) in directing chemotherapy in metastatic breast cancer. *Int J Biol Markers* 2000;15:203–209.
33. Classen S, Kopp R, Possinger K, Weidenhagen R, Eiermann W, Wilmanns W. Clinical relevance of soluble c-erbB-2 for patients with metastatic breast cancer predicting the response to second line hormone or chemotherapy. *Tumor Biol* 2002;23:70–75.
34. Colomer R, Montero S, Lluch A, et al. Circulating HER2 extracellular domain and resistance to chemotherapy in advanced breast Cancer. *Clin Cancer Res* 2000;6:2356–2362.
35. Cook GB, Neamann IE, Goldblatt JL, et al. Clinical utility of serum HER-2/*neu* testing on the Bayer Immuno 1 automated system in breast cancer. *Anticancer Res* 2001;21:1465–1470.
36. Dittadi R, Zancan M, Perasole A, Gion M. Evaluation of HER-2/*neu* in serum and tissue of primary and metastatic breast cancer patients using an automated enzyme immunoassay. *Int J Biol Markers* 2001;16:255–261.
37. Dnistrian AM, Schwartz MK, Schwartz DC, Ghani F, Kish L. Significance of serum HER-2/*neu* oncoprotein, CA 15-3 and CEA in the clinical evaluation of metastatic breast cancer. *J Clin Ligand Assay* 2002;25:215–220.

38. Fehm T, Maimonis P, Weitz S, Teramoto Y, Katalinic A, Jäger W. Influence of circulating c-erbB-2 serum protein on response to adjuvant chemotherapy in node-positive breast cancer patients. *Breast Cancer Res Treat* 1997;43:87–95.

39. Fehm T, Maimonis P, Katalinic A, Jäger W. The prognostic significance of c-erbB-2 serum protein in metastatic breast cancer. *Oncology* 1998;55:33–38.

40. Fehm T, Gebauer G, Jager W. Clinical utility of serial serum c-erB-2 determinations in the follow-up of breast cancer patients. *Breast Cancer Res Treat* 2002;75:97–106.

41. Fontana X, Ferrari P, Namer M, Peysson R, Salanon C, Bussiere F. C-erbB2 gene amplification and serum level of c-erb-B2 oncoprotein at primary breast cancer diagnosis. *Anticancer Res* 1994;14:2099–2104.

42. Harris LN, Lueftner D, Jager W, Robertson JFR. C-erbB-2 in serum of patients with breast cancer. *Int J Biol Markers* 1999;14:8–15.

43. Harris LN, Liotcheva V, Broadwater G, et al. Comparison of methods of measuring HER-2 in metastatic breast cancer patients treated with high-dose chemotherapy. *J Clin Oncol* 2001;19:1698–1706.

44. Hayes DF, Yamauchi H, Broadwater G, et al. Circulating HER-2/erbB-2/c-*neu* (HER-2) extracellular domain as a prognostic factor in patients with metastatic breast. *Clin Cancer Res* 2001;7:2703–2711.

45. Hosona M, Saga T, Sakahara H, et al. Construction of immunoradiometric assay for circulating c-erbB-2 protooncogene product in advanced breast cancer patients. *Jpn J Cancer Res* 1993;84:147–152.

46. Imoto S, Kitoh T, Hasebe T. Serum c-erbB-2 levels in monitoring of operable breast cancer patients. *Jpn J Clin Oncol* 1999;29:336–339.

47. Isola JJ, Holli K, Oksa H, Teramoto Y, Kallioniemi OP. Elevated erbB-2 oncoprotein levels in preoperative and follow-up serum samples define and aggressive disease course in patients with breast cancer. *Cancer* 1994;73:652–658.

48. Kandl H, Seymour L, Bezwoda WR. Soluble c-erbB-2 fragment in serum correlates with disease stage and predicts for shortened survival in patients with early-stage and advanced breast cancer. *Br J Cancer* 1994;70:739–742.

49. Kasimir-Bauer S, Oberhoff C, Sliwinska K, Neumann R, Schindler AE, Seeber S. Evaluation of different methods for the detection of minimal residual disease in blood and bone marrow of patients with primary breast cancer: importance of clinical use. *Breast Cancer Res Treat* 2001;16:123–132.

50. Kath R, Höffken K, Otte C, Metz K, Scheulen ME, Hülskamp F, Seeber S. The *neu*-oncogene product in serum and tissue of patients with breast carcinoma. *Ann Oncol* 1993;4:585–589.

51. Klein B, Levin I, Kfir B, et al. Soluble c-erbB-2 (P185) in breast cancer patients in relation to prognosis. *Oncol Rep* 1995;2:759–761.

52. Krainer M, Brodowicz T, Zeillinger R, et al. Tissue expression and serum levels of HER-2/*neu* in patients with breast cancer. *Oncology* 1997;54:475–481.

53. Kynast B, Binder L, Marx D, et al. Determination of a fragment of the c-erbB-2 fragment translational product p185 in serum of breast cancer patients. *Cancer Res Clin Oncol* 1993;119:249–252.

54. Lipton A, Ali SM, Leitzel K, et al. Elevated serum HER-2/*neu* level predicts decreased response to hormone therapy in metastatic breast cancer. *J Clin Oncol* 2002;20:1467–1472.

55. Lipton A, Ali SM, Leitzel K, Demers L, Harvey HA, Chaudri-Ross HA, Brady C, Wyld P, Carney W. Serum HER-2/*neu* and response to the aromatase inhibitor letrozole versus tamoxifen. *J Clin Oncol* 2003;21:1967–1972.

56. Lueftner D, Schnabel S, Possinger K. c-erbB-2 in serum of patients receiving fractionated paclitaxel chemotherapy. *Int J Biol Markers* 1999;14:55–59.
57. Molina R, Jo J, Filella X, Zanon G, et al. C-erbB-2 oncoprotein in the sera and tissue of patients with breast cancer. Utility in prognosis. *Anticancer Res* 1996;16:2295–2300.
58. Molina R, Jo J, Zanon G, et al. Utility of c-erbB-2 in tissue and serum in the early diagnosis of recurrence in breast cancer patients: comparison with carcino-embryonic antigen and CA 15.3. *Br J Cancer* 1996;74:1126–1131.
59. Molina R, Jo J, Filella X, Bruix J, Castells A, Hague M, Ballesta AM. Serum levels of c-erbB-2 (HER-2/*neu*) in patients with malignant and non-malignant diseases. *Tumor Biol* 1997;18:188–196.
60. Molina R, Jo J, Filella X, et al. C-erbB-2, CEA and CA 15.3 serum levels in the early diagnosis of recurrence in breast cancer patients. *Anticancer Res* 1999;19:2551–2556.
61. Narita T, Funahashi H, Satoh Y, Takagi H. C-erbB-2 protein in the sera of breast cancer patients. *Breast Cancer Res Treat* 1992;24:97–102.
62. Nugent A, Mc Dermott E, Duffy K, O'Higgins N, Fennelly JJ, Duffy MJ. Enzyme-linked immunosorbent assay of c-erbB-2 oncoprotein in breast cancer. *Clin Chem* 1992;38:1471–1474.
63. Revillion F, Hebbar M, Bonneterre J, Peyrat JP. Plasma c-erbB2 concentrations in relation to chemotherapy in breast cancer patients. *Eur J Cancer* 1996;32A:231–234.
64. Schoendorf T, Hoopmann M, Warm M, et al. Serologic concentrations of HER-2/*neu* in breast cancer patients with visceral metastases receiving trastuzumab therapy predict the clinical course. *Clin Chem* 2002;48:1360–1362.
65. Schwartz MK, Smith C, Schwartz DC, Dnistrian A, Neiman I. Monitoring therapy by serum HER-2/*neu*. *Int J Biol Markers* 2000;15:324–329.
66. Streckfus C, Bigler L, Dellinger T, Dali X, Kingman A, Thigpen JT. The presence of soluble c-erbB-2 in saliva and serum among women with breast carcinoma: a preliminary study. *Clin Cancer Res* 2000;6:2363–2370.
67. Sugano K, Kawai T, Ishii M, et al. Clinical evaluation of serum ErbB-2 protein using enzyme immunoassay (ErbB-2 EIA [Nichirei] Gan To Kagaku Ryoho 1994;21:1255–1262.
68. Sugano K, Ushiama M, Fukutomi T, Tsuda H, Kitoh T, Ohkura H. Combined measurement of the c-erbB-2 protein in breast carcinoma tissues and sera is useful as a sensitive tumor marker for monitoring tumor relapse. *Int J Cancer* 2000;89:329–333.
69. Visco V, Bei R, Moriconi E, Gianni W, Kraus MH, Muraro R. ErbB2 immune response in breast cancer patients with soluble receptor ectodomain. *Am J Pathol* 2000;156:1417–1424.
70. Wu JT, Astill ME, Zhang P. Detection of the extracellular domain of c-erbB-2 oncoprotein in sera from patients with various carcinomas: correlation with tumor markers. *J Clin Lab Anal* 1993;7:31–40.
71. Wu JT, Astill ME, Gagon SD, Bryson L. Measurement of c-erbB-2 proteins in sera from patients with carcinomas and in breast tumor tissue cytosols: correlation with serum tumor markers and membrane-bound oncoprotein. *J Clin Lab Anal* 1995;9:151–165.
72. Wu Y, Khan H, Chillar R, Vadgama J. Prognostic value of plasma HER-2/*neu* in African American and Hispanic women with breast cancer. *Int J Oncol* 1999;14:1021–1037.

73. Yamauchi H, O'Neill A, Gelman R, et al. Prediction of response to antiestrogen therapy in advanced breast cancer patients by pretreatment circulating levels of extracellular domain of the HER-2/c-*neu* protein. *J Clin Oncol* 1997;15:2518–2525.

74. Payne RC, Allard JW, Anderson-Mauser L, Humphreys JD, Tenney DY, Morris DL. Automated assay for HER-2/*neu* in serum. *Clin Chem* 2000;46:2:175–182.

75. Wright C, Cairns J, Cantwell BJ, Hall AG, Harris AL, Horne CH. Response to mitoxantrone in advanced breast cancer: correlation with expression of c-erbB-2 protein and glutathione S-transferases. *Br J Cancer* 1992;65:271–274.

76. Leitzel K, Teramoto Y, Konrad K, et al. Elevated serum c-erbB-2 antigen levels and decreased response to hormone therapy of breast cancer. *J Clin Oncol* 1995;13:1129–1135.

77. Hait WN. The prognostic and predictive values of ECD-HER-2. *Clin Cancer Res* 2001;7:2601–2604.

78. Pegram MD, Finn RS, Arzoo K. The effect of c-erbB-2 Her-2/*neu* overexpression on chemotherapeutic drug sensitivity in human breast and ovarian cancer cells. *Oncogene* 1997;15:537–547.

79. Gusterson BA, Gelber RD, Goldhirsch A, et al. Prognostic importance of c-erbB-2 expression in breast cancer. *J Clin Oncol* 1992;10:1049–1056.

80. Muss HB, Thor AD, Berry DA, et al. c-erbB-2 expression and response to adjuvant therapy in women with node-positive early breast cancer. *N Engl J Med* 1994;330:1260–1266.

81. Tsai CM, Yu D, Chang KT, et al. Enhanced chemoresistance by elevations of the levels of p185 *neu* in the HER-2/*neu*-transfected human lung cancer cells. *J Natl Cancer Inst* 1995;87:682–684.

82. Tsai CM, Chang KT, Wu LH, Chen JY, Gazdar AF, Mitsudomi T, Correlations between intrinsic chemoresistance and HER-2/*neu* gene expression, p53 gene mutations, and cell proliferation characteristics in non-small cell lung cancer cell lines. *Cancer Res* 1996;56:206–209.

83. Mehta RR, McDermott JH, Heiken TJ, et al. Plasma c-erbB-2 levels in breast cancer patients: prognostic significance in predicting response to chemotherapy. *J Clin Oncol* 1998;16:2409–2416.

84. Yu D, Jing T, Liu B. Overexpression of Erb2 blocks taxol-induced apoptosis by upregulation of p21Cip1, which inhibits p34 Cdc2 kinase. *Mol Cell* 1998;2:581–591.

85. Pegram M, Hsu S, Lewis G. Inhibitory effects of combinations of HER-2/*neu* antibody and chemotherapeutic agents used for treatment of human breast cancers. *Oncogene* 1999;18:2241–2251.

86. Esteva FJ, Valero V, Booser D, et al. Phase II study of weekly docetaxel and trastuzumab for patients with HER2-overexpressing metastatic breast cancer. *J Clin Oncol* 2002;20:1800–1808.

87. Hoopmann M, Neumann R, Tanasale T, Schoendorf, T. HER-2/*neu* determination in blood plasma of patients with HER-2/*neu* overexpressing metastasized breast cancer: A Longitudinal Study. *Anticancer Res* 2003;23:1031–1034.

88. Mansour OA, Zekri AR, Harvey J, Teramoto Y, Elahmady O. Tissue and serum c-erbB-2 and tissue EGFR in breast carcinoma: three years follow-up. *Anticancer Res* 1997;17:3101–3106.

89. Carney, WP. The emerging role of monitoring serum HER-2/*neu* oncoprotein levels in women with metastatic breast cancer. *Lab Med* 2003;34:58–64.

90. Eskelinen M, Kataja V, Hamalainen E, Kosma VM, Penttila I, Alhava E. Serum tumor markers CEA, AFP, CA15-3, TPS and *neu* in diagnosis of breast cancer. *Anticancer Res* 1997;17:231–234.

91. Joensuu H, Isola J, Lundin M, et al. Amplification of erbB2 and erbB2 expression are superior to estrogen receptor status as risk factors for distant recurrence in pT1N0M0 breast cancer: a nationwide population-based study. *Clin Can Res* 2003;9:923–930.

92. Pegram MD, Lipton A, Hayes DF, et al. Phase II study of receptor-enhanced chemosensitivity using recombinant humanized anti-p185 HER2/*neu* monoclonal antibody plus cisplatin in patients with HER2/*neu*-overexpressing metastatic breast cancer refractory to chemotherapy treatment. *J Clin Oncol* 1998;16:2659–2671.

93. Cobleigh MA, Vogel CL, Tripathy D, Robert NJ, Scholl S, Fehrenhacher L. Multinational study of the efficacy and safety of humanized anti-HER2 monoclonal antibody in women who have HER2 overexpressing metastatic breast cancer that has progressed after chemotherapy for metastatic disease. *J Clin Oncol* 1999;17: 2639–2648.

94. Edgerton SE, Merkel D, Moore DH, Thor AD. HER-2/*neu*/erbB-b2 status by immunohistochemistry and FISH: clonality and progression with recurrence and metastases. *Breast Cancer Res Treat* 2000;64:55 (Abstract 180).

95. De Placido S, De Laurentiis M, Carlomagno C, Gallo C, Perrone F, Pepe S, et al. Twenty-year results of the Naples GUN randomized trial: predictive factors of adjuvant tamoxifen efficacy in early breast cancer. *Clin Can Res* 2003;9:1039–1046.

96. Kostler WJ, Schwab B, Singer C, Neumann R, Marton E, Brodowicz T, et al. Predictive value of serum HER-2/*neu* extracellular domain (ECD) during trastuzumab-based therapies. *Am Assoc for Cancer Res* 93rd Annual Meeting April 2002; p 201 (abstract 2437).

14 Circulating Vascular Endothelial Growth Factor

Methods, Prognostic Significance, and Potential Application for Antiangiogenic Therapy

Roberta Sarmiento, MD,
Roberta Franceschini, MS,
Sabrina Meo, MS,
Massimo Gion, MD,
Raffaele Longo, MD,
and Giampietro Gasparini, MD

CONTENTS

INTRODUCTION
ROLE OF ANGIOGENESIS IN TUMOR GROWTH
    AND PROGRESSION
DETERMINATION OF TISSUE ANGIOGENESIS
    AS A CANCER BIOMARKER
CIRCULATING BIOMARKERS OF ANGIOGENESIS:
    PROMISES AND PITFALLS
CONCLUSIONS
REFERENCES

Cancer Drug Discovery and Development: Biomarkers in Breast Cancer:
Molecular Diagnostics for Predicting and Monitoring Therapeutic Effect
Edited by: G. Gasparini and D. F. Hayes © Humana Press Inc., Totowa, NJ

SUMMARY

Despite significant advances in early detection and treatment, breast cancer still remains the major cause of cancer-related death in women. Many studies suggest a relationship between angiogenesis and breast cancer prognosis. Angiogenesis is the complex process leading to the formation of new blood vessels from pre-existing vascular network. The VEGF is the most active growth factor involved in angiogenesis; more specifically, raised intratumoral VEGF concentrations have been shown to correlate with tumor aggressiveness. VEGF is therefore a promising target for new therapies, but it is still unclear in which blood matrix the determination of VEGF is more accurate as a cancer biomarker and which matrix provides the optimal clinical information. Circulating levels of VEGF have been measured by several investigators who reported conflicting results. However, these studies are not comparable with each other due to a lack of standardization of the pre-analytical phase. The chapter presents the main studies concerning anti-VEGF therapies; several studies evaluated the safety profile and activity of the combination of standard chemotherapy with new antiangiogenic agents. However, to date only a few definitive results on the effect of angiogenesis blood markers have been reported. Determination of circulating VEGF still remains an experimental procedure with no evident application for routine clinical decisions. Data from retrospective studies, however, suggest that VEGF levels may predict clinical outcome of breast cancer.

Key Words: Vascular endothelial growth factor; breast cancer; angiogenesis; therapy; prognosis.

1. INTRODUCTION

Angiogenesis, or neovascularization, is the complex process leading to the formation of new blood vessels from the preexisting vascular network of the tissue. It is necessary for new organ development and differentiation during embryogenesis, wound healing, and reproductive functions in adults *(1)*. Angiogenesis is also involved in pathogenesis of certain chronic diseases, such as rheumatoid arthritis, age-related macular degeneration, proliferative retinopathies, psoriasis, as well as malignant tumors. Angiogenesis is a complex process that, during physiologic tissue growth and repair, is closely regulated by pro- and anti-angiogenic growth factors (Table 1). In cancer, the net balance of pro- and antifactors is altered vs down-regulation of angiogenic inhibitors or up-regulation of angiogenic activators, providing tumor progression and metastasis. Neovascularization occurs in a series of complex and interrelated steps. First, tumor or certain stromal cells (e.g., macrophages, mast cells, and fibroblasts) release endothelial cell

Table 1
Proangiogenic and Antiangiogenic Factors

Proangiogenic factors	Naturally occurring inhibitors
Angiogenin	Angiostatin (plasminogen fragment)
Angiopoietin-1	Antiangiogenic antithrombin III
Del-1	Cartilage-derived inhibitor (CDI)
Fibroblast growth factor, acidic (aFGF)	CD 59 complement fragment
Fibroblast growth factor, basic (bFGF)	Endostatin (collagen XVIII fragment)
Follistatin	Fibronectin fragment
Granulocyte colony-stimulating factor (G-CSF)	Gro-β
Hepatocyte growth factor (HGF)	Heparinases
Interleukin-8 (IL-8)	Heparin hexasaccharide fragment
Leptin	Human chorionic gonadotropin (hCG)
Midkine	Interferon-α, β, γ
Placental-growth factor (PiGF)	Interferon inducible protein (IP-10)
Platelet-derived endothelial cell growth factor	Interleukin-12 (IL-12)
Platelet-derived endothelial cell growth factor-BB	Kringle 5 (plasminogen fragment)
Pleiotrophin (PTN)	Tissue inhibitors of metalloproteinases
Proliferin	2-Methoxyestradiol
Transforming growth factor-α (TGF-α)	Placental ribonuclease inhibitor
Transforming growth factor-β (TGF-β)	Plasminogen activator inhibitor
Tumor necrosis factor-α (TNF-α)	Platelet factor 4 (PF4)
Vascular endothelial growth factor (VEGF)	Prolactin 16-kDa fragment
	Retinoids
	Tetrahydrocortisol-S
	Thrombospondin-1
	TGF-β
	Vasculostatin
	Vasostatin

growth factors, such as vascular endothelial growth factor (VEGF), fibroblast growth factor (FGF), or platelet-derived growth factor (PDGF) into the surrounding tissue. These factors are secreted in response to proteins overexpressed in the microenvironment for example, epidermal growth factor (EGF), insulin growth factor (IGF), FGF, interleukins, PDGF, or in response to several mechanisms as hypoxia, hypoglycemia, inflammation, and genetic alterations. The endothelial growth factors bind to, thereby activating, endothelial cells that form the walls of new blood vessels. Subsequently, activated endothelial cells stimulate proteolytic enzymes that break down the extracellular matrix, allowing endothelial cells to invade the matrix and migrate. The proliferation and migration of activated endothelial cells give origin to new capillary tubes. Endothelial cells differentiate and synthesize a new basement membrane *(2)*. The maturation and differentiation of the new vessel is completed with the formation of the vascular lumen. Finally, the adhesion receptor integrins $\alpha v \beta$, present on the surface of activated endothelial cells, permit the linkage of the new vessels with the preexisting ones to generate the intratumoral vascular network. The angiogenic process is necessary for tumor growth, invasiveness, progression, and metastasis and its determination has multiple important clinical applications as a potentially useful prognostic indicator, or as predictive marker of response to antiangiogenic therapy.

2. ROLE OF ANGIOGENESIS IN TUMOR GROWTH AND PROGRESSION

Despite significant advances in early detection and treatment, breast cancer still remains the major cause of cancer-related death in women.

There are compelling data suggesting a relationship between angiogenesis and breast cancer prognosis. Preclinical studies in vivo have shown that while normal, healthy breast tissue has no angiogenic activity, all breast carcinoma samples have some degree of angiogenesis *(3)*.

The growth of MCF-7 cells transfected to overexpress VEGF in vivo correlates with a significant increased number of microvessels, indicating the importance of neovascularization for tumor growth *(4)*. The experimental findings are supported by clinical studies that have demonstrated the prognostic significance of angiogenesis in breast cancer, either in terms of metastatic potential *(5)*, relapse-free survival *(6)*, or long-term survival *(7)*. Most of the studies have found that an increased level of angiogenesis, as measured by the assessment of microvessel density, is associated with a reduced survival, shorter relapse-free survival, and an increased risk of metastases. Indirect markers of angiogenesis, such as microvessel density, could potentially be used to select those patients with a poor prognosis for whom alternative therapeutic approaches may be necessary.

The "angiogenic switch" is characterized by oncogene-driven tumor expression of pro-angiogenic proteins, such as VEGF, bFGF, interleukin-8, transforming growth factor-β, PDGF, and others *(8–10)*. It has been shown that other mediators of neovascularization such as interleukins, oncogenes, and tumor growth factors may produce their effects by altering the expression of VEGF, suggesting that the VEGF pathway plays a central role in in vivo angiogenesis *(11)*.

Among the endothelial cell growth factors, VEGF is the most active, specific, and potent mitogen for vascular endothelium *(12)*. VEGF is a promising target, as it has been shown to be a potent promoter of endothelial cell proliferation *(13)* and chemotaxis *(14)*, and it also increases vascular permeability *(15)*. VEGF-A is a dimeric 34–42-kDa glycosylated basic protein, encoded in five isoforms; the two larger isoforms (VEGF 189 and VEGF 209) are cell associated, while the two smaller ones (VEGF 121 and VEGF 165) are secreted as soluble molecules. VEGF activation requires the phosphorylation of specific transmembrane tyrosine kinase receptors, which are preferentially expressed on vascular endothelial cells.

Three specific VEGF related tyrosine-kinase receptors have been identified: VEGF-R1 (flt-1 or fms-like-tyrosine kinase), VEGF-R2 (flk-1/KDR), located on vascular endothelial cells (Ecs) and VEGF-R3 (flt-4), located on lymphatic vessels *(16–18)*. Recently, two isoform-specific nontyrosine kinase receptors, neurophilins 1 and 2, involved in neural cells guidance, have also been reported to bind VEGF *(19)*. Neurophilin 1 binds VEGF-165, but not VEGF 121, and neurophilin 2 is correlated to VEGFR-1 *(20)*. Activated VEGFR phosphorylates several signaling cascade proteins, including phospholipase C, phosphoinositol-3 kinase, and ras GTPase activating proteins *(21)*. This cascade of cellular events leads to proliferation, migration, and differentiation of activated endothelial cells *(22)*.

The VEGF family includes at least sequenced isoforms, derived by alternative exone-splicing: VEGF 121 (A), 165 (B), 189 (C), 206 (D), and 145 (E). Three other members—PIGFs 1, 2, and 3—are also described as alternative spliced isoforms of the same gene *(12,23)*. Recently, four independent research groups provided direct evidence that VEGF-C and VEGF-D are important regulators of lymph vessel growth in vivo, both being ligands for the VEGF-3 receptor *(16,17)*. These studies provided the first experimental evidence that tumors are able to promote lymphangiogenesis, a phenomenon that has been neglected for a long time. By using a novel specific marker for lymphatic endothelium, the anti-LYVE-1 antibody *(24)*, a significant correlation of lymphatic vessel immunostaining with over-expression of VEGF-C or VEGF-D was demonstrated. Indeed, tumor lymphangiogenesis was associated to lymph node metastasis. Skobe et al. *(17)* demonstrated the occurrence of intratumoral lymphangiogenesis within human breast cancer after orthotopic transplantation onto nude mice. The degree of lymphatic vessels density was associated with overexpression of VEGF-C and enhanced regional lymph node and lung metastasis. Moreover, another study *(25)* showed that VEGF-C overexpression is detectable only in human invasive breast cancers with histologically proven axillary lymph node metastasis. Makinen et al. *(26)* found in an experimental model that a soluble VEGFR-3 fusion protein inhibits the process of lymphatic vessel development, leads to regression of existing lymphatics in vivo, and reduces lymphedema in transgenic mice expressing soluble VEGFR-3.

Because the evaluation of a blood sample is easier in comparison to immunohistochemical assessments, or immunoassays that involve laborious tissue preparation procedures and it allows for serial measurements, many studies have been published on circulating VEGF, as a surrogate marker of angiogenesis.

VEGF gene expression is regulated by several mechanisms: hypoxia, glucose deprivation, soluble cytokines, oxidative and mechanical stresses, oncogenes, and tumor-suppressor genes mutations (27,28).

3. DETERMINATION OF TISSUE ANGIOGENESIS AS A CANCER BIOMARKER

Studies have confirmed the presence of VEGF gene overexpression in malignant tumors as compared to benign breast tissues. Raised intratumoral VEGF concentrations have also been shown to correlate with tumor aggressiveness. However, there are conflicting reports on the association of VEGF levels with disease-free survival (29–31).

The clinical significance of cytosolic VEGF levels was first tested by Gasparini et al. in two studies published in 1997. The first study (32) evaluated VEGF protein in 260 consecutive patients with node-negative disease not treated with adjuvant therapy, median follow-up of 72 mo. In both univariate and multivariate analysis for RFS and OS, VEGF retained a significant and independent prognostic value. The second study (33) was performed in the same cohort of cases, with prognostic evaluation extended also to other biological factors, such as: cathepsin D, p53 protein, and TP. More recently, Gasparini et al. (34) performed a study to evaluate the clinical significance of co-determination of VEGF and TP in series of node-positive breast cancer patients treated with adjuvant therapy. Two series of patients were evaluated: the first group of patients included 137 patients treated with adjuvant chemotherapy (CMF iv schedule). The second group included 164 patients who received adjuvant hormone therapy (tamoxifen). In the first group of patients, the two angiogenic peptides were found to be significant and independent prognostic factors. In multivariate analysis on RFS only VEGF and the number of involved lymph nodes retained a significant and independent prognostic value. Both estrogen and progesterone receptors were significant prognostic indicators for both RFS and OS in univariate analysis, but they lost their significance in the multivariate model inclusive of VEGF. No statistically significant associations were found between VEGF and the other prognostic factors examined (age, menopausal status, histologic tumor type, tumor size, and hormone receptors). The lack of association of VEGF with hormone receptors suggests that this angiogenic peptide is likely to stimulate the growth of human breast cancer independently of the hormone pathways via direct autocrine/or paracrine stimulation on tumour cells or enhancing intratumoral vascular permeability, thus allowing more oxygen and nutrient to reach the tumor.

It has been recently hypothesized that overexpression of VEGF by estrogen-dependent breast cancer cells could produce an effect on breast cancer progression (acquisition of estrogen-independent growth) similar to the growth stimulation induced by estrogens. Li et al. *(35)* found that overexpression of the VEGF isoforms 121 and 165 by estrogen-dependent MCF-7 breast cells stimulated breast tumor formation in an estrogen-independent fashion in ovariectomized mice, in the absence of estrogen treatment. In addition, VEGF strongly stimulated neovascularization in MCF-7 tumors either in estrogen-treated or untreated mice, as well as enhanced estrogen-dependent tumor growth in estrogen-treated mice. These findings suggest that up-regulation of VEGF indirectly contributes to the acquisition of estrogen-independent cancer growth by stimulating tumor angiogenesis.

4. CIRCULATING BIOMARKERS OF ANGIOGENESIS: PROMISES AND PITFALLS

4.1. Methods of Determination: Factors Impacting on Clinical Value of the Biomarker

4.1.1. PREANALYTICAL REASONS FOR VARIABILITY

Circulating levels of VEGF have been measured by several investigators who reported conflicting results (Table 2). However, these studies are not comparable owing to a lack of standardization of the preanalytical phase *(36)*. In fact, the utility of biomarkers in oncology is closely dependent to the information that comes from its measure. It is therefore necessary to define standardized operative procedures to be used in all the phases of determination (preanalytical, analytical, and postanalytical).

It is still unclear in which blood matrix the determination of VEGF is more accurate as a cancer biomarker and which matrix provides the optimal clinical information. Circulating VEGF has a multicompartmental origin because it is mainly produced by cancer cells and/or transported and released by platelets, lymphocytes, granulocytes, monocytes, and megakaryocytes. Consequently, the different compartments in which VEGF is measured such as serum, plasma, or whole blood, may give different information.

The presence of VEGF in the alpha granules of platelets *(37)* implies that serum VEGF levels not only reflect the circulating VEGF, but also the VEGF released from blood cells during the coagulation process. Normally, plasma of healthy people does not contain relevant quantities of VEGF.

As a consequence, any variation in sample handling may affect the blood cell activation and, thus, the release of VEGF into serum. Activated platelets release VEGF in a rapid discharge reaction, increasing the VEGF content up

Table 2
Summary of Methods for Sample Collection Reported in the Literature

a. Serum

Authors (ref.)	Collection tube	Temperature sample blood	Clotting		Centrifugation			Serum storage	VEGF levels found in health controls	
			Time	Temp.	G	Time	Temp.		Cases	VEGF (pg/mL)
Yamamoto 1996 (49)	NR	NR	NR	NR	3000 rpm	10 min	4°C	−20°C	184	0–227.5 Min–max Mean = 77
Dirix 1997 (94)	Vacutainer system (Becton Dickinson)	RT	NR	NR	3000 rpm	10 min	NR	−80°C	NR	NR
Salven 1997 (42)	Venoject blood collection system (Terumo)	4°C	30 min	4°C	2000 g	10 min	4°C	−70°C	113	1–177 Min–max Median = 15
Verheul 1997 (38)	NR	NR	20–30 min	RT	3000 rpm	NR	NR	−20°C	30	0–287 Min–max
Banks 1998 (39)	Plastic tube Monovette (Sarstedt)	RT	NR	NR	2000g	10 min	NR	−70°C	8	76–854 Min–max
Benoy 1998 (95)	NR	NR	NR	NR	NR	NR	NR	−80°C	6	30–403 Min–max Median = 153
Heer 1998 (47)	NR	NR	NR	NR	NR	NR	NR	−80°C	14	83.1–327.7 Min–max
Maloney 1998 (96)	Plastic tube (Becton Dickinson)	RT	30 min	22°C	750g	10 min	4°C	−70°C	10	230 ± 63 (Mean ± SD)
Webb 1998 (97)	Plain glass (Becton Dickinson)	RT	2 h	NR	NR	NR	NR	−80°C	34	Mean = 249.4
Agrawal 1999 (48)	NR	NR	NR	NR	NR	NR	NR	−80°C	14	1300–7000 Min–max
Balsari 1999 (98)	NR	NR	NR	NR	2000 rpm	20 min	NR	−20°C	30	<230

274

Study	Tube/system		Time before centrifugation	Temp	Centrifugation	Time	Temp	Storage temp	N	Values
Kraft 1999 (99)	NR	NR	NR	NR	16000g	10 min	NR	−80°C	145	30–1752 Min–max Median = 294
Salgado 1999 (37)	Vacutainer system (Becton Dickinson)	NR	NR	NR	3000 rpm	10 min	NR	−80°C	NR	NR
Salven 1999 (43)	Venoject blood collection system (Terumo)	NR	60–240 min	4°C	2000g	10 min	4°C	−70°C	56	12–492 Min–max Median = 66
Salven 1999 (44)	Venoject blood collection system (Terumo)	NR	60–240 min	4°C	2000g	10 min	4°C	−70°C	NR	NR
Wynendaele 1999 (100)	Vacutainer system	NR	30 min	RT	3000g	10 min	20°C	−20°C	32	40–530 Min–max
Adams 2000 (40)	NR	NR	Within 30 min	NR	2000g	10 min	NR	−80°C	63	4–720 Min–max Median = 186
Byrne 2000 (29)	NR	NR	NR	NR	3500g	20 min	NR	−70°C	64	Median = 250 postmenopausal Median = 104 premenopausal
Gunsilius 2000 (101)	Plastic tube Monovette (Sarstedt)	NR	NR	NR	2000g	10 min	4°C	−80°C	3	119.2–282.7 Min–max
Lee 2000 (108)	NR	NR	NR	NR	NR	NR	NR	−80°C	42	232.4 ± 163.6 (Mean ± SD)
Heer 2001 (74)	NR	NR	30 min	NR	3000 rpm	10 min	NR	−80°C	88	201.7 mean Median = 167.5
Benoy 2002 (45)	NR	NR	NR	NR	NR	NR	NR	−80°C	26	250 (95° perc.)
Lantzsch 2002 (102)	NR	NR	NR	NR	3000g	15 min	NR	−80°C	NR	NR
McIlhenny 2002 (50)	Vacutainer system (Becton Dickinson)	NR	60 min	NR	NR	NR	NR	−70°C	20	6.01–774.76 Min–max Median = 261.13
Bachelot 2003 (103)	NR	NR	NR	NR	NR	NR	NR	−80°C	NR	NR

(continued)

275

Table 2 (*continued*) b. Plasma

Authors (ref.)	Anticoagulant Type	Conc.	Temperature of sample handling	Centrifugation g	Time	Temp.	Plasma storage	Cases	VEGF levels found in health controls VEGF (pg/mL)
Verheul 1997 (38)	EDTA	NR	RT	NR	NR	NR	−20°C	30	0–50 Min–max
Banks 1998 (39)	EDTA (K₂) Trisodium citrate	0.12–0.2% (w/v) 0.31% (w/v)	RT RT	2000g 2000g	10 min 10 min	RT RT	−70°C	8	<9–42 Min–max
Maloney 1998 (96)	EDTA	NR	RT	750g	10 min	4°C	−70°C	10	38.2 ± 7.7 Mean ± SD
Webb 1998 (97)	EDTA	7.5% (w/v)	RT	NR	NR	NR	−80°C	34	Mean = 76.1
Salven 1999 (43)	Sodium citrate	NR	4°C	2000g	10 min	4°C	−70°C	56	9–109 Min–max Median = 15
Wynendaele 1999 (100)	K₃ EDTA Sodium citrate: For PRP For PPP CTAD	NR 0.129 M	NR	3000g 180g 3000g 2500g 2000g	10 min 10 min 10 min 30 min 10 min	20°C 20°C 20°C 4°C	−20°C	32	0–28 Min–max
Adams 2000 (40)	Trisodium citrate	0.31% (w/v)	NR	2000g	10 min	NR	−80°C	63	9–92 Min–max Median = 27.3
Gunsilius 2000 (101)	Sodium citrate	0.106 M	NR	2000g	10 min	4°C	−80°C	3	62.3% of value below det. level
Lee 2000 (108)	EDTA (Na)	NR	NR	NR	NR	NR	−80°C	42	48.2 ± 34.7 Mean ± SD
McIlhenny 2002 (50)	EDTA	NR	NR	10,000 rpm	10 min	NR	−70°C	20	0–70.72 Min–max Median = 5.78
Wu 2002 (79)	EDTA	NR	NR	500g	10 min	4°C	−80°C	20	18–77.7 Min–max Median = 24.4
Bachelot 2003 (103)	EDTA	NR	NR	NR	NR	NR	−80°C	NR	NR
Caine 2003 (104)	Sodium citrate	NR	4°C	1000g	20 min	4°C	−70°C	12	25–60 IQR Median = 30

IQR, Interquartile range.

276

to 8–10 times *(38)*. So, serum VEGF concentration mainly reflects platelet counts rather than the tumor burden. For this reason, some authors suggested the use of a specific matrix to avoid the potential hazard for systematic errors.

The majority of studies on the role of VEGF as a circulating tumor marker used serum prepared by different procedures: the time from venipuncture to centrifugation was quite variable, ranging from "immediately" to 30 min at room temperature, and from 30 min to 4 h at 4°C. In a study that standardizes the sampling procedure for the determination of VEGF in different blood fractions, Banks et al. *(39)* demonstrated that in a time range from 0 to 2 h at room temperature, serum VEGF increased from a minimum of 118% to a maximum of 4515%, with respect to the VEGF levels found in the serum obtained 10 min after blood withdrawal. The maximum VEGF released from clotting is reached only after 2 h at room temperature.

Also clinical studies of plasma VEGF levels have been performed using a wide variety of methods for sample collection and handling: as far as the type of anticoagulant is concerned, some authors suggested the use of sodium citrate plasma *(40,41)*. Banks et al. *(39)* demonstrated that sodium citrate does not prevent activation of platelets, and the authors propose the use of CTAD plasma, it being more effective in preventing the release of VEGF by platelets. VEGF has also been investigated in whole blood *(42)*, while others estimated the theoretical VEGF load of platelets as the ratio of VEGF serum concentration related to the platelets number *(39,43–46)*. The biological significance of white blood cell–derived VEGF has yet to be clarified. To date there is only reported a significant association between whole blood VEGF and leukocyte count. Hence, it remains unclear in cancer patients which measurement of circulating VEGF actually represents the fraction of biologically active VEGF in the circulation.

4.1.2. BIOLOGICAL REASONS FOR VARIABILITY

VEGF levels have been studied also in relation to the menstrual cycle. However, contradictory results have been found with some studies suggesting correlation with hormones, some found higher levels of serum VEGF in the follicular phase *(47)*, some in the luteal phase *(48)*, while others did not find consistent changes *(49,50)*.

In a study Meo et al. *(51)* concluded that a difference between serial results can be considered as normal if the variation is less than about 60% in the plasma CTAD, 33% in serum and 43% in whole blood. Moreover, the individuality Index (ratio between intrasubject biological variation and intersubject biological variation) has shown that the range of reference used in some studies could be misleading and that the VEGF determination could be more useful in monitoring the variation within a subject, for example, during therapy, considering the found value of critical difference.

Table 3
Ways of Targeting VEGF

Ligand sequestration
Attack external membrane receptor
Inhibit VEGF-R message
Indirect inhibition

4.2. Clinical Studies

How to best target VEGF has been the subject of several investigative approaches, many of which have been applied in the clinic (Table 3). Several studies are being conducted to evaluate the safety profile and activity of the combination of standard chemotherapy with new antiangiogenetic agents. However, definitive results on the effect on angiogenesis blood markers have been reported only in a few of them to date (Table 4).

4.3. Anti-VEGF Therapy

4.3.1. LIGAND SEQUESTRATION

Ligand sequestration has been approached with the use of monoclonal antibodies directed against VEGF, several of which have been generated and clinical trials are underway. A recombinant humanized monoclonal antibody has been developed that recognizes all VEGF isoforms (rhuMab VEGF) without binding to FGF, HGF, PDGF, or nerve growth factor. It has shown to have indirect and potent antitumor activity in experimental models. The safety of bevacizumab was evaluated in a phase I dose-escalating study involving 25 patients who had a variety of tumors, including sarcomas ($n = 8$), renal cancer ($n = 7$) and breast cancer ($n = 2$) (52,53).

Dose-limiting toxicities were not observed at weekly doses of ≤10 mg/kg, although some patients experienced asthenia, mild headache, fatigue, nausea, and low-grade fever on the day of the administration. In addition, bleeding at tumor sites developed in 3 (12%) of the 25 patients. No objective response was observed; two patients obtained a minor response. Twelve (52%) of the 23 patents had stabilization of disease during the 70-d study period. As a single agent, rhuMAb VEGF has been shown by Sledge et al. (54) to induce remissions and prolonged stabilization of disease in patients with heavily pretreated metastatic breast cancer. A phase III trial has been conducted in advanced breast cancer patients and the results recently published. This study was performed to evaluate the combination of bevacizumab with capecitabine vs capecitabine alone in patients affected by metastatic breast cancer previously treated with anthracycline and taxane. Patients were randomized to either capecitabine alone or in combination with bevacizumab. Treatment was continued until evidence of progression;

Table 4
Clinical Studies

Drug	Mechanism of action	Clinical development
BEVACIZUMAB	Anti-VEGF monoclonal antibody	Phase III: Miller et al. (55)
SU5416	Inhibition of Flk-1 (VEGFR)	Phase I: Stopeck et al. (68)
ZD6474	Inhibition of VEGFR and EGFR	Phase I: Minami et al. (69)
CEP-7055	Inhibition of VEGFR1-2-3	Phase I: Ruggeri et al. (70)
SU6668	Inhibition of tyrosine kinase receptor of VEGF, bFGF, PDGF, c-Kit	Phase I: Hoeckman et al. (71)
PTK 787/ZK 222584	Inhibition of VEGF-R1 (Flt-1) and VEGF-R2 (Flk-1/KDR)	Phase I: Thomas et al. (72)
Angiozyme	Constructs targeting VEGFR Flt-1 mRNA	Phase I–Phase II (105–107)

patients randomized to the combination arm of the study were eligible to receive bevacizumab after progression, either alone or with other therapies. Promising results have been observed in terms of response rate, but no benefit was obtained regarding overall survival *(55)*.

Monoclonal antibodies have also been developed against the external membrane domain of the VEGF-R2 receptor *(56,57)* and clinical trials have recently been initiated with these agents, but there are no published reports are to date.

4.3.2. TYROSINE KINASE INHIBITORS

Several receptor tyrosine kinase inhibitors directed against the internal membrane tyrosine kinase portion of VEGF receptors 1 and/or 2, have been developed *(58–65)*. Many of these compounds target more than one receptor: SU6668 targets the VEGF-R2 as well as the PDGF and FGF-1 receptors; PTK 787/ZK 222584 targets both VEGF-R1 and R2 *(63)*.

SU5416 is a small, lipophilic, highly protein-binding synthetic molecule that inhibits phosphorylation of the selective tyrosine kinase for the VEGF receptor Flk-1 on endothelial cells *(66)*. In addition, it binds to the PFDG receptor, which is also involved in the transduction of angiogenesis signals. Finally, it binds c-Kit, a related tyrosine kinase receptor for stem cell factor and a hematopoietic growth factor that promotes the survival of hematopoietic progenitor cells and in multiple lineages *(52,67)*. SU5416 produces a dose-dependent inhibition of tumor growth in a variety of xenograft models, including malignant melanoma, glioma, fibrosarcoma, and carcinomas of the lung, breast, prostate and skin *(52,66)*. In a human colon cancer xenograft model, SU5416 inhibited tumor metastases, microvessel formation, and cell proliferation *(52)*.

Phase I and II clinical trials have been completed using a twice-weekly dosing regimen with a maximum tolerated dose equal to 145 mg/mq. Stopeck et al. *(68)* performed a phase I dose-escalating study of SU5416 in 22 patients with advanced malignancies, 3 of them were affected by breast cancer. Of the 19 evaluable patients, 1 obtained a partial regression and 3 obtained disease stabilization for at least 12 wk.

ZD6474 is a novel vascular selective endothelial growth factor receptor tyrosine kinase inhibitor that also has activity against epidermal growth factor receptor tyrosine kinase. A phase I study of ZD6474 has been conducted in 18 Japanese patients with solid tumors refractory to standard therapy. Most patients treated had non-small-cell lung cancer (NSCLC) or colorectal cancer (CRC). A dose range of 100–300 mg/d of ZD6474 was well tolerated and considered to be appropriate in terms of efficacy for use in phase II studies of patients with NSCLC *(69)*.

CEP-7055 is a low molecular weight tyrosine kinase inhibitor with activity against VEGF-R1, 2, and 3. In a range of experimental models, CEP-7055 has been shown to induce significant inhibition of both angiogenesis and tumor growth. The clinical activity and tolerability of CEP-7055 has been explored in a phase I study: 19 patients have been recruited at doses of 10, 20, 40, 80, and 120 mg given twice daily. Pharmacodynamic assessments of tumor blood flow by PET, dermal wound angiogenesis, and other blood markers are being performed (70).

SU6668 is a novel compound that competitively inhibits the tyrosine kinase of the receptors of VEGF, bFGF, PDGF, and c-Kit. SU6668 inhibits angiogenesis through several mechanisms, primarily by the induction of apoptosis in both endothelial and tumor cells. Currently, phase I studies are underway to evaluate the potential of SU6668 as anticancer agent for humans (71).

PTK 787/ZK 222584 (PTK/ZK) is an oral potent and selective inhibitor of VEGF-mediated Flt-1 and KDR receptor tyrosine kinases. Phase I studies are underway evaluating the optimum dose and schedule of oral PTK/ZK administered continuously to patients with advanced cancers known to overexpress VEGF. To date, particularly in patients with liver metastases from colorectal cancer treated with PTK/ZK, dynamic contrast-enhanced magnetic resonance imaging has been a useful predictor of the biological response of VEGF-receptor inhibition (72).

At least another five selective anti-VEGF small tyrosine kinase inhibitors are entering clinical evaluation.

4.3.3. Has VEGF Determination a Prognostic–Predictive Value?

Based on the finding that in breast cancer intratumoral VEGF expression and microvessel density significantly correlate with decreased relapse-free survival (73), several studies have been conducted to evaluate the prognostic–predictive value of circulating VEGF in breast cancer (Table 5). The relationship of preoperative serum VEGF with conventional prognostic indicators of breast cancer has been recently studied and serum VEGF was compared with two established tumor markers for breast cancer: CEA and CA 15-3 (74). This prospective study involved 200 patients. Eighty-eight healthy females were also recruited as controls for serum VEGF. This study showed that serum VEGF is significantly high in ductal but not in lobular carcinoma. This study agrees with Dvorak et al. (22), who showed that only lobular carcinoma of the breast and papillary carcinoma of the bladder failed to reveal significant VEGF mRNA expression. Moreover, it has been shown that serum VEGF has a much higher sensitivity (62.1%) in detecting breast cancer than both the tumor markers CA 15-3 (13.6%) and CEA (10.3%), with a specificity of 74%.

A difference in the angiogenic response of different types of breast cancers would allow the selection of patients for whom personalized adjuvant therapy is needed, similarly to the selection of patients for tamoxifen therapy

Table 5
Prognostic/Predictive Value of Circulating VEGF in Breast Cancer

Study	Results
Serum VEGF levels and tumor markers for breast cancer	VEGF shows higher sensitivity when compared to CEA and CA 15-3 in detecting breast cancer *(74)*.
Plasma VEGF levels and progression of breast cancer	Plasma VEGF is an independent predictor of overall survival of local recurrence *(79)*.
Serum VEGF levels and endostatin	Elevated serum VEGF levels are correlated with short free-relapse survival *(81)*.
Serum VEGF levels and response to chemotherapy	Normalization or decline >50% in VEGF levels is significantly higher in patients who responded to chemotherapy then in nonresponders *(83)*.
Serum VEGF levels and response to thalidomide	VEGF levels changes not significantly correlates to response to thalidomide *(87,90)*.

on the basis of the ER status. Various factors such as estrogen, protein kinase C, and cAMP can induce the expression of these gene complexes, which in turn can up-regulate VEGF expression *(75)*. It has been demonstrated that the genetic status of a tumor may determine whether or not estrogen can stimulate VEGF expression *(76)*. However, long term follow-up studies are required to determine whether preoperative serum VEGF levels are of prognostic significance, as has been shown for tumor VEGF levels, and whether serum VEGF will be useful in detecting early recurrence in breast cancer patients *(74)*.

Based on the finding that plasma VEGF shows better discrimination than serum VEGF *(77)* and that no information is so far available on the prognostic relevance of plasma VEGF levels in patients who have had surgery for breast cancer *(78)*, Wu et al. *(79)* performed a study on plasma VEGF to assess whether this biomarker is associated with progression of breast cancer in African-American and Hispanic women. Wu et al. *(79)* measured plasma VEGF of 125 women after adjuvant treatments and examined the association of plasma VEGF levels with other tumor characteristics such as steroid hormone receptors, tumor size, regional nodes, and stage. Plasma VEGF levels were found to be significantly higher in breast cancer patients than in normal subjects and in patients with large tumor size, and stage III/IV disease. Multivariate analysis showed that plasma VEGF was an independent predictor of overall survival of local recurrence. These findings suggest that plasma VEGF should be considered as a tumor marker of breast cancer progression.

However, the dispute whether serum VEGF or plasma VEGF should be used as a surrogate biomarker of angiogenesis is still controversial. Some studies suggest that platelet-poor plasma more accurately reflect tumor progression, whereas others found that serum VEGF gives a better prognostic information. On the basis of the hypothesis that activated platelets in tumor vasculature release thrombopoietin and, thereby, stimulate bone marrow generation of platelets, both plasma VEGF and serum VEGF may be important for tumor activity. Plasma VEGF may be increased because of direct tumor release of VEGF, and by tumor-induced intravascular platelet activation and subsequent VEGF release. Elevated serum VEGF may be the consequence of increased platelet numbers in cancer patient, caused by intratumoral platelet activation and subsequent release of thrombopoietin.

Recently, Nishimura et al. *(80)* have measured plasma VEGF levels in various breast diseases. Fifteen patients had benign breast disease, 187 patients primary breast cancer: 32 patients of whom without postoperative recurrence, and 56 patients with recurrence. Plasma VEGF levels were measured by enzyme-linked immunosorbent assay (ELISA). Plasma VEGF levels were higher in malignant than in benign breast disease, and were also higher in patients with recurrence or distant metastasis.

More recently, Zhao et al. *(81)* also investigated the correlation between serum VEGF and endostatin levels in patients with breast cancer. Serum VEGF and endogenous endostatin levels were detected before surgery and 3 wk after surgery. Preoperatively, the levels of the two biomarkers were significantly elevated and correlated with each other. Postoperatively, VEGF levels decreased significantly while those of endostatin remained high. Patients with both normalized VEGF and elevated endostatin following surgery had a lower risk of relapse. Univariate and multivariate analysis showed a correlation between elevated VEGF level and short free-relapse survival.

A similar study has been conducted to investigate whether increased VEGF serum levels correlate with poor outcome in advanced colorectal cancer patients. Catalano et al. *(82)* investigated in a retrospective study the pretreatment serum levels of VEGF and their correlation with outcome in 140 consecutive colorectal cancer patients and 50 healthy subjects. Fifty-seven patients were staged as locally advanced disease (stage III), while 83 had metastatic disease (stage IV). The median pretreatment VEGF serum levels were significantly higher in colorectal cancer patients as compared to control subjects. Median VEGF serum levels were shown to be significantly higher in stage IV patients than in those with stage III (834 pg/mL vs 435 pg/mL, when basal VEGF serum levels in metastatic patients were analyzed according to response to chemotherapy, responders patients were shown to have significantly lower VEGF serum levels than non-responders: 398 pg/mL vs 734 pg/mL. In univariate analysis basal VEGF serum levels correlated with both overall survival and time to treatment failure. A multivariate analysis included pretreatment serum VEGF levels, ECOG performance status and tumor stage as the independent prognostic factors for overall survival and time to failure. These results suggest that the evaluation of pretreatment serum VEGF levels may be useful for predicting outcome in patients with locally advanced or metastatic colorectal cancer.

The VEGF signaling pathway provides many different levels or targets that could be used to modify or disrupt the transmission of the signal, both upstream or downstream of VEGFR binding. Since VEGF represents the main angiogenic factor, the control of VEGF secretion could represent the most important target for inhibition of angiogenesis-related tumor growth.

In experimental studies, certain chemotherapeutic agents such as paclitaxel inhibit VEGF-induced angiogenesis, while at present there are no data on the possible influence of chemotherapy on VEGF secretion in cancer patients. A preliminary study was conducted by Lissoni et al. *(83)*. The study included 14 patients with metastatic breast cancer treated with paclitaxel. Serum levels of VEGF were measured by ELISA in blood samples collected before and after therapy and at 21-d intervals. The clinical response consisted of partial response (PR) in three and stable disease (SD) in six patients. The percentage of normalization or decline greater than 50% in VEGF levels was significantly higher in patients with PR or SD than in those with progressive disease (PD) (5/9 vs 0/5). This preliminary study suggests that the efficacy of paclitaxel, at least in terms of disease stabilization, may be associated with decreased VEGF blood levels of course, the small size of the study prevents any definitive conclusion.

VEGF is commonly over-expressed in pancreatic cancer and its expression appears to be an important predictor of survival. At the 39th ASCO meeting a study was presented of the combination of bevacizumab plus gemcitabine in patients with advanced pancreatic cancer. Twenty-one patients were enrolled to receive gemcitabine at a dose of 1000 mg/m^2 given intravenously on d 1, 8, and 15, every 28 d and bevacizumab at a dose of 10 mg/kg given intravenously d 1, 15. Pretreatment serum VEGF levels were collected. The study is still ongoing and 16 patients are currently evaluable for response in this trial. There have been 6 confirmed partial responses (38%), 7 patients (44%) had stable disease. Median survival has not been reached. Median time to progression is 5.5 mo. Pretreatment VEGF levels range from 0 to 586 pg/mL and do not correlate with clinical end points. Estimated 1-yr survival is 54% *(84)*.

Bevacizumab has also been tested in patients with advanced melanoma in a study by Carson et al. *(85)*. Patients with metastatic melanoma who had not received prior cytokine therapy were eligible. They were randomized to receive bevacizumab (15 mg/kg intravenously every 2 wk) ± low dose α-interferon (1 million units/m² daily). Patients were restaged after 12 wk and received 12 more wk of therapy if they had a clinical response or stable disease. There were two responses in the combination arm. Four patients (three bevacizumab, one bevacizumab+interferon) had prolonged stabilization of disease. Baseline levels of VEGF were measured by ELISA and ranged from 471 to 2686 pg/mL except for one patient who had levels of >4000 pg/mL. The above patient had the longest period of stabilization of disease. Otherwise, VEGF levels did not correlate with response. By contrast, FGF levels ranged from 0 to 180 pg/mL at baseline and dropped significantly during cycle 1 in the two response patients and two of four SD patients. The accrual is ongoing.

Interesting results have been observed with the use of thalidomide, a drug developed as a sedative, that has shown antitumor activity by various mechanisms of action: inhibition of angiogenesis, cytokine-mediated pathways, modulation of adhesion molecules, inhibition of cyclooxygenase-2, and stimulation of immunoresponse *(86)*. Baidas et al. *(87)* performed a randomized phase II study of thalidomide in patients affected by metastatic breast cancer: 28 patients were randomized to receive either 200 mg/d (arm A) or 800 mg/d (arm B) to be escalated to 1200 mg. No partial or complete responses were observed. Two patients in arm A had stable disease. Changes in serum bFGF, VEGF, and TNF-α levels from baseline to time of removal from study in 26 patients were determined. The results of these analysis indicate mean percentage changes from baseline of –37% for bFGF, +60% for VEGF, and +79% for TNF-α. Of these, only the increase in TNF-α levels was statistically significant.

The vascular pattern of renal cell carcinoma (RCC) suggests that angiogenesis inhibition may be a new biological treatment for patients with this disease *(88,89)*. Several studies have been conducted testing thalidomide in metastatic RCC (MRCC), Minor et al. *(90)* evaluated the toxicity and activity of thalidomide and measured the changes of VEGF 165 plasma levels after therapy. In this phase II study, 29 patients were enrolled and the drug was given using a intrapatient dose escalation schedule, starting at a daily dose of 400 mg and escalated as tolerated up to 1200 mg. Of the 24 patients evaluable for response only 1 partial response, 1 minor response, and 2 stable disease for over 6 mo were observed. VEGF 165 levels were not modified by therapy.

Endostatin, a 20-kDa fragment of collagen XVIII, is an endogenous angiogenesis inhibitor that has been shown to inhibit, in a potent and dose-dependent manner, the growth of a wide variety of human and murine primary metastatic tumors in mice *(91,92)*. Herbst et al. *(93)* have evaluated recombinant human endostatin (rh-Endo) in a phase I study designed to assess safety, pharmacokinetics, and serum markers of angiogenesis in patients with refractory solid tumors. The serum levels of VCAM-1 were assayed before the study and every 28 d, using the ELISA method. Twenty-five patients were treated and a considerable variation in the baseline levels of all four factors was observed. Furthermore, after of therapy with rh-endostatin, there were no consistent changes in the levels of any of these proteins. The absence of a measurable effect on VEGF, bFGF, VCAM, and E-selectin also included the two patients who experienced minor anticancer effects *(93)*.

5. CONCLUSIONS

Determination of circulating VEGF still remains an experimental procedure with no evident application for routine clinical decisions. Data from retrospective studies, however, suggest that VEGF levels may predict clinical outcome of breast cancer. Prospective studies are needed to properly evaluate the method of choice and the clinical significance of preoperative determination of tissue or circulating VEGF for prognostic purposes. Only a minority of phase I studies with selective inhibitors of angiogenesis evaluated the biological activity as antiangiogenic compounds by determination of surrogate biomarkers. Therefore, both the selection of the patients and the prediction of response to anti VEGF therapy still remain unanswered questions. From a biological point of view the pathways regulating tumor hypoxia and VEGF expression seem to be highly correlated, so codetermination of both may allow for more accurate information on the angiogenica status of each single tumor. Clinical prospective studies should be planned to test the value of surrogate markers of angiogenesis as an integral part of the study-design for the testing of a new antiangiogenic compounds.

Properly designed projects of translational research aimed to correlate information from laboratory assays with activity of new therapeutic strategies based on the use of biological response modifiers/molecular-targeting agents should also foresee the use of adequate methods of validation of laboratory methods, with procedures of standardization and quality controls. Recent clinical data on the activity of bevacizumab associated with chemotherapy in colorectal and renal cancers in unselected series of patients are promising, also regarding the expression of the molecular target. The discovery of predictive biomarkers for response are presumed to be the key to improve the selection of the cases to be treated with anti-VEGF compounds in future studies.

REFERENCES

1. Rosen LE. Clinical experience with angiogenesis signalling inhibitors: focus on vascular endothelial growth factor (VEGF) blockers. *Cancer Control* 2002;19:36–44.
2. Gasparini G. Clinical significance of determination of surrogate markers of angiogenesis in breast cancer. *Crit Rev Oncol Hematol* 2001;37:97–114.

3. Linchtenbeld HC, Barendsz-Janson AF, van Essen H, Struijker Boudier H, Griffioen AW, Hillen HF. Angiogenic potential of malignant and non-malignant human breast tissues in an in vivo angiogenesis model. *Int J Cancer* 1998;77:455–459.

4. McLeskey SW, Tobias CA, Vezza PR, Filie AC, Kern FG, Hanfelt J. Tumor growth of FGF or VEGF transfected angiogenic factor. *Am J Pathol* 1998;153: 1993–2006.

5. Weidner N, Semple JP, Welch WR, Folkman J. Tumor angiogenesis and metastasis-correlation in invasive breast carcinoma. *N Engl J Med* 1991;324:1–8.

6. Weidner N, Folkman J, Pozza F, et al. Tumor angiogenesis: a new significant and independent prognostic indicator in early stage breast carcinoma. *J Natl Cancer Inst* 1992;84:1875–1887.

7. Heimann R, Ferguson D, Powers C, Recant WM, Weischelbaum RR, Hellman S. Angiogenesis as a predictor of long-term survival for patients with node negative breast cancer. *J Natl Cancer Inst* 1996;88:1764–1769.

8. Relf M, et al. Expression of the angiogenic factors vascular endothelial growth factor, acidic and basic fibroblast growth factor, tumour growth factor-b-1, platelet-derived endothelial cell growth factor, and pleiotrophin in human primary breast cancer and its relation to angiogenesis. *Cancer Res* 1997;57:963–969.

9. Carmeliet P, et al. Role of HIF-1α hypoxia-mediated apoptosis, cell proliferation and tumour angiogenesis. *Nature* 1998;394:485–490.

10. Fukumura D, et al. Tumour induction of VEGF promoter activity in stromal cells. *Cell* 1998;94:715–725.

11. Ferrara N, Bunting S. Vascular endothelial growth factor, a specific regulator of angiogenesis. *Curr Opin Nephrol Hypertens* 1996;5:35–44.

12. Ferrara N, Alitalo K. Clinical application of angiogenic growth factors and their inhibitors. *Nat Med* 1999;1:120–122.

13. Keck PJ, Hauser SD, Krivi G, et al. Vascular permeability factor, an endothelial cell mitogen related to PDGF. *Science* 1989;246:1309–1312.

14. Pepper MS, Ferrara N, Orci L, Montesano R. Potent synergism between vascular endothelial growth factor and basic fibroblast growth factor and basic fibroblast growth factor in the induction of angiogenesis in vitro. *Biochem Biophys Res Commun* 1992;189:824–831.

15. Roberts WG, Palade GE. Neovasculature induced by vascular endothelial growth factor is fenestrated. *Cancer Res* 1997;57:765–772.

16. Stacker SA, Caesar C, Baldwin ME, et al. VEGF-D promotes the metastatic spread of tumor cells via the lymphatics. *Nat Med* 2001;77:186–191.

17. Skobe M, Hawighorst T, Jackson DG, et al. Induction of tumor lymphangiogenesis by VEGF-C promotes breast cancer metastasis. *Nat Med* 2001;7:192–198.

18. Kliche S, Waltenberger J. VEGF receptor signaling and endothelial function. *JUBMB Life* 2001;52:61–66.

19. Soker S, Takashima S, Miao HQ, et al. Neuropilin-1 is expressed by endothelial and tumor cells as an isoform-specific receptor for vascular endothelial growth factor. *Cell* 1998;92:735–742.

20. Gluzman-Poltorak Z, Cohen T, Shibuya M, et al. Vascular endothelial growth factor receptor-1 (VEGFR-1) and neuropilin-2 form complexes. *J Biol Chem* 2001; 276:18688–18694.

21. Fuh G, Garcia KC, DeVos AM. The interaction of neuropilin-1 with vascular endothelial growth factor and its receptor flt-1. *J Biol Chem* 2000;275:26690–26695.

22. Dvorak HF, Brown LF, Detmar M, et al. Vascular permeability factor/vascular endothelial growth factor, microvascular hyperpermeability and angiogenesis. *Am J Pathol* 1995;146:1029–1039.

23. Ferrara N. VEGF: an update on biological and therapeutic aspects. *Curr Opin Biotechnol* 2000;11:517–524.
24. Banerji S, et al. Lyve-1, a new homologue of the CD44 glycoprotein is a lymph-specific receptor for hyaluran. *J Cell Biol* 1999;144:789–801.
25. Kurebayashi J, Otsuki T, Kunisue H, et al. Expression of vascular endothelial growth factor (VEGF) family members in breast cancer. *Jpn J Cancer Res* 1999; 90:977–981.
26. Makinen T, Jussila L, Veikkola T, et al. Inhibition of lymphangiogenesis with resulting lymphedema in transgenic mice expressing soluble VEGF receptor-3. *Nat Med* 2001;7:199–205.
27. Ferrara N. Vascular endothelial growth factor and the regulation of angiogenesis. *Recent Prog Horm Res* 2000;55:15–35.
28. Neufeld G, Cohen T, Gengrinovitz S, et al. Vascular endothelial growth factor (VEGF) and its receptors. *FASEB J* 1999;13:9–22.
29. Byrne GJ, Bundred NJ. Surrogate markers of tumoral angiogenesis. *Int J Biol Markers* 2000;15:334–339.
30. Solorzano CC, Jung YD, Bucana CD, McConkey DJ, Gallick GE, McMahon G, Ellis LM. In vivo intracellular signaling as a marker of antiangiogenic activity. *Cancer Res* 2001;61:7048–7051.
31. Axelsson K, Ljung BM, Moore DH, et al. Tumor angiogenesis as a prognostic assay for invasive ductal breast carcinoma. *J Natl Cancer Inst* 1996;87:997–1008.
32. Gasparini G, Toi M, Gion M, et al. Prognostic significance of vascular endothelial growth factor protein in node-negative breast carcinoma. *J Natl Cancer Inst* 1997;89:139–147.
33. Toi M, Gion M, Biganzoli E, et al. Co-determination of the angiogenic factors thymidine phosphorylase and vascular endothelial growth factor in node-negative breast cancer: prognostic implications. *Angiogenesis* 1997;1:71–83.
34. Gasparini G, Toi M, Miceli R, et al. Clinical relevance of vascular endothelial growth factor (VEGF) and thymidine phosphorylase (TP) in patients with node-positive breast cancer treated either with adjuvant chemotherapy or hormone therapy. *Cancer J Sci Am* 1999;5:101–111.
35. Li C, Guo B, Bernabeu C, et al. Angiogenesis in breast cancer: the role of trans-forming growth factor beta and CD 105. *Microsc Res Tech* 2001;52:437–449.
36. Hormbrey E, et al. A critical review of VEGF analysis in peripheral blood: is the current literature meaningful? *Clin Exp Metastas* 2002;19:651–663.
37. Salgado R. Platelets and vascular endothelial growth factor (VEGF): a morpho-logical and functional study. *Angiogenesis* 2001;4:37–43.
38. Verheul HMW, Hoekman K, Luykx-de Bakker S, et al. Platelet: transporter of vascular endothelial growth factor. *Clin Cancer Res* 1997;3:2187–2190.
39. Banks RE, Forbes MA, Kinsey SE, et al. Release of the angiogenic cytokine vascular endothelial growth factor (VEGF) from platelets: significance for VEGF measurements and cancer biology. *Br J Cancer* 1998;77:956–964.
40. Adams J, Carder PJ, Downey S, et al. Vascular endothelial growth factor (VEGF) in breast cancer: comparison of plasma, serum and tissue VEGF and microvessel density and effects of tamoxifen. *Cancer Res* 2000;60:2898–2905.
41. Dittadi R, et al. Validation of blood collection procedures for the determination of circulating vascular endothelial growth factor (VEGF) in different blood compart-ments. *Int J Biol Markers* 2001;16:87–96.
42. Salven P, Mäenpää H, Orpana A, et al. Serum vascular endothelial growth factor is often elevated in disseminated cancer. *Clin Cancer Res* 1997;3:647–651.

43. Salven P, Orpana A, Joensuu H. Leukocytes and platelets of patients with cancer contain high levels of vascular endothelial growth factor. *Clin Cancer Res* 1999;5:487–491.

44. Salven P, Perhoniemi V, Tykkä H, et al. Serum VEGF levels in women with a benign breast tumor or breast cancer. *Breast Cancer Res Treat* 1999;53:161–166.

45. Benoy I, et al. Serum interleukin 6, plasma VEGF, serum VEGF, and VEGF platelet load in breast cancer patients. *Clin Breast Cancer* 2002;2:311–315.

46. Poon RT, Fan ST, Wong J. Clinical implications of circulating angiogenic factors in cancer patients. *J Clin Oncol* 2001;19:1207–1225 (Review).

47. Heer K, Kumar H, Speirs V, et al. Vascular endothelial growth factor in premenopausal women—indicator of the best time for breast cancer surgery? *Br J Cancer* 1998;78:1203–1207.

48. Agraval R, Conway GS, Sladkevicius P, et al. Serum vascular endothelial growth factor (VEGF) in the normal menstrual cycle: association with changes in ovarian and uterine Doppler blood flow. *Clin Endocrinol* 1999;50:101–106.

49. Yamamoto Y, Toi M, Kondo S, et al. Concentrations of vascular endothelial growth factor in the sera of normal controls and cancer patients. *Clin Cancer Res* 1996;2:821–826.

50. McIlenny C, George WD, Doughty JC. A comparison of serum and plasma levels of vascular endothelial growth factor during the menstrual cycle in healthy volunteers. *Br J Cancer* 2002;86:1786–1789.

51. Meo S, Dittadi R, Gion M. Biological variation of circulating vascular endothelial growth factor (VEGF). Hamburger Symposium on Tumour Markers. December 3, 2003 (Abstr).

52. Hagedorn M, Bikfalvi A. Target molecules for anti-angiogenic therapy: from basic research to clinical trials. *Crit Rev Oncol Hematol* 2000;34:89–110.

53. Gordon MS, Margolin K, Talpaz M, et al. Phase I safety and pharmacokinetic study of recombinant human antivascular endothelial growth factor in patients with advanced cancer. *J Clin Oncol* 2001;19:843–850.

54. Sledge G, Miller K, Novotny W, et al. A Phase II trial of single-agent rhuMAb VEGF (recombinant humanized monoclonal antibody to vascular endothelial growth factor) in patients with relapsed metastatic breast cancer. *Proc Am Soc Clin Oncol* 19:3a, 2000 (Abstr 5c).

55. Miller KD, Rugo HS, Cbleigh MA, et al. Phase III trial of capecitabine (Xeloda) plus bevacizumab (Avastin) versus capecitabine alone in women with metastatic breast cancer (MBC) previously treated with anthracycline and a taxane. *Breast Cancer Res Treat* 2002;76(Suppl)1:1 (Abstr 36).

56. Zhu Z, Witte L. Inhibition of tumor growth and metastasis by targeting tumor-associated angiogenesis with antagonists to the receptors of vascular endothelial growth factor. *Invest New Drugs* 1999;17:195–212.

57. Kozin S, Boucher Y, Hicklin D, et al. Vascular endothelial growth factor receptor-2-blocking antibody potentiates radiation-induced long-term control of human tumor xenografts. *Cancer Res* 2001;61:39–44.

58. Smolich B, Yuen H, West K, et al. The angiogenic protein kinase inhibitors SU5416 and SU6668 inhibit the SCF receptor (c-kit) in a human myeloid leukemia cell line and in acute myeloid leukemia blasts. *Blood* 2001;97:1413–1421.

59. Mendel D, Laird A, Smolich B, et al. Development of SU5416, a selective small molecule inhibitor of VEGF receptor tyrosine activity, as an anti-angiogenesis agent. *Anticancer Drug Des* 2000;15:29–41.

60. Mendel D, Schreck R, West D, et al. The angiogenesis inhibitor SU5416 has long-lasting effects on vascular endothelial growth factor receptor phosphorylation and function. *Clin Cancer Res* 2000;6:4848–4858.

61. Shaheen R, Tseng W, Davis D, et al. Tyrosine kinase inhibition of multiple angiogenic growth factor receptors improves survival in mice bearing colon cancer liver metastases by inhibition of endothelial cell survival mechanisms. *Cancer Res* 2001;61:1454–1458.

62. Antonian L, Zhang H, Yang C, et al. Biotransformation of the anti-angiogenic compounds SU5416. *Drug Metab Dispos* 2000;28:1505–1512.

63. Drevs J, Hofmann I, Hugenschmidt H, et al. Effects of PTK787/ZK 222584, a specific inhibitor of vascular endothelial growth factor receptor tyrosine kinases, on primary tumor, metastasis, vessel density, and blood flow in a murine renal cell carcinoma model. *Cancer Res* 2000;60:4819–4824.

64. Laird A, Vajkoczy P, Shawver L, et al. SU6668 is a potent antiangiogenic and antitumor agent that induces regression of established tumors. *Cancer Res* 2000;60:4152–4160.

65. Wood J, Bold G, Buchdunger E, et al. PTK787/ZK 222584, a novel and potent inhibitor of vascular endothelial growth factor receptor tyrosine kinases, impairs vascular endothelial growth factor-induced responses and tumor growth after oral administration. *Cancer Res* 2000;60:2178–2189.

66. Fong TAT, Shawver LK, Sun L, et al. SU5416 is a potent and selective inhibitor of the vascular endothelial growth factor receptor (Flk-1/KDR) that inhibits tyrosine kinase catalysis, tumour vascularization, and growth of multiple tumour types. *Cancer Res* 1999;59:99–106.

67. Taylor ML, Metcalfe DD. Kit signal transduction. *Hematol Oncol Clin North Am* 2000;14:517–535.

68. Stopeck A, Sheldon M, Vahedian M, et al. Results of a Phase I dose-escalating study of the antiangiogenic agent, SU5416, in patients with advanced malignancies. *Clin Cancer Res* 2002;8:2798–2805.

69. Minami H, Ebi H, Tahara M, et al. A Phase I study of an oral VEGF receptor tyrosine kinase inhibitor ZD6474, in Japanese patients with solid tumors. *Proc Am Soc Clin Oncol* 2003, Abstr 778.

70. Ruggeri B, Singh J, Gingrich D, et al. CEP-7055: a novel, orally active pan inhibitor of vascular endothelial growth factor receptor tyrosine kinases with potent antiangiogenic activity and antitumor efficacy in preclinical models. *Cancer Res* 2003;63:5978–5991.

71. Hoekman K. SU6668, a multitargeted angiogenesis inhibitor. *Cancer J* 2001; (Suppl. 7)3:S134–138.

72. Thomas AL, et al. Vascular endothelial growth factor receptor tyrosine kinase inhibitor PTK787/ZK 222584. *Semin Oncol* 2003;(Suppl. 6):32–38.

73. Toi M, Inada K, Suzuki H, Tominaga T. Tumour angiogenesis in breast cancer: its importance as a prognostic indicator and the association with vascular endothelial growth factor expression. *Breast Cancer Res Treat* 1995;36: 195–202.

74. Heer K, Kumar H, Read RJ, Fox JN, Monson JRT, Kerin MJ. Serum vascular endothelial growth factor in breast cancer: its relation with cancer type and estrogen receptor status. *Clin Cancer Res* 2001;7:3491–3494.

75. Kolch W, Martiny-Baron G, Kieser A, et al. Regulation of the expression of the VEGF/VPS and its receptors: role in tumour angiogenesis. *Breast Cancer Res Treat* 1995;36:139–155.

76. Shweiki D, Itin A, Neufeld G, et al. Patterns of expression of vascular endothelial growth factor (VEGF) and VEGF receptors in mice suggest a role in hormonally regulated angiogenesis. *J Clin Investig* 1993;91:2235–2243.

77. Adama J, Carder PJ, Downey S, et al. Vascular endothelial growth factor (VEGF) in breast cancer: comparison of plasma, serum, and tissue VEGF and microvessel density and effects of tamoxifen. *Cancer Res* 2000;60:2898–2905.

78. Ferrer FA, Miller LJ, Andrawisi RI, et al. Vascular endothelial growth factor (VEGF) expression in human prostate cancer: in situ and in vitro expression of VEGF by human prostate cancer cells. *J Urol* 1997;157:2329–2333.

79. Wu Y, Saldana L, Chillar R, Vadgama J, et al. Plasma vascular endothelial growth factor is useful in assessing progression of breast cancer post surgery and during adjuvant treatment. *Int J Oncol* 2002;20:509–516.

80. Nishimura R, Nagao K, Miyayama H, et al. Higher plasma vascular endothelial growth factor levels correlate with menopause, overexpression of p53, and recurrence of breast cancer. *Breast Cancer* 2003;10:120–128.

81. Zhao J, Yan F, Yu H, et al. Correlation between serum vascular endothelial growth factor and endostatin levels in patients with breast cancer. *Cancer Lett* 2004; 204:87–95.

82. Catalano G, Orditura M, Galizia G, et al. Increased vascular endothelial growth factor (VEGF) serum levels correlate with poor outcome in advanced colorectal cancer (CRC) patients. *Proc Am Soc Clin Oncol* Abstr 3522.

83. Lissoni P, Fumagalli E, Malugani F, et al. Chemotherapy and angiogenesis in advanced cancer: vascular endothelial growth factor (VEGF) decline as predictor of disease control during taxol therapy in metastatic breast cancer. *Int J Biol Markers* 2000;15:308–311.

84. Kindler HL, Ansari R, Lester E, et al. Bevacizumab (B) plus gemcitabine (G) in patients (pts) with advanced pancreatic cancer (PC). *Proc Am Soc Clin Oncol* 2003; Abstr 1037.

85. Carson WE, Biber J, Shah N, et al. A Phase 2 trial of a recombinant humanized monoclonal anti-vascular endothelial growth factor (VEGF) antibody in patients with malignant melanoma. *Proc Am Soc Clin Oncol* 2003 Abstr 2873.

86. Fanelli M, Sarmiento R, Gattuso D., et al. Thalidomide: a new anticancer drug? *Expert Opin Invest Drugs* 2003;12:1211–1225.

87. Baidas SM, Winer EP, Fleming GF, et al. Phase II evaluation of thalidomide in patients with metastatic breast cancer. *J Clin Oncol* 2000;18:2710–2717.

88. Nanus DM, Schmitz-Drager BJ, Motzer RJ. Expression of basic fibroblast growth factor in primary human renal tumors: correlation with poor survival. *J Natl Cancer Inst* 1993;85:1597–1599.

89. Nathan PD, Eisen G. The biological treatment of renal cell carcinoma and melanoma. *Lancet Oncol* 2002;3:89–96.

90. Minor DR, Monroe D, D'Amico LA, et al. A Phase II study of thalidomide in advanced metastatic renal cell carcinoma. *Invest New Drugs* 2002;20:389–393.

91. O'Really MS, Boehm T, Shing Y, et al. Endostatin: an endogenous inhibitor of angiogenesis and tumor growth. *Cell* 1997;88:277–285.

92. Bohem T, Folkman J, Browder T, et al. Antiangiogenic therapy of experimental therapy of experimental cancer does not induce acquired resistance. *Nature* 1997;390:404–407.

93. Herbst RS, Kenneth RH, Hai TT, et al. Phase I study of recombinant human endostatin in patients with advanced solid tumors. *J Clin Oncol* 2002;20:3792–3803.

94. Dirix LY, Vermeulen PB, Pawinski A, et al. Elevated levels of the angiogenic cytokines basic fibroblast growth factor and vascular endothelial growth factor in sera of cancer patients. *Br J Cancer* 1997;76:238–243.

95. Benoy I, Vermeulen P, Wuyts H, et al. Vascular endothelial Cell Growth Factor (VEGF) serum concentrations change according to the phase of the menstrual cycle. *Eur J Cancer* 1998;34:1298–1299.

96. Maloney JP, Silliman CC, Ambruso DR, et al. In vitro release of vascular endothelial growth factor during platelet aggregation. *Am J Physiol* 1998;275 (*Heart Circ Physiol* 1998;44:H1054–H1061.

97. Webb NJA, Bottomley MJ, Watson CJ, et al. Vascular endothelial growth factor (VEGF) is released from platelets during blood clotting: implications for measurement of circulating VEGF levels in clinical disease. *Clin Sci* 1998;94:395–404.

98. Balsari A, Maier JAM, Colnaghi MI, et al. Correlation between tumor vascularity, vascular endothelial growth factor production by tumor cells, serum vascular endothelial growth factor levels, and serum angiogenic activity in patients with breast carcinoma. *Lab Invest* 1999;79:897–902.

99. Kraft A, Weindel K, Ochs A, et al. Vascular endothelial growth factor in the sera and effusions of patients with malignant and nonmalignant disease. *Cancer* 1999;85:178–187.

100. Wynendaele W, Derua R, Hoylaerts MF, et al. Vascular endothelial growth factor measured in platelet poor plasma allows optimal separation between cancer patients and volunteers: a key to study an angiogenic marker in vivo. *Ann Oncol* 1999;10:965–971.

101. Gunsilius E, Petzer A, Stockhammer G, et al. Thrombocytes are the major source for soluble vascular endothelial growth factor in peripheral blood. *Oncology* 2000;58:169–174.

102. Lantzsch T, et al. The correlation between immunohistochemically-detected markers of angiogenesis and serum vascular endothelial growth factor in patients with breast cancer. *Anticancer Res* 2002;22:1925–1928.

103. Bachelot T, et al. Prognostic value of serum levels of interleukin 6 and of serum and plasma levels of vascular endothelial growth factor in hormone-refractory metastatic breast cancer patients. *Br J Cancer* 2003;88:1721–1726.

104. Caine GJ, Blann AD, Stonelake PS, Ryan P, Lip GYH. Plasma angiopoietin-1, angiopoietin-2, and Tie-2 in breast and prostate cancer: a comparison with VEGF and Flt-1. *Eur J Clin Invest* 2003;33:883–890.

105. Bauer JA, Morrison B, Oates R, et al. Angyozime and interferon α2b synergistically inhibit tumor angiogenesis. *Proc Am Assoc Cancer Res* 2003;44 Abstr 1159.

106. Parry TJ, Bouhana KS, Blanchard KS, et al. Ribozyme pharmacokinetic screening for predicting pharmacodynamic dosing regimen. *Curr Issues Mol Biol* 2000;2: 113–118.

107. Weng DE, Usman N. Angiozyme: a novel angiogenesis inhibitor. *Curr Oncol Rep* 2001; 3:141–146.

108. Lee JK, Hong YJ, Han CJ, Hwang DY, Hong SI. Clinical usefulness of serum and plasma vascular endothelial growth factor in cancer patients: which is the optimal specimen? *Int J Oncol* 2000; 17:149–152.

15 Detection of Early Tumor Dissemination in Patients With Breast Cancer

Debra Hawes, MD
and Richard J. Cote, MD, FRCPATH

CONTENTS

SUMMARY

Women who are newly diagnosed with breast cancer have operable disease, and therefore are potentially curable. Nevertheless, a subpopulation of these patients, who are thought to be disease free after initial treatment, go on to develop recurrent disease. These recurrences are due to early spread of tumor cells, either systemically

Cancer Drug Discovery and Development: Biomarkers in Breast Cancer:
Molecular Diagnostics for Predicting and Monitoring Therapeutic Effect
Edited by: G. Gasparini and D. F. Hayes © Humana Press Inc., Totowa, NJ

(peripheral blood and/or bone marrow) or regionally (lymph nodes) that are not detected by methods routinely employed. To address this problem, more sensitive methodologies of detecting early disseminated tumor cells have been developed over the past decade and a half. This chapter looks at the more important methods and discusses the clinical relevance of these methods.

Key Words: Bone marrow; circulating tumor cells; early tumor dissemination; flow cytometry; immunohistochemistry; immunomagnetic separation; lymph nodes; micrometastasis; occult metastasis; peripheral blood; prognosis; reverse transcriptase-polymerase chain reaction; sentinel lymph nodes.

1. INTRODUCTION

As with most types of cancer, early detection and definitive treatment are the keys to disease-free survival in patients with breast cancer. The majority of patients with newly diagnosed breast cancer have operable disease, and these patients are considered potentially curable. The traditional prognostic indicators for patients with operable disease are the size of the primary tumor and the spread of disease, either regionally to the lymph nodes or systemically to the bone marrow. However, up to 35% of patients, including up to 7–19% of patients with no evidence of metastasis at the time of diagnosis develop recurrent disease after primary therapy *(1,2)*. This rate of disease recurrence in patients with no evidence of regional or systemic metastasis at the time of initial treatment supports the notion that traditional methods are not sensitive enough to detect the earliest metastatic spread of disease, as clearly, these patients had occult systemic spread of disease that was undetectabled. As a result of this, several groups have recommended adjuvant treatment for patients with lymph node negative disease *(1–6)*. While this is controversial (because the majority of node negative patients will be clinically cured without adjuvant therapy), it is in this group of patients who have early disseminated tumor cells either regionally or systemically, that adjuvant therapy should be most successful.

A substantial amount of work has been done over the past decade and a half to develop more sensitive, reproducible and clinically relevant methods of detecting the earliest evidence of tumor cell dissemination *(7)*. Several terms denoting these early-disseminated tumors cells are currently used, most commonly, micrometastases (MMs), occult metastasis (OM), occult micrometastasis (OMM), minimal residual disease (MRD), circulating epithelial cells (CECs), and early-disseminated tumor cells (EDTCs). We will use the term occult metastasis (OM).

This discussion focuses on the detection and significance of occult metastatic tumor cells in the peripheral blood, bone marrow (OMBM), and lymph nodes (OMLM) of patients with breast cancer as well as on the biologic characterization of these cells and potential for the development of specific molecular targets.

1.1. Strategies Employed for the Detection of Occult Metastases

Several techniques have been used to identify occult metastases in the various compartments. The most important of these include immunohistochemistry (IHC), flow cytometry, and molecular methods, usually the reverse-transcriptase polymerase chain reaction (RT-PCR) technique. Each method has its advantages and disadvantages. We will discuss each of the major techniques commonly in use today.

1.1.2. FLOW CYTOMETRY

A flow cytometric assay was developed to detect rare cancer cells in the blood and bone marrow (8). The method has been reported to be extremely sensitive, with an ability to detect as little as one positive cell in ten million blood cells in a model system, although this level of sensitivity has not been universally obtained (9). Leers and associates (10) assessed the utility of multiparameter flow cytometry (MP-FCM) using an anticytokeratin antibody, to determine whether or not it is an effective method for the detection of occult metastases in the lymph nodes in patients with breast cancer. Of the 38 cases they examined in which the lymph nodes were positive by hematoxylin and eosin (H&E) and/or IHC they were able to detect more than 1% cytokeratin-positive cells in 37 cases. They concluded that MP-FCM was a highly specific and sensitive nonmorphological technique and provided several advantages including: (1) almost the entire lymph node is assessed, (2) the technique is able to provide information concerning ploidy, and (3) it may be possible to introduce sorting of metastatic tumor cells for further molecular studies. One major disadvantage of most flow cytometric systems has traditionally been the inability to morphologically characterize the cells constituting the "positive" events. However, by employing sophisticated cell-sorting technologies, in which the extrinsic cell population can be captured for subsequent morphologic evaluation, the specificity of tumor cell detection might be improved.

1.1.3. IHC

IHC was one if the earliest techniques employed for the detection of occult metastases and remains the most important method to date. Pioneering studies at the Ludwig Institute and Royal Marsden Hospital in London, England (11), helped to establish specific IHC procedures to identify occult metastatic cancer cells in the peripheral blood and bone marrow of patients with cancer. The initial focus was on the study of breast cancer (11–15), although many other tumor types have subsequently been studied including colon *(16–19)*, prostate *(20–23)*, lung *(24–32)*, esophagus *(33–37)*, and melanoma *(38–40)*. IHC methods are based on the ability of monoclonal antibodies to distinguish between cells of different histogenesis (i.e., epithelial cancer cells vs the hematopoietic cells of the peripheral blood, bone marrow, and lymph nodes). The results indicate that it is possible to identify occult metastatic cancer cells in these compartments prior to their detection by routine histologic analyses, and that the presence of these cells may be an important risk factor for disease recurrence.

The most widely used antibodies to detect occult metastatic tumor cells are monoclonal antibodies to epithelial-specific antigens. These antibodies do not react with hematopoietic cells normally present in the peripheral blood, bone marrow, and lymph nodes. None of the antibodies used in any study is specific for cancer; all react with normal and malignant epithelial cells. They are useful because they can identify an extrinsic population of epithelial cells in the blood and bone marrow, where there are normally no epithelial elements. The reported sensitivity of the IHC method ranges from the detection of one epithelial cell in 10,000 *(41)* to that of two to five epithelial cells in a million hematopoietic cells *(14,41,42)*.

Because current methods used to detect occult metastases generally involve epithelial markers that are not specific for malignant cells, concerns have been raised over interpreting artifactually present epithelial cells as tumor cells *(43)*. Certainly, keratin-positive epithelial cells have been found on the surface of "clean" slides and floating on water baths and in staining solutions. Perhaps a greater danger is the possibility that tumor cells may be mechanically shed from the primary tumor to the lymph nodes as a result of manipulation of the tumor, for example as a result of fine needle aspiration or core biopsy. The danger exists that these cells could be overinterpreted as occult metastatic cells by an inexperienced observer. However, normally exfoliated epithelial cells lack the morphologic features of tumor cells and can be differentiated from metastatic malignant cells on the basis of size, nuclear hyperchromasia, nuclear to cytoplasmic ratio, and location on the slide by an experienced pathologist. In addition, the number of positive events and their pattern of distribution in the lymph node can give valuable clues as to their origin.

1.1.4. MOLECULAR METHODS

While IHC methods are effective in identifying occult metastases in the peripheral blood, bone marrow and lymph nodes of patients with operable breast cancer, these methods are laborious and require considerable technical expertise to perform and interpret. Efforts are under way to develop molecular techniques for the detection of occult metastases. The method usually employed is RT-PCR, which differentiates gene expression between epithelial and lymphoid cells to identify epithelial cancer cells. RT-PCR entails the isolation and reverse-transcription of epithelial-specific messenger RNA to complementary-DNA (cDNA), and thereafter, involves PCR-based amplification of the cDNA template between specific primers. This results in a several thousand-fold amplification of the signal, and makes the method theoretically extremely sensitive. Keratin 18 or 19 (CK-18, CK-19) mRNA that is expressed in epithelial cells has been the most frequent target for amplification to detect occult metastases. Studies have *(44)* used the CK-19 transcript to identify cancer cells in the bone marrow and peripheral blood of breast cancer patients. However, it is known that a pseudogene for CK-19 exists that shares a very high homology with the mature mRNA from the *CK-19* gene. Contamination of DNA in the RNA sample used for reverse transcription can result in amplification of the pseudogene, giving rise to specific "background" bands in the negative controls (known negative bone marrow and blood) *(23)*. Furthermore, the nonepithelial cells may have a low level of expression of epithelial transcripts, leading to background bands. To evaluate the specificity and sensitivity of RT-PCR in detecting occult metastases, transcripts were amplified from epithelial and breast cell-specific genes including carcinoembryonic antigen (CEA), cytokeratin 19 (CK-19), cytokeratin-20 (CK-20), mucin-1 (MUC-1), and gastrointestinal tumor-associated antigen 733.2 (GA733.2), from the blood of healthy donors and lymph nodes from patients without cancer by RT-PCR. CK-20 was the only marker not detected in the lymph nodes or blood from patients without cancer *(45)*. Similarly, the specificity of RT-PCR assays was studied *(46)* using primers specific for various tumor-associated and organ-specific mRNA species including prostate-specific antigen (PSA), epithelial glyco-protein-40 (EGP-40) desmoplakin I (DPI I) CEA, erb-B2, erb-B3 prostate-specific membrane antigen (PSM), and CK-18. The bone marrow from 53 subjects with no epithelial malignancy as well as bone marrow samples from 53 patients with prostate cancer and 10 patients with breast cancer were examined. It was found that seven of the eight markers tested could be detected in a considerable number of bone marrow samples from control patients. In this study only PSA mRNA was not detected in any of the 53 control bone marrow samples *(46)*.

The known relative nonspecificity of epithelial cell markers has prompted the search for even more specific breast cancer markers. One such candidate currently under investigation is mammaglobin (hMAM). Mammaglobin, a glycoprotein expressed in the mammary glands of women, as well as in breast cancer cell lines, has been investigated as a potential marker to detect early metastatic breast cancer in the peripheral blood *(47–49)* of patients with breast cancer. The specificity and sensitivity of hMAM will be discussed in detail later. In summary, blood samples from patients with breast cancer and other malignancies tested for hMAM by RT-PCR showed the marker to be relatively sensitive but lacked specificity when analyzed alone *(47)*.

Metastatic melanoma has been successfully detected by RT-PCR using mRNA markers for tyrosinase, p 97 and MelanA/MART1.

In summary, the drawbacks of molecular methods include the chance of low level of epithelial gene expression from lymphoid cells that could result in high background, as well as the inability to employ morphologic criteria to confirm the presence of metastatic cells. However, RT-PCR has been successfully used for the detection of occult metastases to the bone marrow in melanoma and carcinoma of the prostate and colon.

Techniques to detect occult metastases are neither easy to perform nor simple to evaluate. We therefore, recommend that these tests be preformed by laboratories that are experienced in doing large numbers of them and that they be evaluated by specialists who are thoroughly trained in their interpretation.

2. DETECTION OF OCCULT METASTASES IN THE PERIPHERAL BLOOD

Clearly a technique that could reliably detect the presence of early tumor in the peripheral blood would be a great practical advantage over one in which a sample of bone marrow was required. There have been a number of studies designed to explore this possibility. Unfortunately, the yield of occult metastatic cells from peripheral blood is extremely low. Redding et al. *(11)* found that 28.2% patients with breast cancer showed extrinsic cancer cells in their bone marrow, but only 2.7% of these patients had detectable cells in their peripheral blood. It is not clear why tumor cells are detected less commonly in peripheral blood than in bone marrow. For this reason most of the studies looking for the presence of early metastases in the blood have focused on using molecular methods. Nevertheless important work continues to examine occult metastases in the peripheral blood by a variety of methods and markers especially in the area of breast cancer.

2.1. IHC vs RT-PCR

To compare the sensitivity of OM in blood by molecular and IHC methods, both peripheral blood and bone marrow samples from women with primary breast cancer using RT-PCR and IHC have been analyzed *(50)*. The study demonstrated that the peripheral blood is a less sensitive compartment than the bone marrow (9% vs 43%) *(51)*. The reason for this difference in sensitivities is not known. It has been suggested that this lack of sensitivity in detecting tumor cells in the blood may be, at least in part, because tumor cells are likely to only be shed intermittently into the circulation *(51)*. Therefore, the lack of sensitivity in blood is a real reflection of the biology of tumor dissemination and not a failure of the detection methods used. The rates of sensitivity of detecting occult metastasis in the blood using RT-PCR vs IHC methodologies was also compared. There was only a small gain in sensitivity using RT-PCR over IHC *(51)*. In summary, it appears that while the methods may not detect an identical population of positive patients and that molecular detection methods may be slightly more sensitive, the number of circulation tumor cells in the blood is less than in the bone marrow.

2.2. RT-PCR

The studies referenced above all examined the peripheral blood for cytokeratin transcripts and/or protein. Molecular (RT-PCR) detection of other markers have been tested in an attempt to improve the sensitivity and specificity of the detection of OM in the blood. Among the most well studied and promising of the new markers are mammaglobin (hMAM) described in Section 1.1.4., and epidermal growth factor receptor (EGFR) *(47,49,52)*. One study found 25% positivity for hMAM in the blood from patients with breast cancer, and in 5% of patients tested with malignancies other than breast cancer, indication that the marker is probably sensitive, but not entirely specific for breast cancer. As many as 43% of patients with metastatic breast cancer who were positive for hMAM by RT-PCR in the peripheral blood have been detected *(52)*. Variations in rates of positivity have been found using the different markers. In a comparison of hMAM, EGFR, and CK-19 in the blood by RT-PCR from patients with breast cancer the rates of positivity were found to be 8%, 10%, and 48%, respectively *(47)*. It was also determined that there is a lack of specificity in some of the markers. None of the blood samples from patients without cancer was positive for hMAM, while CK-19 mRNA was found in the blood of 39% healthy volunteers and transcripts for EGFR and CK-19 were detectable in 25% and 10%, respectively, of the patients with hematological malignancies *(47)*. The lack of sensitivity and specificity found in the markers may indicate that a panel of markers (i.e., CK-19, hMAM, EGFR) may yield superior results than any single marker. Further studies with clinical follow-up is required to test this hypothesis.

2.3. Immunomagnetic Separation

Another method currently under investigation for detecting OM in the blood is the use of immunomagnetic separation techniques. This technology uses antibodies to separate and concentrate the epithelial cells from the hematopoietic cells to improve detection sensitivity. Several enrichment methods are currently available. By the use of various antibody-coupled magnetic particles, tumor cells have been enriched by several orders of magnitude in model tests *(42,53)*. Enrichment can be achieved by positive or negative selection. Tumor cells can be selected with beads coated with antibodies against tumor-associated antigens (positive selection), or normal blood cells in the preparation can be depleted by use of beads coated with antibodies against hematopoietic cell antigens (negative selection) *(54–58)*. The peripheral blood samples from 21 patients with primary operable breast cancer, 29 patients with metastatic breast cancer, and 21 healthy women have been analyzed by IHC following immunomagnetic separation *(59)*. Tumor cells were not detected in either the healthy women or the women with operable breast cancer. Conversely, 28% women with metastatic breast did have tumor cells in their peripheral blood *(59)*.

2.4. Prognostic Significance of OM in the Blood

The goal of detecting OM in the blood is to us the results to predict patient outcome and develop more patient-specific treatment regimens. Stathopoulou et al. *(60)* looked at the peripheral blood for the presence and prognostic significance of CK-19–positive cells in patients with breast cancer using the nested RT-PCR assay for CK-19 mRNA. Detection rates for CK-19 mRNA-positive cells in the blood of patients with early or metastatic breast cancer were 74% and 52% respectively. For stage I and II breast cancer, detection of CK-19–positive cells in the peripheral blood before adjuvant therapy was associated with reduced disease-free survival ($p = 0.0007$) and overall survival ($p = 0.01$). Finally, the hypothesis that the number, not just the presence of circulating tumor cells, was tested using fluorescently labeled monoclonal antibodies cytokeratins *(61)* from peripheral blood samples from patients with breast cancer. It was found that the levels of circulating tumor cells were significant predictors of progression-free overall survival *(61)*. These data support the hypothesis that OM in the peripheral blood may be prognostically important

In summary, because of the advantage of ease of accessibility of obtaining the peripheral blood over bone marrow, efforts are underway to optimize currently available detection techniques and to develop new methods of assessing the blood for the presence of early-disseminated tumor. To date, while progress has been made, the peripheral blood continues to be a less sensitive compartment for the assessment of OM than the bone marrow (or lymph nodes). Several markers have been used to detect OM in the peripheral blood of patients with breast cancer including CK-19, hMAM, and EGF-R While none of the markers is entirely specific for the detection of metastatic breast cancer, and the sensitivity of the peripheral blood continues to be less than that of the bone marrow, there is growing evidence that the detection of OM cells in the peripheral blood has a negative impact on prognosis. New techniques such as immunomagnetic cell separation may have an impact in future, but current available data are too preliminary and no clinical follow-up data is available. Further studies are needed with long-term clinical follow-up to determine the clinical utility of OM detection in the peripheral blood.

3. DETECTION OF OCCULT METASTASES IN THE BONE MARROW (OMBM)

The bone marrow vasculature consists of a unique sinusoidal system that may simply act as a filter that traps or concentrates malignant cells. The marrow environment may provide a more favorable support system for tumor cell proliferation than does the blood. One may also speculate that cancer cells that are released into the systemic circulation represent a small subpopulation of cells with altered expression of cell adhesion molecules. Whatever the reason, bone marrow appears to offer the maximum opportunity to detect cancer cells that have been released into the blood. Therefore, the majority of studies to detect occult metastatic cells in the systemic circulation have investigated bone marrow as a site of spread.

Bone marrow in general is the single most common site of breast cancer metastasis, and up to 80% of patients with recurrent tumors will develop metastatic lesions in the bone marrow at some point during evolution of their disease *(62)*; it is also the most frequent initial site of clinically detectable breast cancer metastasis *(63)*. Tumor cells are estimated to be present in the bone marrow of 10 to 45 percent of patients with primary operable breast cancer *(11,14,15,64–66)*, and 20% to 70% of patients with metastatic breast cancer *(67)*. As with most cancers, the most widely used method to detect occult metastatic cells is IHC.

Because IHC is the most widely used (and currently, the most reliable) method for the detection of occult metastases in the bone marrow (OMBM) in breast cancer patients, we have summarized the results from several groups performing IHC assays using monoclonal antibodies.

The percentage of patients with early stage breast cancer in whom extrinsic cells were detected in the bone marrow ranges from 10% to 45%. The possible reasons for some of the variations observed include: (1) use of single antibodies to detect extrinsic cells in some of the studies; (2) differences in patient populations, although all the results were from patients with early stage disease; (3) differences in the antibody reactivity with breast cancer cells; and (4) the presence of antigenic heterogeneity. However, what is evident and striking is that occult metastases in the bone marrow were detected in all of the studies. Furthermore, it is becoming apparent that the rate of detection of occult metastases in the bone marrow in patients with operable breast cancer is decreasing when appropriate antibodies are used. In recent years we have noticed a marked decline in the number of occult metastases–positive cases. We believe that this may, at least in part, be due to the stage migration that has occurred. With the success of early breast cancer detection methods have enabled women to be diagnosed sooner. The latest figures show more than 90% of breast cancer deaths are now diagnosed at a local or regional stage when 5-yr survival rates are 97% and 79%, respectively (68,69). These patients will thus be expected to have a low rate of occult metastases.

Because methods of detecting occult metastases do not specifically target tumor cells, there has been some controversy over whether or not malignant cells are being detected. To help to answer this question, a study was performed by Fehm et al. (70) in which they looked at the blood and primary tumor from patients with cancer (breast, kidney, prostate, and colon) and who had known circulating epithelial cells identified by anticytokeratin antibody. These were analyzed by enumerator DNA probes for chromosomes 1, 3, 4, 7, 8, 11, or 17 by fluorescence in situ hybridization and compared to the primary tumor. The pattern of aneusomy matched a clone in the primary tumor in 10 of 13 patients, indicating that the vast majority of these circulating tumor cells were anuesomic and derived from the primary tumor.

3.1. Detection of Occult Metastases in the Bone Marrow in Patients with Early Stage Breast Cancer: Clinical Significance

OMBM have been correlated with known predictors of prognosis in several studies. In our studies (14), the lymph node–negative group had fewer extrinsic cells than the lymph node–positive group, suggesting a trend toward a greater metastatic tumor burden in patients with lymph node metastases.

The presence of OMBM has been correlated with pathologic Tumor–Node–Metastasis (TNM) stage in breast cancer. Several other investigators have obtained similar results. In the original study from the Ludwig Institute (11), the presence of OMBM was correlated with the tumor stage ($p = 0.05$), and vascular invasion ($p < 0.01$), both of which are known predictors of poor prognosis.

While the presence of OMBM appears to be correlated with known features of disease progression, the ultimate utility of this test will be determined by whether it can predict breast cancer recurrence. Several studies now show that, in fact, the presence of occult metastases in the bone marrow identifies a population of patients at high risk for recurrence (Table 1) (14,71–76). Our own studies (14) have revealed that the presence of occult metastases in the bone marrow significantly predicts recurrence; the 2-yr recurrence rate for patients with no evidence of OMBM was 3% compared with 33% for patients with detectable OMBM. Diel and associates (71) studied 727 patients with primary operable breast cancer. They were able to detect tumor cells in the bone marrow of 55% of lymph node-positive

Table 1
Detection of Occult Bone Marrow Metastases in Breast Cancer

	No. of patients	Clinical follow-up[a]	OMBM⁻ (number)	OMBM⁺ (number)	p-value
Dearnaley 1991 (77)	39	9.5	31% (8/26)	85% (11/13)	<0.05
Mansi 1991 (78)	350	2.3	25% (64/261)	48% (43/89)	<0.05
Cote 1991 (14)	49	2[b]	16% (5/31)	54% (7/13)	<0.04
Diel 1992 (80)	211	2	3% (4/130)	27% (22/81)	0.0001
Diel 1996 (79)	727	3	8% (34/412)	35% (109/315)	<0.001
Braun 2000 (73)	552	4	8% (28/353)	40% (79/199)	
Gebauer 2001 (75)	393	6	20% (46/227)	35% (59/166)	<0.001
Gerber 2001 (74)	554	4.5	9%	24%	0.0001
Wiedswang 2003 (76)	817	4	9% (60/709[c])	26% (28/108[c])	<0.001

[a]Years.
[b]Estimated 2 yr of recurrence rate.
[c]Overall survival.

patients and in 31% of lymph node negative patients. They found that OMBM was an independent prognostic indicator for both distant disease-free survival and overall survival that was superior to axillary lymph node status, tumor stage, and tumor grade. In a more recent study, Mansi and associates (72) looked at bone marrow aspirates from 350 women with primary breast cancer. While they found that patients with OMBM did have shorter relapse-free and overall survival times, it was not found to be an independent prognostic indicator when tumor size, lymph node status and vascular invasion were taken into account (72). Braun and associates (73), analyzed the bone marrow samples from 552 patients with stage I, II, or III breast cancer by IHC. They found cytokeratin positive cells in 36% (199/552) of the patients studied. Forty-nine of the 199 (25%) patients with OMBM died of cancer-related causes, while only 49 of 353 (14%) patients without OMBM died ($p < 0.001$). They concluded that OMBM was an independent prognostic indicator of the risk of death from cancer (73). Gebauer and associates (75) examined the bone marrow from 393 patients with primary breast cancer. They were able to detect the presence of epithelial cells in 42% of these bone marrow samples. After a median follow-up of 75 months they found that 27% of all patients in the study developed distant metastases. Multivariate analysis showed that, in this study, the presence of bone marrow occult metastasis was an independent prognostic parameter of tumor recurrence or cancer-related death. Gerber and associates (74) looked at 484 patients with pT1-2N0M0 breast cancer. Occult tumor cells were detected in 37.2% of patients, of these 26% had positive bone marrows only, 6.4% had positive lymph nodes only and 4.8% had tumor cells found in both compartments. Patients who had occult metastases in and any compartment showed a decreased disease-free survival and the overall survival rates were found to be comparable top those patients who had one positive lymph node. It appears that occult metastatic tumor cells detected by simultaneous IHC analysis of axillary lymph nodes and bone marrow demonstrate independent metastatic pathways. Finally, Wiedswang et al. *(76)* examined the bone marrow aspirates from 817 patients with breast cancer. OMBM were detected by IHC using anticytokeratin antibodies. OMBM were detected in 13.2% of all patients and were associated with poor prognosis in node-positive patients and in node-negative patients not receiving adjuvant therapy.

These large studies provide strong evidence that the detection of occult metastases by IHC methods is prognostically important. The presence of OMBM predicts a higher risk for recurrence in bone as well as in other sites. Of particular importance in all of these findings is the fact that the presence of OMBM identifies patients with node-negative disease who are at a higher risk for recurrence; this subset of patients can therefore be the target of more aggressive adjuvant therapy. The studies by both Diel *(71)* and Braun *(73)* have shown that bone marrow metastasis is a more powerful predictor of recurrence than histologic node status.

In fact, several studies have now shown that the bone marrow status can be combined with other prognostic factors such as axillary lymph node status. This allows groups of patients to be stratified *(14,26,71,77,78)* as follows: (1) those with very low recurrence rates (lymph node negative, bone marrow negative); (2) those with moderate rates of recurrence (lymph node negative, bone marrow positive, and lymph node positive, bone marrow negative); and (3) those with high recurrence rates (lymph node positive, bone marrow positive) *(14,78–80)*.

3.1.1. Detection of Bone Marrow Occult Metastases: Effect of Tumor Burden

The number of carcinoma cells detected in the bone marrow (the bone marrow tumor burden) may be significantly associated with disease recurrence *(14)*. In our study, the bone marrow aspirates were processed so that the concentration of bone marrow elements was equal for each patient. Consequently, the number of extrinsic cells counted for each case could be compared among patients; the number of extrinsic cells identified in the bone marrow was considered to be reflective of the peripheral tumor burden in each patient. Among patients with OMBM, those who did not recur had on an average, fewer extrinsic cells in their marrow than those who recurred (15 vs 43 cells respectively). In addition, the estimated 2-yr recurrence rate of patients with 10 or more cells (46%) was significantly higher than that of patients with fewer than 10 cells. Further, the number of extrinsic cells detected in the bone marrow was an independent predictor of prognosis.

4. DETECTION OF OCCULT METASTASES IN THE LYMPH NODES

Despite the explosion on our knowledge of the biology of cancer, the single most important prognostic factor for most solid tumors is the presence of histologically detectable regional lymph node metastases: patients with tumors that have not metastasized to the regional lymph nodes tend to do far better than patients with lymph node metastases. A significant proportion of node-negative patients will, however, develop distant metastasis. As we have seen, systemic dissemination takes place by routes other than lymphatic spread; the presence of bone marrow occult metastases in node-negative patients demonstrates this. Nevertheless, a proportion of node-negative patients without the evidence of bone marrow metastases will experience recurrence. It has now become clear that another possible site for occult tumor spread in histologically node-negative patients is the regional lymph nodes.

Routine histopathological examination of lymph nodes is in reality only a lymph node sampling; in fact, it has been calculated that a pathologist has only a 1% chance of identifying a metastatic focus of cancer with a diameter of three cells in cross-section occupying a lymph node *(81)*. It has also been clearly shown that reexamination of lymph node sections initially considered negative for tumor after routine histopathologic screening frequently shows metastatic deposits, demonstrating that even when tumor cells are present in the section, they can be missed *(82)*. It is evident that routine processing and histologic examination of regional lymph nodes is inadequate to detect the presence of tumor in all cases.

Most studies have involved the detection of regional (axillary) lymph nodes occult metastases in patients with breast cancer *(82–89)*. These studies can be classified into two major categories: (1) detection of metastasis after more intensive histological examination of the lymph node, including analysis of multiple serial sections and (2) studies which use IHC to take advantage of the differential expression of antigens between normal lymph node constituents and epithelial carcinoma cells in order to detect occult tumor in lymph nodes. In fact, this is the same principle as that used for detecting occult tumor in bone marrow. Attempts have also been made to use molecular techniques to detect lymph node occult metastatic cells *(89–102)*.

4.1. Detection of Occult Metastases in Lymph Nodes (OMLN) by Histological Review

Studies undertaken to detect occult lymph node metastases by routine histologic methods have generally been performed by cutting serial sections from all paraffin blocks containing lymph nodes, followed by routine staining and microscopic review *(93)*. However, several studies have simply rereviewed the original histologic slides. All of these studies have demonstrated that deposits of tumor can be detected using these methods. Between 7% and 33% of previously node-negative cases convert to node-positive after review. As reviewed by Neville *(96)*, the mean conversion rate is approx 13%.

4.2. Detection of OMLN by IHC

Several investigators have used various antibodies in order to detect occult lymph node metastases in patients with breast cancer using IHC methods. In general, most studies have used antibodies specific for low molecular weight intermediate filament proteins to distinguish the epithelial tumor deposits from normal node elements. Other studies have used antimucin antibodies raised against human mammary carcinoma cells *(100)*. In our own studies, we have used a cocktail of two anticytokeratin antibodies, AE1 and CAM5.2 (which in combination recognize CK-18 and CK-19, the predominant intermediate filament proteins in simple epithelial cells). While antibodies to cytokeratins have been reported to react with dendritic reticulum cells (with the possibility of producing false positive results) this has not been a significant problem in our own studies. Furthermore, as with the bone marrow examination previously described, the morphologic evaluation of the "positive" cells is critical; cells that do not possess the morphologic characteristics of malignant epithelial cells are not considered tumor cells in our studies.

Unlike routine histological evaluation for the detection of occult metastases in which multiple sections from each block are studied, most of the studies employing immunohistochemical techniques have tested only a single section. When a single section is studied, the percentage of patients who convert from node-negative to node-positive ranges from 14% to 30% with a mean conversion rate of 16% *(82,96)*.

4.3. Detection of Occult Lymph Node Metastases by RT-PCR

Although it may at some point be possible to detect occult metastases in the lymph nodes of patients with breast cancer using PCR methods, this procedure continues to have major drawbacks compared with IHC. In addition to the problems of identifying appropriately sensitive and specific markers discussed above, the lymph nodes used must be fresh (or fresh frozen), and all lymph nodes in their entirety must be disaggregated to undergo RNA extraction (as we have shown that metastases in node-negative cases usually occurs to only one lymph node). Therefore, these lymph nodes will be unavailable for histologic review, and the method will test for both histologic and occult positives. This is in contrast to immunohistochemical techniques, which can be done on formalin-fixed, paraffin-embedded tissue that has been routinely prepared for histologic evaluation.

4.4. Clinical Significance of OMLN in Patients with Breast Cancer

Although virtually all studies have demonstrated that lymph node metastases can be overlooked, there is a surprising disagreement about the prognostic importance of these occult tumor deposits. Many of the studies using routine histologic review of sections have found that the presence of OMLN does not influence the recurrence rates in a statistically significant way *(84–86)*; several studies using immunohistochemical techniques have reported similar findings *(90,91,98)*. To begin to understand this, a few basic observations need to be made. Many earlier studies have involved fewer than 100 patients; in fact some have involved even fewer than 50 patients. Cote and Groshen have demonstrated that even if the finding of occult lymph node metastases is prognostically important, there is no possibility that studies of the clinical impact of occult lymph node metastases involving few patients will provide statistically significant data (unpublished data). In fact, Fisher et al. *(85)* were the first to clearly point this out: "it has been mathematically estimated that differences in survival of 10%, if indeed they occur between the two groups (true lymph node negative versus occult lymph node positive), would require a study of approx 1400 cases." Therefore, studies involving a few patients are not suitable to address the issue of prognostic significance of occult lymph node metastases.

Investigators from the Ludwig Institute and International Breast Cancer study group have performed a definitive study of the importance of occult lymph node metastases in patients with node-negative breast cancer *(87)*. They examined serial sections of 921 node-negative breast cancer patients by routine histological methods. Nine percent of these patients were found to have OMLN; these patients had a poorer disease-free ($p = 0.003$) and overall survival ($p = 0.002$) after 5 yr median follow-up, compared with patients whose nodes remained negative after serial sectioning. Six-year median follow-up data give even more conclusive evidence of the prognostic significance of occult lymph node metastases. Another large-scale study was performed *(88)*. These investigators studied the lymph nodes from 1121 patients with primary operable breast cancer, by serial macroscopic sectioning; they found single OMLN in 120 patients. A significant difference in recurrence ($p = 0.005$) and survival ($p = 0.04$) was found between node-negative patients and those with single occult metastases. Immunohistochemical methods have also shown the prognostic significance of occult lymph node metastases *(92,94,100)*. Trial V of the International (Ludwig) Breast Cancer Study for the presence of metastases showed that in lymph nodes from patients with breast cancer, occult metastases were associated with significantly poorer disease-free and overall survival in postmenopausal patients but not in premenopausal patients. Immunohistochemically detected OMLN remained an independent and highly significant predictor of recurrence, even after control for tumor grade, tumor size, estrogen-receptor status, vascular invasion, and treatment (*p* = 0.007) *(103)*.

It can be seen by these recent studies that the evidence is mounting that when sufficiently large patient populations are analyzed, OMLN is an independent indicator of the likelihood of disease progression. In addition, it appears that OMLN is a biologic event independent of bone marrow status and has an intermediate risk of recurrence associated with it *(74)*.

4.4.1. SENTINEL LYMPH NODES

Axillary lymph node dissection (ALND) is the standard in care for patients with breast cancer. In more recent years the sentinel lymph node dissection (SLND) technique has been extensively studied. The technique uses isosulfan blue dye, a radiopharmaceutical, or a combination of both to locate and remove the first few lymph nodes that drain the tumor. These sentinel lymph nodes are considered the most likely to contain cancer cells. This procedure has the advantage of potentially saving patients with early stage breast cancer from having a complete axillary lymph node dissection and the subsequent morbidity that is associated with this procedure. Several studies have shown that this technique is highly accurate in staging patients. Giuliano et al. *(104)* showed a false-negative rate for patients who had an ALND performed after SLND of only 2%. Veronesi et al. *(105)* reported no false-negative sentinel lymph nodes among 45 patients with T1 breast cancer that measured less than 1.5 cm. The overall accuracy rate that included T3 tumors was 97%. In a more recent study they *(106)* examined 516 patients with breast cancer who had tumors that measured 2 cm or less in diameter. The overall accuracy of sentinel node status was 96.9%, the sensitivity was 91.2% and the specificity was 100%. They concluded that sentinel-node biopsy is an accurate screening of axillary node status in women with early-stage breast cancer. Furthermore, Alex and Krag *(107)* were able to identify the sentinel lymph nodes in 50 of the 70 patients they studied. Of these 50 patients 18 were found to have positive sentinel nodes that were predictive of the axillary status. Albertini et al. *(108)* were able to identify the sentinel lymph nodes in 57 of 62 (92%) patients. All patients with axillary nodal metastases were identified by the sentinel lymph node examination. However, a trial that looked at the sentinel lymph nodes from multiple institutions using only the radioisotope technique alone showed somewhat less promising results *(109)*. In this study of 443 patients a sentinel lymph node was identified in 405 patients. These 405 then underwent a completion axillary lymph node dissection. Of these 405 there were 114 node-positive cases with 13 false-negative nodes for a false-negative rate of 11%.

In cases in which the routine histologic examination of the sentinel lymph node is negative, immunohistochemical evaluation for the presence of occult metastases may play an important role in the histopathologic evaluation of these patients. The reported rate of positivity for occult metastases in these histologically negative nodes ranges from 5% to 15% *(92)*. It is clear that large-scale clinical trials are needed to determine the clinical relevance of these occult metastases positive sentinel lymph nodes.

4.4.2. OCCULT METASTASES IN LYMPH NODES IN PATIENTS WITH DCIS

The significance of finding occult metastases in patients with small tumors or comedo carcinoma is less clear than for patients with invasive carcinoma. The purpose for detecting occult metastases in lymph nodes, or in any other site for that matter, is to assess the risk for distant metastasis and death due to breast cancer. While most measures of DCIS outcome are focused on rates of local recurrence and the incidence of development of invasive disease, the critical issue with regard to lymph node analysis in DCIS is the distant outcome for the patient.

A number of studies have now addressed this issue. In an analysis from the NSABP Project B-17, it was found that for 814 patients with ductal carcinoma *in situ* followed for a median time of 7.5 yr, that the rate of distant metastasis was 1.8%, and deaths due to breast cancer was 1.8% *(110)*. In another study 1002 women who were diagnosed with DCIS between 1986 and 1996 were followed for a median time of 4.25 yr. The rate of distant metastasis in this group was 2.4%, and deaths due to breast cancer was 1.5% *(111)*. Finally, it should be noted that in all of these studies, a number of women subsequently developed invasive carcinoma and these women are included in the distant metastasis and death due to breast cancer rate. There is no question that some of the incidence of metastasis and death due to breast cancer is due to the subsequent development of either ipsilateral or contralateral invasive carcinoma. However, for the purposes of this evaluation, we have not separated out these patients, but have rather taken a "conservative" approach to the data analysis. Nevertheless, the data are virtually noncontroversial; systemic events in patients with DCIS are rare, under any circumstances. Therefore, detection of lymph node metastases, including occult metastases, does not appear to be an important procedure in patients diagnosed with DCIS overall.

However, all of the studies indicated above were performed in all patients with DCIS, without regard to subtype. Because the incidence of DCIS is increasing, and the proportion of women being diagnosed with breast cancer who have the diagnosis of pure DCIS is increasing as well, this subtype analysis may in fact become increasingly important. The question then becomes, do occult metastases occur in any patients with DCIS, and are there particular subtypes in which the risk for occult metastasis, and subsequent systemic events, is substantial?

There are preliminary data to support the idea that occult metastases may be detectable in at least in some types of DCIS *(112,113)*. A positivity rate of up to 5% of nodal metastases in level 1 and 2 axillary dissections from patients with DCIS has been reported *(114)*. However, because of the high morbidity associated with axillary lymph node dissections, and the low rate of recurrent disease in patients with DCIS, axillary lymph node dissection is not recommended as routine practice *(115)*. The advent of the sentinel lymph node (SLN) biopsy technique has greatly reduced the morbidity associated with axillary lymph node sampling, offers a low-risk way of assessing lymph node status in DCIS. This may be of particular importance in patients that are more likely to have nodal involvement such as those with DCIS with an extensive intraductal component or comedo type *(113,114)*. There is evidence that SLN biopsy complimented by IHC detection of occult metastases on these nodes may add to the relevance of the initial diagnosis and subsequent management of patients with DCIS *(113,116)*. Studies to date show that a percentage of patients initially diagnosed with DCIS have tumor cells present in the sentinel nodes and that IHC evaluation of sentinel nodes is more sensitive than routine histology with serial sections at identifying these cases *(113,116)*.

The prognostic significance of finding tumor cells in the sentinel nodes in patients with DCIS is not known. It is certain that not all positive cases will progress to more advanced disease; we know that in invasive cancer with overt nodal positivity, not all patients go on the develop recurrent disease. Nevertheless, large-scale prospective studies are needed to determine what clinical advantage, if any, exists in routinely analyzing sentinel lymph nodes for occult metastases in patients with DCIS.

5. OCCULT METASTASES IN THE BONE MARROW AND LYMPH NODES

While there is strong evidence to suggest that detection of either bone marrow or lymph node metastasis is clinically significant, it is possible that the detection of occult systemic (bone marrow) and regional (lymph node) metastases may provided complementary information in assessing the risk of an individual patient. Preliminary reports exist that support the hypothesis that occult metastases in the bone marrow and lymph nodes represent separate biologic pathways and are present in different subgroups of patients may have different prognostic significance. We studied 90 patients with node-negative breast cancer for the presence of both occult bone marrow and lymph node metastases (Table 2). OMLN were detected in 12 patients (13%) while OMBM were detected in 16 patients (18%). Both lymph node and bone marrow metastases were detected in only one patient (1%). Stratification showed that the presence of OMBM identified patients most likely

Table 2
Lymph Node vs Bone Marrow Occult Metastases

OMLN/OMBM status	Patients	5-yr probability of recurring (± SE)	Relative risk of recurring	p-value
OMLN⁻/OMBM⁻	62/90 (69%)	0.09 ± 0.04	1.00	<0.00001
OMLN⁺	12/90 (13%)	0.31 ± 0.16	2.96	
OMBM⁺	16ᵃ/90 (18%)	0.50 ± 0.13	7.17	

OMLN, Occult metastases in the lymph nodes; OMBM, occult metastases in the bone marrow; –, no occult metastases detected; +, occult metastases detected; SE, standard error.
ᵃIncludes one OMLN⁺ patient.

to recur. Bone marrow negative patients could be stratified into risk groups based on their lymph node status (lymph node negative vs lymph node positive). Thus, three distinct groups were identified; those with detectable OMBM (high risk for recurrence), those with detectable occult metastases in the lymph nodes but none in the bone marrow (intermediate risk for recurrence), and those with no detectable occult metastases in either the lymph nodes or bone marrow (low risk for recurrence).

Gerber et al. *(74)* reported in their study that looked at 484 patients with pT1-2N0M0 breast cancer. Occult tumor cells were detected in 180 (37.2%) of the 484 patients; of these 126 (26%) patients had positive bone marrows only, 31 patients (6.4%) had positive lymph nodes only, and 23 patients (4.8%) had tumor cells found in both compartments. Patients who had occult metastases in and any compartment showed a decreased disease-free survival and the overall survival rates were found to be comparable top those patients who had one positive lymph node. Therefore, it is possible that occult metastatic tumor cells detected by simultaneous immunohistochemical analysis of axillary lymph nodes and bone marrow demonstrate independent metastatic pathways.

6. FUTURE DIRECTIONS

While the detection of occult metastases and the prognostic significance of their presence has been the primary focus to date, it is clear that this represents the tip of the iceberg in terms of the clinical applications possible. First, it is known that not all patients with overt metastases will suffer disease recurrence therefore, it is not reasonable to expect that all patients with occult metastases will recur. This is thought to occur because a proportion if the early-disseminated tumor cells are not viable or may be amenable to being destroyed by the patients immune system. Molecular markers that will predict which cells are likely to progress and which are not are currently being investigated. The relevance of erb-B2 overexpression on disseminated CK-18–positive breast cancer cells in the bone marrow of 52 patients with early-stage breast cancer using immunohistochemical double labeling to the p185erbB2 oncoprotein was examined *(117)*. Expression of p185erb-B2 on cytokeratin-positive cells was detected in 60% of patients. It was determined that patients with p185erb-B2 positive bone marrow occult metastases developed fatal metastatic relapses more frequently than patients with p185erb-B2–negative bone marrow occult metastases. In addition, these markers may prove to be useful as specific targets to deliver chemotherapeutic agents *(118)*. The analysis of occult metastatic cells opens a new avenue by which molecular determinants of both early tumor cell dissemination and subsequent outgrowth into overt metastases can be assessed. The identification of therapeutic targets such as HER2/neu MAGE-1 and E-Cadherin, for example, monitoring the elimination of bone metastases, and assessing treatment resistant tumor cell clones might help us to understand the current limitations of adjuvant systemic therapy.

The *MAGE-A* genes, genes that encode peptide antigens that can be recognized by autologous CTLs in the surface of the tumor cells in association with various classical HLA molecules, have been the subject of investigation *(119)*. Because the *MAGE-A* genes are expressed in a variety of malignant tissues and absent in normal tissues other than the placenta and testis *(120,121)*, their tumor-associated peptides could be used as targets for active immunotherapy. In addition, their expression analysis in malignancies could be of diagnostic and/or prognostic relevance. Preferential expression of *MAGE-A* has been observed in patients who are at a higher risk of recurrence: those harboring tumors with high levels of protease urokinase-type plasminogen activator and its inhibitor plasminogen activator inhibitor 1, high score of Ki-67 proliferation antigen, and a lesser degree if differentiation *(119)*. These findings suggest a potential involvement of *MAGE-A* in tumor progression, with potential implications for active immunotherapy.

Another major concern, especially in terms of breast cancer, in which the disease is known to recur even after many years of remission even if adjuvant therapy was given, is that of tumor cell dormancy. Investigators at the Norwegian Radium Hospital *(122)* have examined the bone marrow aspirates from patients with breast cancer using IHC to detect cytokeratin positive cells before treatment, at the time of surgery and after treatment. At the time of primary diagnosis 22.5% of patients had OMBM, at the time of surgery 16.9% showed OMBM and after treatment 31.9% were positive. They found that 17.2% of patients who were initially negative for OMBM, became positive at the last aspiration, while 14.0% with an initially positive bone marrow remained positive and only 12.9% with initially positive bone marrow results became negative *(122)*. The theory behind this is that a population of tumor cells may exist in a "dormant" state, and these dormant cells may not be responsive to traditional tumor cytotoxic therapies that act on proliferating or actively metabolizing cells. Thus, the study of dormancy in the early-disseminated tumor cell population may have important implications regarding the use (and specific type) of adjuvant therapy in patients with cancer. Dormancy is defined as the maintenance of a balance between proliferation and apoptosis, or a state of "quiescence." Dormant tumor cells may not be effectively treated by cytotoxic regimens that require actively metabolizing or proliferating cells. Studies are underway that will examine individual occult metastatic tumor cells detected for characteristics associated with tumor cell

According to some *(123)*, the cytotoxic agents currently used for chemotherapy in high-risk breast cancer patients do not completely eliminate CK-positive tumor cells in the bone marrow. The presence of these tumor cells after chemotherapy is associated with poor prognosis. Thus bone marrow monitoring might help predict the response to systemic chemotherapy.

7. ONGOING PROSPECTIVE STUDIES

The true test of the prognostic importance of occult metastasis detection in both the bone marrow and lymph nodes will come from large-scale multiinstitutional studies. In the case of breast cancer, such a study is now well underway, under the auspices of the American College of Surgeons Oncology Group (ACOSOG), protocol Z0010 "A prognostic study of sentinel node and bone marrow micrometastases in women with clinical T1-2 N0 breast cancer." This study should provide definitive evidence of the prognostic significance of occult metastases in patients with breast cancer.

We have suggested a new concept in the staging of cancers using the TNM classification, where the traditional T (tumor), N (node), and M (metastasis) may be complemented by n and m (nodal and systemic occult metastases); that is TNnMm *(28,124)*. With the results of larger studies on prognostic significance of occult metastases, either in bone marrow or lymph nodes, this staging may be applied clinically. The estimates of outcome for populations of patients may be narrowed down to those for subpopulations of patients (i.e., those with or without occult metastases).

8. PATIENT-SPECIFIC TREATMENT

The establishment of new techniques that can identify patients who are at risk of recurrence earlier coupled with the ability to determine the molecular profiles of the individual tumors may well enable patient specific treatment regimens to be developed. Treatment will be able to be tailored with regard to dormancy/proliferation state and biological markers of tumor progression that may be present. In addition, the development of therapeutic agents designed to be delivered specifically to the tumor cells will enable more effective elimination of the tumor cells while decreasing the morbidity associated with conventional chemotherapeutic agents that target proliferating cells. Thus more effective and less toxic adjuvant therapy may be provided for women with primary breast cancer.

REFERENCES

1. Wallgren A, Bonetti M, Gelber RD, et al. Risk factors for locoregional recurrence among breast cancer patients: results from international breast cancer study group trials I through VII. *J Clin Oncol* 2003;21:1205–1213.
2. Kuru B, Camlibel M, Gulcelik MA, Alagol H. Prognostic factors affecting survival and disease-free survival in lymph node-negative breast carcinomas. *J Surg Oncol* 2003;83:167–172.
3. Asagoe T, Hanatani Y, Doi M, et al. The indications for postoperative adjuvant therapy in node-negative breast cancer patients. *Jpn J Cancer Chemother* 1996;23:311–316.
4. Abrams JS. Adjuvant therapy for breast cancer—results from USA consensus conference. *Breast Cancer* 2001;8:298–304.
5. Russell CA. Adjuvant systemic therapy for lymph node-negative breast cancer less than or equal to 1 cm. *Curr Women's Health Rep* 2002;2:134–139.
6. Group IBCS. Endocrine responsiveness and tailoring adjuvant therapy for postmenopausal lymph node-negative breast cancer; a randomized trial. *J Natl Cancer Inst* 2002;94:1054–1065.
7. Hawes D, Neville AM, Cote RJ. Detection of occult metastasis in patients with breast cancer. *Semin Surg Oncol* 2001;20:312–318.
8. Gross HJ, Verwer B, Houck D, Hoffman RA, Recketenwald D. Model study detecting breast cancer cells in peripheral blood mononuclear cells at frequencies as low as 10-7. *Proc Natl Acad Sci USA* 1995;92:537–541.
9. Leslie DS, Johnston WW, Daly L, et al. Detection of breast carcinoma cells in human bone marrow using fluorescent-activated cell sorting and conventional cytology. *Am J Clin Pathol* 1990;94:8–13.
10. Leers MPG, Schoffelen RHMG, Hoop JGM, et al. Multiparameter flow cytometry as a tool for the detection of micrometastatic tumour cells in the sentinel lymph node procedure of patients with breast cancer. *J Clin Pathol* 2002;55:359–366.
11. Redding WH, Monaghan P, Imrie SF. Detection of micrometastases in patients with primary breast cancer. *Lancet* 1983:1271–1274.
12. Osborne MP, Wong GY, Asina S, et al. Sensitivity of immunocytochemical detection of breast cancer cells in human bone marrow. *Cancer Res* 1991;51:2706.
13. Ellis G, Fergusson M, Yamanaka E. Monoclonal antibodies for detection of occult carcinoma cells in bone marrow of breast cancer patients. *Cancer* 1989;63:2509–2514.
14. Cote RJ, Rosen PP, Lesser ML, Old LJ, Osborne MP. Prediction of early relapse in patients with operable breast cancer by detection of occult bone marrow micrometastases. *J Clin Oncol* 1991;9:1749–1756.

15. Cote RJ, Rosen PP, Hakes TB, et al. Monoclonal antibodies detect occult breast carcinoma metastases in bone marrow of patients with early-stage disease. *Am J Surg Pathol* 1988;12:333.

16. Schlimok G, Funke I, Bock B, Schweiberer B, Witte J, Riethmuller G. Epithelial tumor cells in bone marrow of patients with colorectal cancer: immunocytochemical detection, phenotypic characterization, and prognostic significance. *J Clin Oncol* 1990;8:831–837.

17. Lindeman F, Schlimok G, Dirschedl P, Witte J, Reithmuller G. Prognostic significance of micrometastatic tumor cells in bone marrow of colorectal cancer patients. *Lancet* 1992;340:685–689.

18. Silly H, Samanigg H, Stoger H, Brezinschek HP, Wilders-Trusching M. Micrometastatic tumor cells in bone marrow in colorectal carcinoma. *Lancet* 1992;340:1288.

19. Calaluce R, Miedema BW, Yesus YW. Micrometastasis in colorectal carcinoma: a review. *J Surg Oncol* 1998;67:194–202.

20. Moreno JG, Croce CM, Fischer R, et al. Detection of hematogenous micrometastases in patients with prostate cancer. *Cancer Res* 1992;52:6110–6112.

21. Oberneder R, Riesenberg R, Kriegmair M, et al. Immunocytochemical detection and phenotypic characterization of micrometastatic tumour cells in bone marrow of patients with prostate cancer. *Urol Res* 1994;22:3–8.

22. Bretton PR, Melamed MR, Fair WR, Cote RJ. Detection of occult micrometastases in the bone marrow of patients with prostate carcinoma. *Prostate* 1994;25:108–114.

23. Wood DPJ, Banks ER, Humphreys S, McRoberts JW, Rangnekar VM. Identification of bone marrow micrometastases in patients with prostate cancer. *Cancer* 1994;74:2533–2540.

24. Frew AJ, Ralkaier N, Ghosh AK, Gatter KC, Mason DY. Immunohistochemistry in the detection of bone marrow micrometastases in patients with primary lung cancer. *Br J Cancer* 1986;53:555–556.

25. Leonard RCF, Duncan LW, Hay FG. Immunocytological detection of residual marrow disease at clinical remission predicts metastatic relapse in small cell lung cancer. *Cancer Res* 1990;50:6545–6548.

26. Pantel K, Izbicki JR, Angswurm M, et al. Immunocytological detection of bone marrow micrometastasis in operable non-small cell lung cancer. *Cancer Res* 1993;53:1027–1031.

27. Pantel K, Isbicki J, Passlick B, et al. Frequency and prognostic significance of isolated tumour cells in bone marrow of patients with non-small cell lung cancer without overt metastases. *Lancet* 1996;347:649–653.

28. Cote RJ, Hawes D, Chaiwun B, Beattie EJ. Detection of occult metastases in lung carcinomas: Progress and implications for staging. *J Surg Oncol* 1998;69: 265–274.

29. Osaki T, Oyama T, Gu C-D, et al. Prognostic impact of micrometastatic tumor cells in the lymph nodes and bone marrow of patients with completely resected stage I non-small-cell lung cancer. *J Clin Oncol* 2002;20:2930–2936.

30. Zheng R, Ge D, Qiao Y, Shin M. Impact of micrometastasis in pathologically negative lymph node on staging and prognosis of non-small cell lung cancers. *Clin J Oncol* 2002;24:41–43.

31. Ohta Y, Oda M, Wu J, et al. Can tumor size be a guide for limited surgical intervention on patients with peripheral non-small cell lung cancer? Assessment from the point of view of nodal micrometastasis. *J Thorac Cardiovasc Surg* 2001; 122:900–906.

32. Gu C-D, Osaki T, Oyama T, et al. Detection of micrometastatic tumor cells in pN0 lymph nodes of patients with completely resected nonsmall cell lung cancer: impact on recurrence and survival. *Ann Surg* 2002;235:133–139.

33. Doki Y, Ishikawa O, Mano M, et al. Cytokeratin deposits in lymph nodes show distinct clinical significance from lymph node micrometastasis in human esophageal cancers. *J Surg Res* 2002;107:75–81.

34. Tanabe T, Nishimaki T, Watanabe H, et al. Immunohistochemically detected micrometastasis in lymph nodes from superficial esophageal squamous cell carcinoma. *J Clin Oncol* 2003;82:153–159.

35. Chen Z, Lu X, Huang R. Detection of occult tumor cells in resected lymph nodes of patients with stage I carcinoma and its clinico-pathological significance. *Chin J Oncol* 1997;19:69–71.

36. Hosch SB, Stoecklein NH, Pichlmeier U, et al. Esophageal cancer: the mode of lymphatic tumor cell spread and its prognostic significance. *J Clin Oncol* 2001;19:1970–1975.

37. Komukai S, Nishimaki T, Watanabe H, Ajioka Y, Suzuki T, Hatakeyama K. Significance of immunohistochemically demonstrated micrometastases to lymph nodes in esophageal cancer with histologically negative nodes. *Surgery* 2000; 127:40–46.

38. Ross GL, Shoaib T, Scott J, et al. The impact of immunohistochemistry on sentinel node biopsy for primary cutaneous malignant melanoma. *Br J Plast Surg* 2003;56:153–155.

39. O'Reilly FM, Brat DJ, McAlpine BE, Grossniklaus HE, Folpe AL, Arbiser JL. Microphthalmia transcription factor immunohistochemistry: a useful diagnostic marker in the diagnosis and detection of cutaneous melanoma, sentinel lymph node metastases, and extracutaneous melanocytic neoplasms. *J Am Acad Dermatol* 2001;45:414–419.

40. Reintgen DS, Shivers S. Sentinel lymph node micrometastasis from melanoma. *Cancer* 1999;86:551–552.

41. Osborne MP, Asina S, Wong GY. Immunofluorescent monoclonal antibody detection of breast cancer in bone marrow: sensitivity in a model system. *Cancer Res* 1989;49:2510.

42. Chaiwun B, Saad AD, Chen S-C, et al. Immunohistochemical detection of occult carcinoma in bone marrow and blood. *Diag Oncol* 1992;2:267.

43. Page DL, Anderson TJ, Carter BA. Minimal solid tumor involvement of regional and distant sites. *Cancer* 1999;86:2589–2592.

44. Datta YH, Adams PT, Drobski WR, et al. Sensitive detection of occult breast cancer by reverse-transcriptase polymerase chain reaction. *J Clin Oncol* 1994;12:475–482.

45. Bostick PJ, Chatterjee S, Chi DD, et al. Limitations of specific reverse-transcriptase polymerase chain reaction markers in the detection of metastases in the lymph nodes and blood of breast cancer patients. *J Clin Oncol* 1998;16:2632–2640.

46. Zippelius P, Kufer P, Honold G, et al. Limitations of reverse-transcriptase polymerase chain reaction analysis for detection of micrometastatic epithelial cancer cells in bone marrow. *J Clin Oncol* 1997;15:2701–2708.

47. Grunewald K, Haun M, Urbanek M, et al. Mammaglobin gene expression: a superior marker of breast cancer cells in peripheral blood in comparison to epidermal-growth-factor receptor and cytokeratin-19. *Lab Invest* 2000;80:1071–1077.

48. Watson MA, Dintzis S, Darrow CM, et al. Mammaglobin expression in primary, metastatic, and occult breast cancer. *Cancer Res* 1999;59:3028–3031.

49. Zach O, Kasparu H, Krieger O, Hehenwarter W, Girschikofsky M, Lutz D. Detection of circulating mammary carcinoma cells in the peripheral blood of breast cancer patients via nested reverse transcriptase polymerase chain reaction assay for mammaglobin mRNA. *J Clin Oncol* 1999;17:2015–2019.
50. Slade MJ, Smith BM, Sinnett D, Cross NCP, Coombes RC. Quantitative polymerase chain reaction for the detection of micrometastases in patients with breast cancer. *J Clin Oncol* 1999;17:870–879.
51. Smith BM, Slade MJ, English J, et al. Response of circulating tumor cells to systemic therapy in patients with metastatic breast cancer: comparison of quantitative polymerase chain reaction and immunocytochemical techniques. *J Clin Oncol* 2000;18:1432–1439.
52. Zach O, Kasparu H, Wagner H, Krieger O, Lutz D. Mammoglobin as a marker for the detection of tumor cells in the peripheral blood of breast cancer patients. *Ann NY Acad Sci* 2000;923:343–345.
53. Pantel K, Schlimok G, Angstwurm M, et al. Methodological analysis of immunocytochemical screening for disseminated epithelial tumor cells in bone marrow. *J Hematother* 1994;3:165–173.
54. Naume B, Borgen E, Beiske K, et al. Immunomagnetic techniques for the enrichment and detection of isolated breast carcinoma cells in bone marrow and peripheral blood. *J Hematother* 1997;6:103–114.
55. Martin VM, Siewert C, Scharl A, et al. Immunomagnetic enrichment of disseminated epithelial tumor cells from peripheral blood by MACS. *Exp Hematol* 1998;26.
56. Naume B, Borgen E, Nesland JM, et al. Increased sensitivity for detection of micrometastases in bone-marrow/peripheral-blood stem-cell products from breast-cancer patients by negative immunomagnetic separation. *Int J Cancer* 1998;78:556–560.
57. Racila E, Euhus D, Weiss AJ, et al. Detection and characterization of carcinoma cells in the blood. *Proc Natl Acad Sci USA* 1998;95:4589–4594.
58. Fodstad O, Trones GE, Forus A, et al. Improved immunomagnetic method for detection and characterization of cancer cells in blood and bone marrow (abstract). *Proc Am Assoc Cancer Res* 1997;38:(abstr 172).
59. Kim SJ, Ikeda N, Shiba E, Takamura Y, Noguchi S. Detection of breast cancer micrometastases in peripheral blood using immunomagnetic separation and immunocytochemistry. *Breast Cancer* 2001;8:63–39.
60. Stathopoulou A, Vlachonikolis I, Mavroudis D, et al. Molecular detection of cytokeratin-19-positive cells in the peripheral blood of patients with operable breast cancer: evaluation of their prognostic significance. *J Clin Oncol* 2002;20:3404–3412.
61. Cristofanelli M, Budd GT, Ellis MJ, et al. Circulating tumor cells, disease progression, and survival in metastatic breast cancer. *N Engl J Med* 2004;351:781–791.
62. Theriult RL, Hortobagy GN. Bone metastases in breast cancer. *Anticancer Drugs* 1992;3:455–462.
63. Body JJ. Metastatic bone disease: clinical and therapeutic aspects. *Bone* 1992;13:857–862.
64. Berger U, Bettelheim R, Mansi JL, Easton D, Coombes RC, Neville AM. The relationship between micrometastases in the bone marrow, histopathologic features in the primary tumor in breast cancer and prognosis. *Am J Clin Pathol* 1988;90:1–6.

65. Osborne MP, Rosen PP. Detection and management of bone marrow micrometastases in breast cancer. *Oncology (Huntingt)* 1994;8:25–31.
66. Mansi JL, Berger U, Easton D, et al. Micrometastases in bone marrow in patients with primary breast cancer: evaluation as an early predictor of bone metastases. *Br Med J* 1987;295:1093–1096.
67. Porro G, Menard S, Tagliabue E, et al. Monoclonal antibody detection of carcinoma cells in bone marrow biopsy specimens from breast cancer patients. *Cancer* 1988;61:2407.
68. Cancer Statistics. *Ca-A Cancer J Clin*, 1990:40.
69. Society AC. Breast Cancer Facts and Figures 2003–2004. Vol. 2003: American Cancer Society, 2003.
70. Fehm T, Sagalowsky A, Cliffird E, et al. Cytogenetic evidence that circulating epithelial cells in patients with carcinoma are malignant. *Clin Cancer Res* 2002;8:2073–2084.
71. Diel IJ, Kaufmann M, Costa SD, et al. Micrometastatic breast cancer cells in bone marrow at primary surgery: prognostic value in comparison with nodal status. *J Natl Cancer Inst* 1997;88:1652–1658.
72. Mansi JL, Gogas H, Bliss JM, Gazet J-C, Berger U, Coombes RC. Outcome of primary-breast-cancer patients with micrometastases: a long-term follow-up study. *Lancet* 1999;354:197–202.
73. Braun S, Pantel K, Muller P, et al. Cytokeratin-positive cells in the bone marrow and survival of patients with stage I, II, or III breast cancer. *N Engl J Med* 2000;342:525–533.
74. Gerber B, Krause A, Muller H, et al. Simultaneous immunohistochemical detection of tumor cells in lymph nodes and bone marrow aspirates in breast cancer and its correlation with other prognostic factors. *J Clin Oncol* 2001;19:960–971.
75. Gebauer G, Fehm T, Merkle E, Beck EP, Lang N, Jager W. Epithelial cells in bone marrow of breast cancer patients at time of primary surgery: clinical outcome during long-term follow-up. *J Clin Oncol* 2001;19:3669–3674.
76. Wiedswang G, Borgen E, Karesen R, et al. Detection of isolated tumor cells in bone marrow is an independent prognostic factor in breast cancer. *J Clin Oncol* 2003;21:3469–3478.
77. Dearnaley DP, Ormerod MG, Sloane JP. Micrometastases in breast cancer: long-term follow-up of the first patient cohort. *Eur J Cancer* 1991;27:236.
78. Mansi JL, Easton U, Berger JC, et al. Bone marrow micrometastases in primary breast cancer: prognostic significance after six years' follow-up. *Eur J Cancer* 1991;27:1552.
79. Diel IJ, Kaufman M, Costa SD, et al. Micrometastatic breast cancer cells in bone marrow at primary surgery: prognostic value in comparison with nodal status. *J Natl Cancer Inst* 1996;88:1652–1658.
80. Diel IJ, Kaufman M, Goener R, et al. Detection of tumor cells in bone marrow of patients with primary breast cancer: a prognostic factor for distant metastases. *J Clin Oncol* 1992;10:1534–1539.
81. Gusterson BA, Ott R. Occult axillary lymph node micrometastases in breast cancer. *Lancet* 1990;336:434–435.
82. Neville AM. Breast cancer micrometastases in lymph nodes and bone marrow are prognostically important. *Ann Oncol* 1989;2:13–14.
83. Saphir O, Amromin GD. Obscure axillary lymph node metastases in carcinoma of the breast. *Cancer* 1948;1:238–241.

84. Pickren JW. Significance of occult metastases. A study of breast cancer. *Cancer* 1961;14:1266–1271.
85. Fisher ER, Saminoss S, Lee CH, et al. Detection and significance of occult axillary node metastases in patients with invasive breast cancer. *Cancer* 1978;42:2025–2031.
86. Wilkinson EJ, Hause LL, Hoffman RG, et al. Occult axillary lymph node metastases in invasive breast carcinoma: characteristics of the primary tumor and the significance of metastases. *Pathol Ann* 1982;17:67–91.
87. International (LUDWIG) Breast Cancer Study Group. Prognostic importance of occult lymph node micrometastases from breast cancers. *Lancet* 1990;335:1565–1568.
88. de Mascarel I, Bonichon F, Coindre JM, Trojani M. Prognostic significance of breast cancer axillary lymph node micrometastases assessed by two special techniques: reevaluation with longer follow-up. *Br J Cancer* 1992;66:523–527.
89. Wells CA, Heryt A, Brochier J, et al. The immunohistochemical detection of axillary micrometastases in breast cancer. *Br J Cancer* 1984;50:193–197.
90. Bussolati G, Gugliotta P, Morra Z, et al. The immunohistochemical detection of lymph node micrometastases from infiltrating lobular carcinoma of the breast. *Br J Cancer* 1986;54:631–636.
91. Byrne J, Waldron R, McAvinchy D, et al. The use of monoclonal antibodies for the histological detection of mammary axillary micrometastases. *Eur J Surg Oncol* 1987;13:409.
92. Trojani L, Mascarel I, Bonichon F, et al. Micrometastases to axillary lymph nodes from carcinoma of the breast: detection by immunohistochemistry and prognostic significance. *Br J Cancer* 1987;55:303–306.
93. Apostolikas N, Petraki C, Agnantis NJ. The reliability of histologically negative axillary lymph nodes in breast cancer. *Pathol Res Pract* 1989;184:35–38.
94. Sedmak DD, Meinke TA, Knechtges DS, et al. Prognostic significance of cytokeratin-postive breast cancer metastases. *Mod Pathol* 1989;2:516–520.
95. Cote RJ, Chaiwun B, Qu J, Agnantis NJ, et al. Prognostic importance of occult lymph node metastases in patients with breast cancer. *Proc Am Assoc Cancer Res* 1992;33:202.
96. Neville AM. Prognostic factors and primary breast cancer. *Diag Oncol* 1991;1:53.
97. Neville AM, Price KN, Gelber RD, et al. Axillary lymph node micrometastases and breast cancer. *Lancet* 1991;337:110.
98. Elson CE, Kufe D, Johnston WW. Immunohistochemical detection and significance of axillary lymph node micrometastases in breast cancer- a study of 97 cases. *Anal Quant Cytol Histol* 1993:171–178.
99. Nasser IA, Lee AKC, Bosari S, Saganich R, Heatly G, Silverman ML. Occult axillary lymph node metastases in "node-negative" breast cancer. *Hum Pathol* 1993;24:950–957.
100. Hainsworth PJ, Tjandra JJ, Stillwell RG, et al. Detection and significance of occult metastases in node-negative breast cancer. *Br J Surg* 1993;80:459–463.
101. Schoenfeld A, Luqmani Y, Smith D, et al. Detection of breast cancer micrometastases in axillary nodes using polymerase chain reaction. *Cancer Res* 1994;54:2986–2990.
102. Noguchi S, Aihara T, Nakamori S, et al. The detection of breast cancer micrometastases in axillary lymph nodes by means of reverse-transcriptase polymerase chain reaction. *Cancer* 1994;74:1595–1600.

103. Cote RJ, Peterson HF, Chaiwun B, et al. Role of immunohistochemical detection of lymph-node metastases in management of breast cancer. *Lancet* 1999;354:896–900.
104. Giuliano AE, Jones RC, Brennan M, Statman R. Sentinel lymphadenectomy in breast cancer. *J Clin Oncol* 1997;15:2345.
105. Veronesi U, Paganelli G, Galimberti V, et al. Sentinel-node biopsy to avoid axillary dissection in breast cancer with clinically negative lymph-nodes. *Lancet* 1997;349:1864–1867.
106. Veronesi U, Paganelli G, Viale G, et al. A randomized comparison of sentinel-node biopsy with routine axillary dissection in breast cancer [comment]. *N Engl J Med* 2003;349:603–605.
107. Alex JC, Krag DN. The gamma-probe-guided resection of radiolabeled primary lymph nodes. *Surg Oncol Clin North Am* 1996;5:33–41.
108. Albertini JJ, Lyman GH, Cox C, et al. Lymphatic mapping and sentinel node biopsy in the patient with breast cancer. *JAMA* 1996;276:1818–1822.
109. Krag DN, Weaver D, Ashikaga T, et al. The sentinel node in breast cancer: a multicenter validation study. *N Engl J Med* 1998;339:941–995.
110. Fisher B, Dignam J, Walmark N. Lumpectomy and radiation therapy for the treatment of intraductal breast cancer: findings from national adjuvant breast and bowel project B-17. *J Clin Oncol* 1998;16:441–452.
111. Julien J-P, Bijker N, Fentiman IS. Radiotherapy in breast-conserving treatment for ductal carcinoma in situ: first results of the EORTC randomised phase III trial 10853. *Lancet* 2000;355:528–533.
112. Dowlatshahi K, Fan M, Snider HC. Lymph node micrometastases from breast carcinoma: reviewing the dilemma. *Cancer* 1997;80:1188–1197.
113. Pendas S, Dauway E, Giuliano R, Ku N, Reintgen DS. Sentinel node biopsy in ductal carcinoma in situ patients. *Ann Surg Oncol* 2000;7:15–20.
114. Frykberg ER, Bland KI. In situ breast carcinoma. *Adv Surg* 1993;26:29–72.
115. Schwartz GF, Lawrence JS, Olivotto IA, Ernster VL, Pressman PI. Consensus Conference on the treatment of in situ ductal carcinoma of the breast. *Cancer* 2000;88:946–954.
116. Cox CE, Pendas S, Cox J. Guidelines for sentinel node biopsy and lymphatic mapping of patients with breast cancer. *Ann Surg* 1998;227:645–653.
117. Braun S, Schlimok G, Heumos I, et al. erbB2 overexpression on occult metastatic cells in bone marrow predicts poor clinical outcome of stage I-III breast cancer patients. *Cancer Res* 2001;61:1890–1895.
118. Pantel K, Braun S. Molecular determinants of occult metastatic tumor cells in bone marrow. [Review]. *Clin Breast Cancer* 2001;2:222–228.
119. Otte M, Zafrakas M, Riethdorf L, et al. MAGE-A gene expression pattern in primary breast cancer. *Cancer Res* 2001;61:6682–6687.
120. De Plaen E, Arden K, Traversari C, et al. Structure, chromosomal localization, and expression on 12 genes of the MAGE family. *Immunogenetics* 1994;40:360–369.
121. Takahashi K, Shichijo S, Noguchi M, Hirohata M, Itoh K. Identification of MAGE-1 and MAGE-4 proteins in spermatogonia and primary spermatocytes. *Cancer Res* 1995;55:3478–3482.
122. Tossvik S, Trane A, Lonning PE, et al. Persistence of occult metastatic cells in bone marrow of breast cancer patients despite systemic neoadjuvant taxol/epidriamycin treatment., 4th International Symposium on Minimal Residual Cancer, Oslo, Norway, November 13–16, 2003, 2003.

123. Braun S, Kentenich C, Janni W, et al. Lack of effect of adjuvant chemotherapy on the elimination of single dormant tumor cells in bone marrow of high-risk breast cancer patients. *J Clin Oncol* 2000;18:80–86.
124. Chaiwun B, Saad A, Chatterjee SJ, Taylor CR, Beattie EJ, Cote RJ. Advances in the pathologic staging of lung cancer: detection of regional and systemic occult metastases. In: Marchevsky AM, Koss MN, eds. State of the Art Reviews. Vol. 4. Philadelphia: Hanley & Belfus, 1996:155–168.

VI FUTURE DIRECTIONS

16   New Technologies/ New Markers/ New Challenges

Daniel F. Hayes, MD
and Giampetro Gasparini, MD

CONTENTS

Key Words: Biomarkers; technologies; development.

1. INTRODUCTION

The field of tumor markers is enigmatic. On the one hand, the explosion of technology in medicine has provided an enormous number of complex tools that might be used to screen for, diagnose, or prevent a newly diagnosed cancer and/or its metastases. Indeed, the preceding chapters have highlighted remarkable progress in these technologies, and potential areas in which they might be useful. On the other hand, very few markers have actually been accepted for routine clinical use in breast cancer. The American Society of Clinical Oncology Tumor Marker Expert Guidelines Panel has issued three sets of guidelines since its inception in 1996. In the initial set of guidelines, the use of estrogen and progesterone receptors (ERs, PgRs) to select patients for hormone therapy and the use of circulating CA15-3 and/or carcinoembryonic antigen (CEA) to monitor selected patients with

Cancer Drug Discovery and Development: Biomarkers in Breast Cancer: Molecular Diagnostics for Predicting and Monitoring Therapeutic Effect
Edited by: G. Gasparini and D. F. Hayes © Humana Press Inc., Totowa, NJ

metastatic disease were the only recommended markers *(1)*. In subsequent updates, the Panel recommended routine measurement of *HER2* in cancer tissue to select trastuzumab for patients with metastatic disease *(2,3)*. None of the other markers that have been reported and proposed for breast cancer was felt to be sufficiently validated for routine use by the Panel. Similar recommendations have been made by the College of American Pathologists *(4)*.

Why are these guidelines so conservative? There are several answers to this question, and each of these questions should serve as the basis for future studies *(5)*.

1. A marker is helpful only if it separates an entire population into two different groups whose outcome is likely to be so different that one group might be treated differently than another. Both ER and *HER2* are classic examples of this category. Patients with ER-negative tumors appear very unlikely to benefit from hormone therapy *(6)*, and, likewise, it appears that patients with *HER2*-low or -negative cancers are very unlikely to benefit from trastuzumab *(5,7)*.

Therefore, future studies should be focused on identifying markers with sufficient strength that outcomes of patients who are "positive" (by whatever criteria used) have sufficiently different outcomes that a clinician would treat them differently than those who are "negative." It is certainly possible that selected, single-gene or single-protein markers might fall into this category. For example, data from Europe support the notion that patients whose tumors do not express urokinase plasminogen activator (uPA) and the plasminogen activator inhibitor 1 (PAI-1) proteins have a sufficiently favorable prognosis that the benefits from chemotherapy would be so low that they might forego this toxic form of therapy *(8,9)*.

The new technologies that permit high-throughput analysis may well identify such a marker. These technologies have two promises: new gene or protein identification and pattern recognition. Currently, the latter has achieved the most notoriety. High-profile publications and presentations have suggested that selected combinations of multiplex gene expressions are associated with very good or poor prognosis *(10–12)*. However, although promising, these observations require validation in prospective, properly designed clinical trials.

Proteomics also offers great promise in identifying specific patterns that might be helpful in the clinic *(13,14)*. However, this field is in its infancy, with many methods and techniques, and at this writing there have been few if any studies that suggest any clinical utility for proteomic pattern recognition in breast cancer.

The use of high-throughput technologies also provides the opportunity to identify new, previously unrecognized genes and their products that might be of value. However, so far, none has been recognized that appear to be of clinical value.

2. The assay must be reliable and reproducible. With few exceptions, tumor markers seem to pass through a "life cycle" in which the original report is extraordinarily positive with great acclaim, but subsequent studies fail to live up to the promise. There are fundamentally three reasons for this conundrum: (1) technical variability of the assay; (2) variations in the manner in which different assays for the same marker are performed; and (3) inadequate and differences in study design. These effects of these concerns are often underestimated in the excitement of apparently "positive" results, but ultimately they are paramount in the consideration of whether a new marker is or is not helpful in caring for patients. Thus, as new techniques and assays are developed, it is important to demonstrate that not only are the result promising, but that they are reproducible. The first of these three requirements, technical variability, is perhaps the most easily accomplished, although even this issue is not always demonstrated. The latter two issues are more common, and perhaps more important, reasons that new markers are so slowly adopted. Because of competition among scientists and commercial interests, different assays are often developed to evaluate the same marker. For example, *HER2* status can be determined by examination of breast cancer tissue amplification of the *erb*-B2 gene using a variety of techniques including Southern blotting, slot-blot quantification, or fluorescence *in situ* hybridization, and by evaluation of the protein using Western blotting, immunohistochemistry, immunofluorescence, or enzyme-linked immunosorbent assays (ELISA). Moreover, circulating extracellular domain of *HER2* can be quantified in human serum using ELISA *(15)*. Although they are all correlated, each of these assays, which in one way or another provides an indication of overproduction of *HER2*, appears to differ from the other and to provide different results in regards to prediction of outcome. Thus, it is not surprising that results from study to study are not validated, if the assays that are being compared are not identical.

Another technical issue that hinders reproducibility is related to selection of the cutoff that distinguishes positive from negative populations. Several means of doing so are employed. One method is to arbitrarily select a cutoff, based on some preconceived reason, such as the mean level of the assay in an affected population or the mean plus two standard deviations of the level in an unaffected population. A second method is to test several potential cutoffs in one population, selecting the one that appears most robust in regard to separation of the outcomes of the two groups or in regards to apparent statistical significance. Regardless of the method used, it is essential to validate the results in a separate group of patients.

Finally, the results are most likely to be valid if they are studied in the context of a plausible hypothesis that is prospectively addressed. Many published studies report results related to hypotheses that are retrospectively derived from the observed data. Although such studies are valuable to generate hypotheses, these observations must be prospectively validated in subsequent, well-designed studies *(5,16)*. Unfortunately, most tumor marker studies are performed using archived specimens collected for reasons unrelated to the study under question. Therefore it is difficult to validate observations, requiring and time-consuming prospective studies. Nonetheless, failure to do so often leaves the marker hanging, with the original exciting results, generated from the retrospective exploratory study, lacking validation.

2. FUTURE DIRECTIONS

The previous caveats notwithstanding, technological advances do offer great promise for individualization of therapy for breast cancer. We believe the following areas of research are particularly exciting.

2.1. Genomics/Proteomics

The ability to examine abnormalities in multiple genes and/or their products simultaneously has permitted avenues of discovery that are unprecedented. Clearly, multiplex gene amplification and gene expression, studying tens, hundreds, and even thousands of genes and/or proteins simultaneously have the potential to move the field exponentially when compared to a gene-by-gene approach. These methods lead to two possible advances: Discovery of new, single genes that may play an important role in breast cancer; and identification of patterns of genes that, even if their individual roles and contributions are uncertain, can act as a single tumor marker when considered in aggregate. The former approach offers the promise not only of improving diagnostics, but of providing clues to potential targets for therapeutic research. The latter, if reproducible and validated, may become the *sine que non* for powerful markers that clearly separate populations with favorable from unfavorable outcomes to the extent that they would be treated much differently. Most of the currently available and promising data have come from genomic studies, either of frozen *(10,11,17)* or fixed tissue *(12)*. However, studies of multiple proteins, including evaluation of posttranslational modification, may well be a much more powerful and accurate strategy in the long run, although the methodologies of this approach are still in their infancies.

2.2. Minimal Detectable Disease

Identification of apparently malignant cells in the circulation or bone marrow has been possible for >130 yr *(18)*. Recent technologies have substantially improved the accuracy and reliability of enumerating such cells, using immunoseparation techniques or reverse transcriptase-polymerase chain reaction (RT-PCR) *(19–21)*. Perhaps even more exciting is the ability to genotype and phenotype these cells once they are identified *(22–25)*. Although clinical utility of this technology has not been shown, the ability to perform "real time" evaluation of the current biology (e.g., *HER2* status or the level of apoptosis) of a patient's cancer is of great promise.

2.3. Pharmacogenomics

Nearly all of this volume has addressed somatic changes within the cancer itself that might predict its natural or treated history. Increasingly, technological advances in genomics and proteomics have permitted studies of inherited, germ-line polymorphisms that may affect response to or toxicity from therapy. These single-nucleotide polymorphisms (SNPs) result in subtle but often important amino acid substitutions within genes that are important for activation and/or metabolism of the drug, or within genes that may serve as the target for the drug *(26)*. Only preliminary studies of these pharmacogenomic (or pharmacogenetic) changes have been reported, both for chemotherapy and for endocrine treatments, such as tamoxifen *(27,28)*.

3. CONCLUSIONS

In summary, incredible technological advances have opened the door for a potential sea change of evaluation and treatment of patients with breast cancer. These advances should help to improve the ability to evaluate risk, screen for new cancers, estimate prognosis and prediction of response to therapy, monitor patients during therapy, and even serve as targets for novel treatments. However, for any of these to take its place in clinical medicine, it will need to be carefully studied in rigorously designed clinical trials based on preexisting hypotheses, with sophisticated statistical analyses, taking into account other factors and treatment effects.

REFERENCES

1. ASCO Expert Panel. Clinical Practice Guidelines for the Use of Tumor Markers in Breast and Colorectal Cancer: Report of the American Society of Clinical Oncology Expert Panel. *J Clin Oncol* 1996;14:2843–2877.
2. ASCO Expert Panel. 1997 Update of recommendations for the use of tumor markers in breast and colorectal cancer. *J Clin Oncol* 1998;16:793–795.
3. Bast RC Jr, Ravdin P, Hayes DF, et al. 2000 Update of recommendations for the use of tumor markers in breast and colorectal cancer: Clinical Practice Guidelines of the American Society of Clinical Oncology. *J Clin Oncol* 2001;19:1865–1878.
4. Fitzgibbons PL, Page DL, Weaver D, et al. Prognostic factors in breast cancer. College of American Pathologists Consensus Statement 1999. *Arch Pathol Lab Med* 2000;124:966–978.
5. Hayes DF, Bast R, Desch CE, et al. A tumor marker utility grading system (TMUGS): a framework to evaluate clinical utility of tumor markers. *J Natl Cancer Inst* 1996;88:1456–1466.

6. Early Breast Cancer Trialist's Collaborative Group. Tamoxifen for early breast cancer: An overview of the randomised trials. *Lancet* 1998;351:1451–1467.

7. Vogel CL, Cobleigh MA, Tripathy D, et al. Efficacy and safety of trastuzumab as a single agent in first-line treatment of *HER2*-overexpressing metastatic breast cancer. *J Clin Oncol* 2002;20:719–726.

8. Janicke F, Prechtl A, Thomssen C, et al. Randomized adjuvant chemotherapy trial in high-risk, lymph node-negative breast cancer patients identified by urokinase-type plasminogen activator and plasminogen activator inhibitor type 1. *J Natl Cancer Inst* 2001;93:913–920.

9. Look M, van Putten W, Duffy M, et al. Pooled analysis of prognostic impact of uPA and PAI-1 in breast cancer patients. *Thromb Haemost* 2003;90:538–548.

10. van't Veer LJ, Dai H, van de Vijver MJ, et al. Gene expression profiling predicts clinical outcome of breast cancer. *Nature* 2002;415:530–536.

11. van de Vijver MJ, He YD, van't Veer LJ, et al. A gene-expression signature as a predictor of survival in breast cancer. *N Engl J Med* 2002;347:1999–2009.

12. Paik S, Shak S, Tang G, et al. Multi-gene RT-PCR assay for predicting recurrence in node negative breast cancer patients-NSABP B-20 and B-14. *Breast Cancer Res Treat* 2003;82:S11 (Abstr 16).

13. Celis JE, Gromov P. Proteomics in translational cancer research: toward an integrated approach. *Cancer Cell* 2003;3:9–15.

14. Petricoin EF, Ardekani AM, Hitt BA, et al. Use of proteomic patterns in serum to identify ovarian cancer. *Lancet* 2002;359:572–577.

15. Yamauchi H, Stearns V, Hayes DF. When is a tumor marker ready for prime time? A case study of c-erbB-2 as a predictive factor in breast cancer. *J Clin Oncol* 2001;19:2334–2356.

16. Simon R, Altman DG. Statistical aspects of prognostic factor studies in oncology. *Br J Cancer* 1994;69:979–985.

17. Perou CM, Sorlie T, Eisen MB, et al. Molecular portraits of human breast tumours. *Nature* 2000;406:747–752.

18. Ashworth TR. A case of cancer in which cells similar to those in the tumours were seen in the blood after death. *Austr Med J* 1869;14:146–149.

19. Cristofanilli M, Budd GT, Ellis MJ, et al. Circulating tumor cells, disease progression, and survival in metastatic breast cancer. *N Engl J Med* 2004;351:781–791.

20. Pantel K, Muller V, Auer M, Nusser N, Harbeck N, Braun S. Detection and clinical implications of early systemic tumor cell dissemination in breast cancer. *Clin Cancer Res* 2003;9:6326–6334.

21. Sabbatini R, Federico M, Morselli M, et al. Detection of circulating tumor cells by reverse transcriptase polymerase chain reaction of maspin in patients with breast cancer undergoing conventional-dose chemotherapy. *J Clin Oncol* 2000;18:1914–1920.

22. Braun S, Schlimok G, Heumos I, et al. ErbB2 overexpression on occult metastatic cells in bone marrow predicts poor clinical outcome of stage I-III breast cancer patients. *Cancer Res* 2001;61:1890–1895.

23. Kufer P, Zippelius A, Lutterbuse R, et al. Heterogeneous expression of MAGE-A genes in occult disseminated tumor cells: a novel multimarker reverse transcription-polymerase chain reaction for diagnosis of micrometastatic disease. *Cancer Res* 2002;62:251–261.

24. Fehm T, Sagalowsky A, Clifford E, et al. Cytogenetic evidence that circulating epithelial cells in patients with carcinoma are malignant. *Clin Cancer Res* 2002;8:2073–2084.

25. Hayes DF, Walker TM, Singh B, et al. Monitoring expression of HER-2 on circulating epithelial cells in patients with advanced breast cancer. *Int J Oncol* 2002;21:1111–1117.
26. Weinshilboum R. Inheritance and drug response. *N Engl J Med* 2003;348: 529–537.
27. Stearns V, Davidson NE, Flockhart DA. Pharmacogenetics in the treatment of breast cancer. *Pharmacogenomics J* 2004;4:143–153.
28. Stearns V, Johnson MD, Rae JM, et al. Active tamoxifen metabolite plasma concentrations after coadministration of tamoxifen and the selective serotonin reuptake inhibitor paroxetine. *J Natl Cancer Inst* 2003;95:1758–1764.

Index

333